MEDICAL RADIOLOGY

Diagnostic Imaging and Radiation Oncology

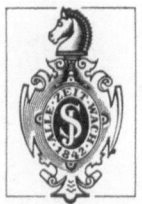

Lung Cancer

Diagnostic Procedures and Therapeutic Management
With Special Reference to Radiotherapy

Contributors

R.H. Choplin · Ch.S. Faulkner, II ·
Ch.J. Kovacs · S.G. Mann · Th. O'Connor · S.K. Plume
F. Richards, II · Ch.W. Scarantino

Edited by

Charles W. Scarantino

With 42 Figures

Springer-Verlag
Berlin Heidelberg New York Tokyo

CHARLES W. SCARANTINO, Ph.D.
Associate Professor
Department of Radiation
Bowman Gray School of Medicine
Wake Forest University
300 South Hawthorne Road
Winston-Salem, NC 27103
USA

New Address:
Professor and Chairman
Department of Radiation Oncology
East Carolina University
School of Medicine
Greenville, NC 27834
USA

MEDICAL RADIOLOGY · Diagnostic Imaging and Radiation Oncology

Continuation of
Handbuch der medizinischen Radiologie
Encyclopedia of Medical Radiology

ISBN-13: 978-3-642-82236-0   e-ISBN-13: 978-3-642-82234-6
DOI: 10.1007/978-3-642-82234-6

Library of Congress Cataloging in Publication Data. Main entry under title: Lung cancer. (Medical radiology) Includes bibliographies and index. 1. Lungs – Cancer. 2. Lungs – Cancer – Radiotherapy. I. Choplin, R.H. (Robert H.) II. Scarantino, Ch.W. (Charles W.), 1942–   . III. Series. [DNLM: 1. Lung Neoplasms. WF 658 L96028   RC280.L8L766   1985   616.99′424   85-8073

2122/3130-543210

To
Our Families, Friends and Colleagues
for Their Encouragement and Patience

List of Contributors

ROBERT H. CHOPLIN, M.D.
Associate Professor of Radiology
Bowman Gray School of Medicine
Wake Forest University
300 South Hawthorne Road
Winston-Salem, NC 27103
USA

CHARLES S. FAULKNER II, M.D.
Associate Professor of Clinical Pathology
Department of Pathology
Dartmouth Medical School
Hanover, NH 03756
USA

CHARLES J. KOVACS, Ph.D.
Associate Professor of Radiology
Director, Radiation Oncology
Laboratories
Bowman Gray School of Medicine
300 South Hawthorne Road
Winston-Salem, NC 27103
USA

STEVEN G. MANN, M.D.
Santa Cruz Radiation Oncology
Medical Group, Inc.
1575 Soquel Drive
Santa Cruz, CA 95065
USA

THOMAS O'CONNOR, M.D.
Director, Radiation Oncology
Community Hospital of Indianapolis,
Inc.
1500 North Ritter Avenue
Indianapolis, Indiana 46219
USA

STEPHEN K. PLUME, M.D.
Associate Professor
Department of Surgery
Dartmouth-Hitchcock Medical School
Hanover, NH 03756
USA

FREDERICK RICHARDS, II, M.D.
Associate Professor of Medicine
Bowman Gray School of Medicine
Wake Forest University
300 South Hawthorne Road
Winston-Salem, NC 27103
USA

CHARLES W. SCARANTINO, Ph.D.
Associate Professor
Department of Radiation
Bowman Gray School of Medicine
Wake Forest University
300 South Hawthorne Road
Winston-Salem, NC 27103
USA

Preface

At first glance it appears that little has happened in our understanding of bronchogenic carcinoma, since five year survival rates have not changed appreciably over the past ten years. This is partially true, however the depth of our understanding has increased and will continue to do so at a rapid pace over the next five to ten years. Information on the basic tumor biology, identification of important groups at high risk and improved delivery of cytotoxic agents in the treatment of lung cancer, will all add to improve the outcome.

The purpose of this text is to provide useful background information and to serve as a reference for approaching the patient with lung cancer. Therefore it will serve as a review for some and as a beginning for others.

An important starting point in any discussion of lung cancer is an epidemiological survey of the topic (Chapter I). For those who do not avoid the hazards and present with symptoms, what is the most logical approach in determining the diagnosis (Chapter II). This chapter is intended to provide a general overview of the subjects covered in detail in the remainder of the text.

A review of the embryological development of the lung (Chapter III) provides an excellent starting point in understanding the natural history and patterns of failure as they relate to the pathways of spread. In addition, it provides useful information which must be considered when formulating a surgical or radiotherapeutic plan of treatment. Histological information is also important in influencing the therapeutic approach. The pertinent characteristics of each sub type as well as recent information which suggest considerable heterogeneity within each tumor are presented in Chapter IV. Following the establishment of a diagnosis, it is important to determine the extent or stage of the disease. Which studies have been shown to provide most pertinent information are discussed in Chapter V.

Surgery, radiation and drug therapy have been and will continue to be the important therapeutic maneuvers in lung cancer. Surgery continues to offer the best chance for cure. However, when the tumor is found to be unresectable or metastatic, radiation or chemotherapy respectively are usually employed. The radiotherapeutic approach as well as the results of clinical trials using radiation and drugs are presented in Chapters VI and VII. In addition, Chapter VII argues for a more rational basis for combined modality therapy and offers half-body irradiation as an example for reconsidering the application of basic experimental findings to the clinical arena. The basic and applied experimental information form the cornerstone for the past and certainly the future therapeutic maneuvers. The most important and pertinent principles are presented in Chapter VIII.

A wealth of information exists from past experience with lung cancer. It is imperative that we learn from our experience and utilize this information to plan for the future.

CHARLES W. SCARANTINO

Acknowledgements. The editor wishes to thank RALPH HICKS and NINA HAYNES for their enthusiastic support in preparing this book.

Contents

Chapter I Epidemiology of Lung Cancer

Steven G. Mann

1 Introduction

Cancer is the second leading cause of death in the United States. One out of every five people dies from cancer. In 1978, in the United States, cancer caused 396,992 deaths, after heart disease which caused 729,510. In 1983, lung cancer will have been responsible for 35% of all cancer deaths in men and 17% in women. For all ages, 71,000 people died of lung cancer in 1978; 113,000 will have succumbed in 1983 (American Cancer Society, 1983).

2 Epidemiology

2.1 Sex

The number of women who smoke has increased dramatically. Smoking among teenage girls increased to 23 percent from 1969 to 1975 due to advertising and social pressure (Jick et al., 1979). As more women join the work force this should increase further. The age-adjusted annual incidence rate per 100,000 population of lung cancer in women increased from 4.1 to 14.9 for 1937–1971, 260%.

Steven G. Mann, M.D.
1575 Soquel Drive, Santa Cruz, CA 95065, USA

Lung cancer is rapidly approaching breast cancer as a leading cause of female death. It is responsible for 17% of all cancer deaths in women and causes 24,000 deaths a year, third behind breast at 34,000 and colorectal at 27,000. (In women between the ages of 15 and 34, the most common cause of cancer death is breast cancer.) In 1978, for ages 5–74, breast cancer caused 17,403 deaths and lung cancer 14,463 (American Cancer Society) (Table 1).

There are few clinical studies of lung cancer occurrence in women. Forty-one percent of the U.S. work force were women in 1978, and occupational exposure to carcinogens is becoming more important. Asbestos, for example, is used in the manufacture of certain textiles, which is predominantly a female industry.

Although occupational exposure and hereditary effects are important, the increased incidence of lung cancer among women appears to be more closely related to smoking habits (Jick et al., 1979). This is true among ethnic subsets such as Spanish women in Texas (Lee et al., 1976), and Hawaiian and Japanese in Hawaii, who did not have a high incidence of lung cancer prior to immigration to the USA.

In Hong Kong, lung cancer incidence among women is high (15% of female cancers). Fifty-six percent of women with lung cancer smoke there. The other half may be due to chronic exposure to kerosene stove fumes in small, unventilated kitchens. However, only 11% of the lung cancer cases among Chinese who have immigrated to Hawaii can be explained by smoking (Hinds et al., 1981). Lung cancer is at least as lethal among women as it is among men (Huhti et al., 1981).

2.2 Age

The incidence of lung cancer peaks in the sixth decade. About two percent of patients are under 40 years of age, however (Wynder, 1972). These younger patients are heavy smokers predominant-

Table 1. Mortality for the five leading cancer sites for females by age group, United States 1978[a]

All ages	Under 15	15–34	35–54	55–74	75+
34,329 Breast	411 Leukemia	585 Breast	8,205 Breast	17,403 Breast	12,626 Colon and rectum
27,573 Colon and rectum	275 Brain and Central Nervous System	493 Leukemia	4,679 Lung	14,463 Lung	8,129 Breast
24,080 Lung	45 Bone	347 Brain and central nervous system	2,210 Colon and rectum	12,551 Colon and rectum	4,819 Lung
10,842 Uterus	44 Kidney	295 Uterus	2,111 Uterus	5,992 Ovary	3,939 Pancreas
10,651 Ovary	43 Connective tissues	223 Hodgkin's disease	2,029 Ovary	5,480 Uterus	2,954 Uterus

[a] Taken from Silverberg and Lubera, 1982 CA – A Cancer Journal for Clinicians, 32:17.

ly; they have the same survival as older patients (Kyriakos and Webber, 1974).

Lung cancer in children occcurs, but is rare (Fontenelle, 1976). In 1976, 39 cases were in the literature; they were all adeno or undifferentiated carcinoma, except for one squamous cell carcinoma.

From age 35 to 54, lung cancer is the leading cause of cancer death at 10,124 per year compared to 2,462 for colo-rectal (American Cancer Society, 1983). For ages 55 to 74, it is over 46,000, colorectal being 13,717. For ages 75 and over, it is 14,646, with prostate second at 12,292.

2.3 Geography

Out of 163 countries in which 98% of the world's population lives, 88 had a life expectancy greater than 55 years, and of these, 62 have life expectancy greater than 65 years. Cancer is a geriatric disease and the higher the life expectancy (or the more civilized the country) the greater the death rate from cancer (Benjamin, 1977). The male/female ratio of lung cancer in countries with a lower life expectancy is 2:1; in more civilized countries, it jumps to 10:1, implying the increased importance of environmental carcinogens. The age adjusted incidence of lung cancer for the ten leading countries is shown in Table 2.

The incidence of lung cancer in Scotland is the highest at 101/100,000. Age adjusted mortality from lung cancer has increased in the past 20 years in many countries. In Hong Kong, mortality in-

Table 2. Age adjusted incidence of lung cancer per 100,000 population for the 10 countries with greatest incidence of lung cancer

Men	Women	Country
83.9	17.1	Scotland
73.7	14.8	England and Wales
70.6	4.4	Netherlands
67.5	5.6	Belgium
66.4	5.5	Czechoslovakia
64.4	4.2	Finland
54.1	3.8	Luxembourg
53.0	11.0	Northern Ireland
51.8	7.0	Austria
51.2	12.2	Unites States

Adapted from Silverberg E and Luben J, *Cancer* (1983) Vol. 33, No. 1, p. 20.

creased 80%; adenocarcinoma was the most common type in females (Chan and MacLennan, 1977). Because of an increased number of females smoking in Hong Kong in the past 20 years, it was thought that adenocarcinoma there was due to smoking.

3 Etiology of Lung Cancer

3.1 Tobacco

The evidence that cigarette smoking causes cancer is inferential, but so strong that is universally accepted among the scientific community (Wynder, 1972). Lung cancer among non-smokers is uncommon. The risk of developing lung cancer is proportional to total cigarette exposure (age at initiation, duration of smoking, total lifetime number, depth of inhalation and tar levels) (REIF, 1976).

As the number of cigarettes smoked increases, the chance of getting lung cancer increases. A study by the American Cancer Society of 200,000 interviewees over seven years and the review of 12,000 death certificates indicated that the incidence of lung cancer per 100,000 population is 3.4 for non-smokers, 51.4 if less than half pack per day, 143.9 for one to two packs a day, and 217.3 for greater than two packs a day. The chance was 11.4 for cigar smokers and 28.1 for pipe smokers. As cigarette comsumption increased in the U.S. after World War I, so did lung cancer following a 20-year latency period. In 1930 there were 2500 deaths in the U.S. from lung cancer; in 1950, 16,000; in 1964, 43,000; and in 1972, 75,000 (OCHSNER, 1973). The cigarette consumption/cancer relationship has also been analyzed among British physicians. When a smoker stops smoking, the risk of developing lung cancer decreases progressively for 15 years, after which the chance of getting lung cancer is close to the chance of that of a non-smoker. In a study of British physicians who smoked, those who continued had an annual mortality 16 times that of lifetime non-smokers (EBERT, 1978). The death rate of ex-smokers abstinent five to nine years was six times that for non-smokers, and those abstinent greater than 15 years had a death rate from lung cancer twice that of non-smokers.

The most important pulmonary carcinogen in cigarette smoke is tar; tar contains polynuclear aromatic hydrocarbons which are the major contributors to tumorogenicity in animals (BURRASCANO, 1978). Cigarette filters reduce tar content but smokers can eliminate this effect by taking deeper inhalation in order to absorb more nicotine (EBERT, 1978).

More urban dwellers get lung cancer than rural dwellers. This has been used to implicate air pollution as a cause for lung cancer. When tobacco use is standardized, this difference disappears (WYNDER, 1972). A study examining non-smoking Seventh Day Adventists in an urban population and their very low lung cancer rate made this clear (OCHSNER, 1973).

A recent argument by proponents of smoking, fostered by the tobacco industry, is that the genetic predisposition of the need to smoke and lung cancer are linked on the same gene, and that there is no cause and effect relationship. This has been rebutted by Reif (ATUKORALA et al., 1980), who summarized the evidence that lung cancer is caused by tobacco.

3.1.1 Passive Smoking

The ability of secondary cigarette smoke to produce lung cancer is pertinent to the development of regulations for smoking in public places and to the health of the smoker's immediate family. In 1981 HIRAYAMA reported the lung cancer mortality rates of 91,000 non-smoking wives in Japan over age 40, followed from 1966–1979, and related this to the smoking habits of their husbands. The risk of developing lung cancer increased with the number of cigarettes and the time smoked to a maximum relative risk of 4.6 if the husband smoked more than one pack a day. It was 3.17 for 1–19 cigarettes a day (HIRAYAMA, 1981). Other factors, such as Japanese women's exposure to charcoal and wood stoves partially invalidated HIRAYAMA's findings (GRUNDMANN 1981). The American Tobacco Institute also refuted Hirayama and refers to GARFINKEL's article (1981) to indicate his inability to prove such a relationship. However, there is strong support for further research on passive smoking. In one study quoted in the *British Medical Journal,* wives of smokers die on the average four years earlier than wives of non-smokers (MILLER, 1978). Rebreathing one's own smoke might be harmful and someone living in a family where several people smoked could be harmed; even good ventilation might not decrease the incidence of lung cancer (SUTTON, 1981). TRICHOPOULOS examined 51 women with lung cancer and 163 other female patients in a hospital in Athens. Forty of the 51 women and 149 of the 163 other patients did not smoke. The husbands of the 40 women in the first group smoked considerably more than the spouses of the 149 other female patients. Relative risk for getting lung cancer was estimated at 2.4 if the husband smoked less than one pack a day to 3.4 for greater than one pack a day. Present evidence indicates passive smoking may produce lung cancer (TRICHOPOULOS et al., 1981).

Decreasing or stopping cigarette consumption is the most effective way of eliminating lung cancer. The only time cigarette smoking decreased in the U.S. was from 1965–1971, when the media advertised the dangers of smoking. In 1970, there were 29,000 ex-smokers in the U.S. and in 1976, about 45,000,000 smoking adults. Numerous groups have emerged claiming success in helping smokers to stop. Smoke-stopping developed into a $ 50,000,000 business by the mid-70's. The American Health Foundation has stated that the usual way of presenting results is poor and should be standardized (Shewchuck, 1975).

3.2   Occupation

There is an increased incidence of lung cancer among miners and a variety of other occupations.

Nickel workers are at higher risk for contracting lung cancer, particularly in Wales, Canada and the Soviet Union (Sunderman, 1976). In 1976, there were 400 cases of lung cancer in the literature secondary to nickel exposure. The increased risk is *not* related to metallic nickel or nickel carbonyl, but to a refining process of the calcination of impure nickel copper sulfide to nickel copper oxide (Doll et al., 1977). As the refining process changed in Wales from 1914 to 1929, the incidence decreased.

Chromate workers have a similar increased risk. In the United States, it is 10–20 times greater than in the general population (Sunderman, 1976). The risk has decreased since the 1950's due to changes in the refining process (Hill and Ferguson, 1979). Lung cancer due to chromate exposure has been reported in Great Britain, Czechoslovakia, Italy, Japan, Norway and the Soviet Union (Sunderman, 1976).

Foundry workers (metal, ceramic, glass, stone and other industries) exposed to dust have a 1.5–2.0 fold greater risk of lung cancer than the general population (controlled for age, sex and smoking). Within the foundry, it is confined to molders, casters, and clean room operators (Newman et al., 1976). Uranium workers, regardless of whether they smoke, are at increased risk for squamous cell carcinoma (Newman et al., 1976; Hill and Ferguson, 1979). Areas with phosphate mines have elevated rates of lung cancer (Fleisher, 1981). Exposure to high levels of radon and its radioactive daughters in mines leads to lung cancer. Radon is expelled after it is inhaled and the radiation exposure comes from alpha active plutonium attached to aerosols that can be inhaled. Very low doses can theoretically cause lung cancer; doses in U.S. homes in the range of 0.8 pc/liter may be enough to affect several thousand people a year (Fleisher, 1981).

Copper miners have an increased risk which is not due to radiation from radon products in the mines. Arsenic exposure causes not only skin cancer, but respiratory tract cancer; it is as high as eight-fold among men who worked in copper refineries more than 15 years and were heavily exposed to arsenic oxide. A six-fold increase is present among Rhodesian gold miners.

Female beauticians are exposed to potentially noxious substances in sprays and hair dyes (Menck et al., 1977). A six-fold chance of developing lung cancer was found in a retrospective study of death certificates in California (Garfinkel et al., 1977). A second study for LA county area indicated a two-fold risk (Menck et al., 1977), but neither study could control for smoking habits.

Chemical workers exposed to bischloromethyl ether have an increased risk of developing lung cancer (Weiss et al., 1976) with an induction period of 10–24 years. The more intense the exposure, the greater the change. Eighty percent of the lung cancers were squamous cell carcinoma among heavy smokers. In vinyl chloride workers there is an association with large cell carcinoma and adenocarcinoma (Weiss et al., 1980).

Benzopyrene is a component of soot from the inefficient combustion of coal. It is responsible for scrotal cancer; its concentration in England has decreased ten-fold in the past few decades. Benzopyrene is carcinogenic in animals, but its effect on humans, due to its small concentration in the air, is undetermined; roofers do have an increased risk (Hammond et al., 1976). Urban air pollution has been implicated to cause lung cancer. Those areas of Philadelphia that are highly industrialized have a greater incidence of lung cancer, but this is uncontrolled for smoking (Weiss et al., 1978b). Coal fires, industrial emmisions and automobiles are sources of pulmonary carcinogens.

Asbestos is a potent carcinogen. It produces bronchogenic carcinoma as well as mesothelioma. All types of asbestos can cause any type of lung cancer; it usually occurs peripherally and in the lower lobes. Fibers primarily 5–10 millimeters in length are responsible (Frank, 1982).

3.3   Vitamin A and Lung Cancer

Vitamin A is necessary for the differentiation of epithelial tissue (Mettlin et al., 1979). Rodents deficient in vitamin A have an increased susceptibility to respiratory tract cancer. High doses of vitamin A inhibit cancer in hamsters (Harris, 1974). In humans, those with lung cancer have a lower level of serum vitamin A, (Atukorala et al., 1980) and vitamin A intake among smokers is less than among the general population (METT-LIN et al., 1979).

4 Screening for Lung Cancer

Once the diagnosis of lung cancer has been made, staging evaluation eliminates 85–90% of patients from curative resection because of metastatic disease. Early detection is necessary for cures; therefore, annual chest x-ray screening and/or sputum cytology has been advised, particularly in high risk populations. However, lung cancer may have already metastasized in the presence of a small primary, and even if screening x-rays identified early lesions, there is no proof it increases survival.

In the U.S. two large projects have been organized to answer the screening question. The first, called the Philadelphia Pulmonary Neoplasm Research Project, is a prospective study of over 6,000 men that started in December of 1951 and was completed in 1965 (WEISS et al., 1982; 1978a). Volunteers over the age of 45 underwent a semi-annual chest x-ray, questionnaires and ten-year follow-ups. Eighty-six percent were smokers or ex-smokers. Two percent of the men developed lung cancer over the ten year period. One hundred and twenty-one new cases of lung cancer were discovered, after eliminating 84 cases found at first chest x-ray examination. Ninety-four of 121 were eventually confirmed. The chance of getting two succesive semi-annual chest x-rays was 57%, and 45% of new cases had greater than 7.5 month interval from diagnosis to time of the last chest x-ray. The five year "cure rate" was eight percent.

Incidence increased with age and was three times higher in non-whites compared to whites. Eight hundred and thirty of 6,027 men never smoked regularly and none developed lung cancer. The incidence among cigar and pipe smokers was 1/8 that of cigarette smokers. Incidence increased with cigarette consumption to 7 of 103 men who smoked more than two packs a day; all three major histologic types correlated with smoking (squamous cell, adeno and small cell carcinoma).

After elimination of men with metastasis and those who where medically inoperable, only 19 were eligible for thoracotomy and they had a 16% five-year survival. WEISS concluded survival is due to the nature of the disease, rather than treatment, and that screening, at least in his population, is ineffective for increasing survival.

A retrospective study was reported from Germany (Cooperative Study Group, 1978) where, since 1962, it has been obligatory to get an annual chest x-ray. Ninety percent of the adult population have had annual chest x-rays and there has been a steady increase in the number of asymptomatic patients found. They found 36% five year survival in 1,915 screened cases and 293 in 785 clinically symptomatic cases and recommended screening on this basis (WIDOW, 1979).

In 1971 the National Cancer Institute (NCI) organized a "Cooperative Early Lung Cancer Group". This consisted of long-term, prospective screening programs conducted by the Mayo Clinic (Mayo Lung Project), Memorial Sloan Kettering (Memorial Hospital) in New York and Johns Hopkins Hospital in Baltimore.

The Mayo Lung Project selected outpatients over the age of 45 who had no known lung cancer but were at high risk because of chronic excessive cigarette smoking (greater than one pack a day). Each had a chest x-ray and three pooled sputa samples. If the chest x-ray were negative, the patient was randomized to a control group versus a test group which had chest x-ray and sputa samples every four months (FONTANA et al., 1972). Of 11,000 persons screened, 9,200 cases were initially negative and eligible for continued screening. Ninety-one cases of lung cancer were identified at the time of the first chest x-ray (prevalence group) and 43% of the 91 were squamous cell histology. Almost half of these were clinical Stage I (American Joint Committee Staging), and after resection, all but two remained Stage I. Chest x-ray was better for detecting peripheral tumors, whereas sputum cytology have a higher yield for central lesions. Sixty-five percent of the prevalence group was detected by chest x-ray and 19% by sputum cytology only. When cytology alone identified the cancer (occult cancer), the resectability rate was 94%.

Data is available through the end of 1979 for 9,000 cases, half of whom were screened. In the screening group, over a six year period, 98 new cases were found, 67 by screening and 31 patients reporting symptoms or having a chest x-ray for another reason. Sixty-four new cases were identified from the controls. Lung cancer mortality was 39 for study patients and 41 for controls. They concluded that up to March of 1983, there was no proof that screening and subsequent early case finding decreased mortality. They do not advocate large screening programs but do follow high risk patients on an individual basis.

The New York Cancer Detection Program was organized by Memorial-Sloan Kettering Hospital. According to their 1981 update (Melamed et al., 1981), 169 cases were identified among 10,040 men at high risk. Sixty-five (40%) were Stage I. Sixty-two of 65 had Stage I, even after surgery which included mediastinal node dissection. Eighty-seven percent were alive with minimum three year follow-up; follow-up was insufficient to determine if this program would effect long term survival.

Neither of these large prospective screening programs in the U.S. has shown an increase in survival among patients at high risk for lung cancer yet who are screened at yearly or semi-annual rates. Although the Mayo Clinic study is not yet complete, there is no indication thus far that mass screening is effective. Mass screening for lung cancer with chest x-ray and/or sputum cytology offers no advantage in early detection and increased survival. However since the studies are not yet closed, individual high risk patients who are reliable should probably be screened.

4.1   Occult Lung Cancer

By definition, this is a lung cancer detected by sputum cytology, but with a negative chest x-ray. It arises as a problem in screening programs and in the evaluation of hemoptysis – 30% of these patients are found to have head and neck cancer. If worked-up aggressively, these patients can do well. At Memorial Hospital, of 54 occult lung cancers, 33 had Stage I and 14 had Stage II or III disease. Of 27 with early disease treated with resection, none has had recurrence after follow-up of two months to twenty years; however, 21 of 47 (45%) developed a second carcinoma and 71% were from the lung (Martini et al., 1980).

The recommended work-up for occult carcinoma is head and neck examination, chest x-ray, rigid bronchoscopy, fiberoptic bronchoscopy with separate lobar and segmental sampling by washings and brushings and bronchoscopy, if necessary. In the event that bronchoscopy is negative for a gross lesion, Marsh et al. (1972) have suggested lavage through a cuffed rigid bronchoscope, awaking the patient to stimulate the cough reflex and then repeating the opposite side to lateralize the lesion. All branches to the fifth generation subsegmental bronchi are recorded on color videotape. Biopsy is done after re-introducing the rigid scope.

References

American Cancer Society (1981) Cancer statistics, 1981, 31:13–28.

American Cancer Society (1983) Cancer statistics, CA 33:9–25.

Atukorala S, Basu TK, Dickerson JWT (1979) Vitamin A, zinc and lung cancer, Br J Cancer 40:927–931.

Benjamin B (1977) Trends and differentials in lung cancer mortality, World Health Stat Q Rep 30:188–145.

Burrascano JJ (1978) Lung cancer etiology – critical appraisal, NY State J Med 78(1):924–934.

Chan WC, MacLennan R (1977) Lung cancer in Hong Knog Chinese: mortality and histological types, 1960–1972, Br J Cancer 35:226–231.

Cooperative Study Group for the Early Detection of Lung Cancer in the German Democratic Republic (1978) Roentgenographic chest screening in the detection and survival of patients with lung cancer, Ann Thorac Surg 26:406–412.

Doll R, Matthews JD, Morgan LJ (1977) Cancers of the lung and nasal sinuses in nickel workers: a reassessment of the period of risk, Br J Ind Med 34:102–105.

Ebert RV (1978) Cessation of cigarette smoking and pulmonary disease, JAMA 240:2159–2161.

Enterline PE (1978) Asbestos and cancer: the international lag, Am Rev Respir Dis 118:975–978.

Fleisher RL (1981) A possible association between lung cancer and phosphate mining and processing, Health Phys 41:171–175.

Fontana RS, Sanderson DR, Miller WE (1972) The Mayo Lung Project: preliminary report of "early cancer detection" phase, Cancer 30:1373–1382.

Fontenelle LJ (1976) Primary adenocarcinoma of lung in a child: review of the literature, Am Surg 42:296–299.

Frank AL (1982) The epidemiology and etiology of lung cancer, Clin Chest Med 3:219–228.

Garfinkel J, Selvin S, Brown SM (1977) Brief communication; possible increased risk of lung cancer among beauticians, JNCI 58:141–143.

Garfinkel L (1981) Time trends in lung cancer mortality among nonsmokers and a note on passive smoking, JNCI 66:1061–1066.

Grundmann E, Müller KM, Winter KD (1981) Non-smoking wives of heavy smokers have a higher risk of lung cancer, Br Med J 282:1156.

Hammond EC, Selikoff IJ, Lawther PL, et al (1976) Inhalation of benzpyrene and cancer in man, Ann NY Acad Sci 271:116–124.

Harris CC (1974) Cause and prevention of lung cancer, Semin Oncol 1:163–166.

Hill WH, Ferguson WS (1979) Statistical analysis of epidemiological data from a chromium chemical manufacturing plant, J Occup Med 21:103–106.

Hinds MW, Stemmermann GN, Yang HY, et al (1981) Differences in lung cancer risk from smoking among Japanese, Chinese and Hawaiian women in Hawaii, Int J Cancer 27:297–302.

Hirayama T (1981) Non-smoking wives of heavy smokers have a higher risk of lung cancer: a study from Japan, Br Med J 282:183–185.

Huhti E, Sutinen S, Saloheimo M (1981) Survival among patients with lung cancer: an epidemiologic study, Am Rev Respir Dis 124:13–16.

Jick H, Porter J, Morrison AS (1979) Lung cancer in young women, Arch Intern Med 139:745–746.

Kyriakos M, Webber B (1974) Cancer of the lung in young men, J Thorac Cardiovasc Surg 67:634–648.

Lee ES, Roberts RE, Labarthe DR (1976) Excess and deficit lung cancer mortality in three ethnic groups in Texas, Cancer 38:2551–2556.

Leung JS (1977) Cigarett smoking, the kerosene stove and lung cancer in Hong Kong, Br J Dis Chest 71:273–276.

Marsh BR, Frost JK, Erozan YS, et al (1972) Occult bronchogenic carcinoma, Cancer 30:1348–1352.

Martini N, McLamed MR (1980) Occult carcinomas of the lung, Ann Thorac Surg 30:215–223.

Melamed MR, Flehinger BJ, Zaman MB, et al (1981) Detection of true pathologic stage I lung cancer in a screening program and the effect on survival, Cancer 47:1182–1187.

Menck HR, Pike MC, Henderson BE, et al (1977) Lung cancer risk among beauticians and other female workers: brief communication, JNCI 59:1423–1425.

Mettlin C, Graham S, Swanson M (1979) Vitamin A and lung cancer, JNCI 62:1435–1438.

Miller G (1978) Passive smoking, J Breathing 41:5–9.

Newman JA, Archer VE, Saccomanno G, et al (1976) Histologic types of bronchogenic carcinoma among members of copper-mining and smelting communities, Ann NY Acad Sci 271:260–268.

Ochsner A (1973) Cancer of the lung, J Am Diet Assoc 62:249–252.

Palmer WG, Scott WD (1981) Lung cancer in ferrous foundry workers: a review, Am Ind Hyg Assoc J 42:329–340.

Reif AE (1976) Public information on smoking: an urgent responsibility for cancer research workers, JNCO 57:1207–1210.

Reif AE (1981) Effect of cigarette smoking on susceptibility to lung cancer, Oncology 38:76–85.

Shewchuck LA (1975) Problems of high-risk populations and high-risk non-responders: smoking behavior. In: Cullen JW, Fox BH, Isom RU (eds) Cancer: the behavioral dimensions, Raven Press, New York, pp 93–99.

Stellman SD, Stellman JM (1981) Women's occupations, smoking and cancer and other diseases, CA 31:29–43.

Sunderman FW, Jr. (1976) A review of the carcinogenicities of nickel, chromium and arsenic compounds in man and animals, Prev Med 5:279–294.

Sutton GC (1981) Correspondence: passive smoking and lung cancer, Br Med J 282:733.

Trichopoulos D, Kalandidi A, Sparros L, et al (1981) Lung cancer and passive smoking, Int J Cancer 27:1–4.

Wald NJ (1976) Mortality from lung cancer and coronary heart-disease in relation to changes in smoking habits, Lancet 1:136–138.

Weiss W, Figueroa WG (1976) The characteristics of lung cancer due to chloromethyl ethers, J Occup Med 18:623–627.

Weiss W, Seidman H, Boucot KR (1978a) The Philadelphia Pulmonary Neoplasm Research Project. Symptoms in occult lung cancer, Chest 73:57–61.

Weiss W (1978b) Lung cancer mortality and urban air pollution, Am J Public Health 68:773–775.

Weiss W, Moser RL, Auerbach O (1979) Lung cancer in chloromethyl ether workers, Am Rev Respir Dis 120:1031–1037.

Weiss W, Boucot KR, Seidman H (1980) The prognosis of lung cancer originating as an infiltrate. Data from the Philadelphia Pulmonary Neoplasm Research Project, Am Rev Respir Dis 121:805–812.

Weiss W, Boucot KR, Seidman H (1982) The Philadelphia Pulmonary Neoplasm Research Project, Clin Chest Med 3:243–256.

Whittemore A, Atlshuler B (1976) Lung cancer incidence in cigarette smokers; further analysis of Doll and Hill's data for British physicians, Biometrics 32:805–816.

Widow W (1979) Zur Bedeutung von jährlichen Röntgenreihenuntersuchungen für die Erfassung und Behandlung des Bronchialkarzinoms (Eng. Abstract). Early detection of bronchial carcinoma by annual mass x-ray screening, Zentralbl Chir 104:81–90.

Wynder EL (1972) Etiology of lung cancer – reflections on two decades of research, Cancer 30:1332–1339.

Chapter II Approach to the Patient with Lung Cancer

Steven G. Mann

CONTENTS

Approach to the Patient with Lung Cancer

This chapter will outline the general approach to the patient with lung cancer, beginning with diagnosis and staging, and proceeding to management and prognosis. The unique problems of small cell cancer and bronchiolo-alveolar histologies are discussed separately, as well as particular clinical problems, such as superior vena caval obstruction and Pancoast tumor.

Steven G. Mann, M.D.
1575 Soquel Drive, Santa Cruz, CA 95065, USA

1 Diagnosis

Sputum cytology, bronchoscopy and percutaneous needle biopsy are the most commonly used tests to diagnose lung cancer.

Sputum cytology is effective in diagnosing lung cancer because of its endobronchial origin. When three consecutive specimens are obtained and read by an experienced cytologist, it gives a 30% yield in the absence of symptoms, 50% when cough is present and 70% when hemoptysis is present (Martini and Burton, 1981). Since distinguishing between small cell and non-small cell cancer is so important, histology is preferred, even though sputa specificity is accurate 80–90% of the time in determining small cell type (Suprun et al., 1980; Jay et al., 1980).

Bronchial brushing and biopsy give a yield of about 70%. In patients presenting with anterior or middle mediastinal masses on chest x-ray, over two-thirds will have positive yield after bronchoscopy if the mass is due to lung cancer and there is some deviation of the tracheo-bronchial tree (Mohsenifar et al., 1979). Bronchial washings do not appear to add to this yield (Chopra et al., 1977). Blind biopsy of the carina should be done in most cases for staging at the time of diagnosis and ten percent of these will have positive yield, mostly due to submucosal tumor. There is no correlation between the presence of carinal involvement and its proximity to the endobronchial tumor (Robbins et al., 1979).

If bronchoscopy is negative, percutaneous needle biopsy is usually the procedure of choice. Implantation at the site of the chest wall penetration is rare (Sinner and Zailcek, 1976). Recently, needle biopsy of mediastinal masses has been reported. Lesions as small as 1.5 cm, when using CT guidance and fluoroscopy can be sampled (Gobien et al., 1981). Westcott reported 91 patients with percutaneous needle aspiration biopsy of hilar and mediastinal masses with no major complication despite puncture of great vessels. Eighty-three patients had malignant tumor and 96% had the diagnosis established. Seventy-two patients were able to avoid mediastinoscopy or surgery (Westcott, 1981). Needle aspiration biopsy agrees with histology 80–90% of the time (Thornbury et al., 1981).

1.1 Atypical Teratoma Syndrome

In evaluating a mediastinal mass with a pulmonary component in a young man in which the histology is undifferentiated carcinoma, it is important to be aware of the "atypical teratoma syndrome". Particularly in men under the age of 40, whether or not they smoke, a primary midline germinal tumor arising from the mediastinum may simulate lung cancer. Diagnosis can be made by elevated tumor markers, viz. serum human chorionic gonadotrophin titers and alpha-fetoprotein markers; this is a potentially chemo-curable disease (Fox et al., 1979).

2 Association of Lung Cancer with Other Diseases

2.1 Tuberculosis

Tuberculosis not uncommonly exists together with primary lung cancer. Each appears to run a separate course without affecting the other. Among 64 cases of patients who had simultaneous diagnoses of lung cancer and active tuberculosis, 94% underwent successful sputum conversion. There was no case of disseminated TB (Mok et al., 1978). Active TB does not seem to be a contraindication to irradiation so long as the patient is receiving anti-TB therapy.

2.2 Scar Cancer

Except for scar cancers, previous damage does not appear to increase vulnerability to lung cancer. Among patients with chronic unilateral lung disease who eventually develop lung cancer, over 80% arise from the contralateral uninvolved lung, probably due to impaired ventilation and decreased contact with carcinogenic aerosols in the impaired side. Of adenocarcinomas, however, 7 out of 15 occurred in the impaired side (Yoneyama et al., 1976). Among patients with asthma, only 10% as many developed lung cancer as among the general population without asthma (Ford,

1978). The incidence of "scar" cancer or primary lung cancer arising peripherally in association with the scar is 3–15% (McDonnell and Long, 1981). Patients of cancer age with large blebs or bullae are at increased risk for lung cancer since these are frequently associated with subpleural scars (Scannell, 1980). Over three-fourths of scar cancer are found in the upper lobes and over one-half are limited to infarcts. Less than one-fourth are related to TB scars. About 45% of all peripheral lung cancers arise in a scar (Auerbach et al., 1979).

2.3 Second Primary

Lung cancer has been reported in association with a group of miscellaneous entities. It has been reported in higher incidence among men under 40 years of age with severe bilateral bullous lung disease (Aronberg et al., 1980). Among patients with Chilaiditi Syndrome (interposition of colon and small bowel between liver and diaphragm), and in higher incidence among patients with lymphoma or chronic leukemia (Libshitz et al., 1978).

Among the entire lung cancer population, one-half percent will develop a second primary before death. Two percent of those who undergo resection and ten percent of long-term survivors will also develop a second primary lung cancer. Most of these occur within the first five years after diagnosis (Shields, 1979). Patients who have survived their treatment for lung cancer should have annual head and neck exams, since tobacco is the causative agent for each (Shankar, 1981). If a patient treated curatively for one lung cancer develops a second primary lung cancer, there is a good basis for being aggressive. Among 58 patients with metachronous primaries, 36% cumulative survival was found with aggressive surgery for the second primary at five years. There was a 9.3% postoperative mortality (Jensik et al., 1981).

Primary lung cancer, primarily adenocarcinoma, is rare in animals, but has been reported in the dog, ox, horse, sheep, cat, chicken and water buffalo (Kharole et al., 1975).

3 History and Physical

The radiation oncologist usually sees the patient with lung cancer for the first time after the diagnosis is made. The first decision to be made is whether the tumor is curatively resectable since surgery offers the best chance for cure among those patients eligible for it. Eligibility for surgery depends on the histologic subtype, stage and general medical status (including pulmonary status) of the patient. The process starts with the history and physical examination.

The history and physical is oriented toward eliminating patients with extra-thoracic or locally advanced disease from curative resection. Symptoms of systemic involvement should be elicited. These include anorexia and weight loss; a loss of taste for food can be a sign of liver involvement or secondary to metabolic effects of tumor. Bony pain is sufficient to obtain a bone scan; headache, blurred vision, unilateral weakness, memory, reading or speech difficulty are all signals to obtain a contrast-enhanced CT scan of the brain. A brain scan is not indicated routinely in the absence of neurologic deficit or symptoms; however, in one study of 50 pre-operative patients without symptoms, 3 out of 50 were found to have solitary metastatic lesions (JACOBS et al., 1977).

Every patient with lung cancer should have a careful head and neck examination. The scalp and soft tissue is examined for subcutaneous nodules; these are usually painless, purplish red, well-demarcated and rapidly growing. Positive excisional biopsy can eliminate the need for bronchoscopy. Careful palpation for lymph nodes, particularly in the cervical and supraclavicular region is important. Left lower lobe lesions drain to the right supraclavicular fossa. In 1.5% of lung cancer patients, the tumor spreads to the cervical nodes (DAVIS et al., 1977).

Fifteen percent of patients with lung cancer will develop a separate head and neck primary if they live long enough, but lung cancer can metastasize to head and neck sites. Lung cancer is the most common primary to metastasize to soft tissues of the oral cavity; the gingiva and tongue are the two most common sites (KIM et al., 1979). Occasionally, a precocious metastasis from lung cancer will present this way. Very rapidly growing non-ulcerative and high grade tumors should heighten the index of suspicion for metastasis, rather than a primary. The most common primary site to metastasize to the nose is kidney; lung is second (SHANMUGHAM, 1976). Examination of the vocal cords for a separate primary and mobility is important. Unilateral paralysis can be due to direct invasion or involvement of the left or right recurrent laryngeal nerve; this indicates T_3, usually unresectable disease.

Fundoscopic examination may reveal choroidal metastasis. Lung is the most common primary

in men and the second most common in women, with breast first to metastasize to the choroid. This is usually a late finding but is occasionally precocious.

Examination of the skin may reveal pallor if the patient is anemic. Jaundice, if due to liver involvement, is usually accompanied by other signs of liver failure; it may be due to extra-hepatic biliary obstruction from peri-portal lymph nodes (SMITH, 1980). A "dirty" tan color in a patient who is becoming weaker may be due to increased ACTH production secondary to adrenal metastasis. It is important to differentiate this weakness from that due to ectopic ADH secretion since they are both accompanied by hyponatremia; but serum potassium is elevated in the former. Up to 27% of lung cancer patients have adrenal metastases at autopsy, but the diagnosis is not usually made during life, partly due to low index of suspicion and the need for 90% replacement of the adrenals before clinical symptoms appear (ZIMM et al., 1981). Iodocholesterol scanning has not been as effective as CT scanning in pre-mortem diagnosis of adrenal metastasis (QURAISHI et al., 1981).

Gastrointestinal symptoms may be due to direct involvement by tumor. Two-thirds of patients with GI tract involvement have symptoms, but the majority is not diagnosed pre-mortem. Twelve percent of patients have metastases and 33% of large cell cancers metastasize to the GI tract (BURBIGE et al., 1980). Perforation of the bowel can occur (RAMANATHAN et al., 1976), it is uncommon but indicates ominous prognosis; most cases are from the right lower lobe (WINCHESTER et al., 1977).

4 Laboratory – Blood Markers

A number of chemicals have been measured in the blood of lung cancer patients as tumor markers.

About 70% of patients have elevated levels of carcino-embryonic antigen (CEA) (VINCENT et al., 1975). If the CEA level is greater than 15–20 mg/ml, the prognosis is uniformly poor; in one series, it was three months (DENT et al., 1978). It is not specific enough to use as a screening agent, but can be used as a tumor marker to monitor therapy. In one study, every patient with a CEA level greater than 50 with squamous cell carcinoma had liver involvement (GOSLIN et al., 1981). Ferritin and alpha 2 PAG are elevated in lung cancer, but alpha fetoprotein is not (GROPP et al., 1977) although a case report was published of a tumor which did secrete alpha fetoprotein (Yasunami et al., 1981).

Plasma calcitonin is elevated in about 85% of patients with extensive oat cell lung cancer, but not in those with limited disease. It can be used serially to follow treatment (Wallach et al., 1981) and it is produced by the tumor rather than the parathyroid gland. Extracts of tumor tissue show immunoreactive calcitonin (Hillyard et al., 1976).

Lung cancer patients overall have an elevated serum copper level, but not sufficiently high to be of clinical use. Levels are in the range of 1.4 mg/liter for malignant, versus 1.03 mg/liter for non-malignant controls (Huhti et al., 1980).

Issell et al., (1981) found that serum zinc was lowered in 24 out of 26 patients with advanced lung cancer. The average blood level was 43.2 ng/100 ml with the normal being 80–100. The zinc level did not correlate with response to chemotherapy, but did correlate with triceps fold thickness, a measurement of fat stores.

5 Pathology

The histologic classification used most often is from the World Health Organization. There are four distinct types: squamous cell carcinoma, adenocarcinoma (includes bronchioalveolar), large cell (or large cell anaplastic, which includes giant cell), and small cell (or small cell anaplastic) carcinoma. The latter includes oat cell type (the size of lymphocytes) and intermediate cell, which is larger than oat cell (but not as large as large cell anaplastic). The intermediate cell type includes the two sub-types formerly designated polygonal and spindle cell.

Giant cell carcinoma is clinically separated from other large cell anaplastic tumors. It occurs in younger ages with more rapid course from initial symptoms to death. The primary is more peripheral and median survival is only four and a half months (Kallenberg and Jaqué, 1979).

The distribution of histologic subtypes varies among institutions. Larsson and Zettergren (1976) reviewed 479 cases in Sweden and found 48.2% epidermoid, 25% small cell, 21.9% adenocarcinoma and 3.1% large cell carcinoma. If the pathologist accepts individual cell keratinization as evidence of squamous cell carcinoma, then a larger proportion of squamous cell, compared to large cell tumors, will be reported.

The distribution of histologic types has changed over the past 20 years. In review of over 1,000 patients in New York State from 1962–1975, no change was found in the incidence of large or small cell or bronchio-alveolar carcinoma. Adenocarcinoma increased from 17.6 to 29.8%, while squamous cell dropped from 48.6 to 25.5% (Vincent et al., 1977).

Lung cancers caused by chronic radiation exposure in uranium mines is associated with a small cell type (Horacek et al., 1977).

6 Staging

Once the diagnosis is made, staging evaluation is done to detect extrathoracic metastases which render the patient incurable. For the clinical TNM staging system, T is defined by bronchoscopy and chest x-ray. N (mediastinal lymph nodes) is defined by mediastinoscopy, mediastinotomy and, in some institutions, gallium scanning. N (hilar lymph nodes) are best identified with 55 degree hilar tomography.

Radioisotope brain and liver scans will detect most symptomatic brain and liver metastases. They have too low a yield to perform in asymptomatic subjects. Hooper et al. (1978) had no positive scans in asymptomatic patients among 225 patients studied who presented with lung cancer. Kelly et al. (1979) identified occult liver disease in 5.3% of 38 patients and occult brain disease in 6.6% of 58 neurologically intact patients.

Turner and Haggith (1981) found three positive scans among bone, brain and liver scans done in 57 asymptomatic patients. Two of the three lived over $2^1/_2$ years without metastasis, indicating a false positive; he concluded that he would not get any scans without symptoms. Wittes and Yeh (1977) studied 56 asymptomatic patients with oat cell cancer and found only three positive scans.

In the neurologically intact patient, a brain scan should not be done; in the absence of pain, a bone scan need not be done. In the presence of normal alkaline phosphatase and no palpable liver, a liver scan will most likely be negative.

Sequential extensive evaluation for small cell cancer yields such a large number of patients with extra-thoracic metastases at presentation that surgery is no longer used except for the uncommon solitary peripheral lesion. In addition to scanning, if symptoms are present, bone marrow aspirate or biopsy will be positive 17–40% of the time (Hirsch et al., 1977). Thrombocytopenia (less

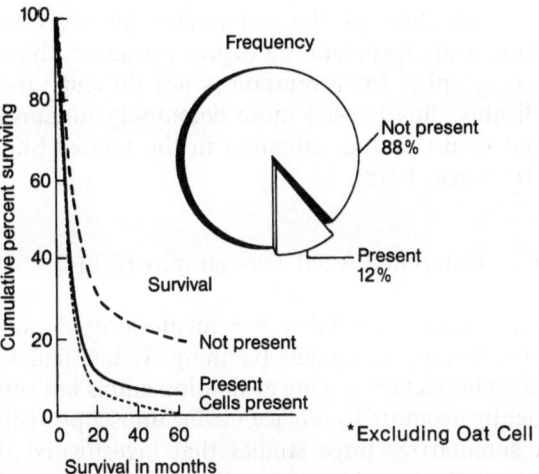

Fig. 1. Lung cancer: Frequency and survival – effect of pleural effusion (excluding oat cell). From Mountain, CF et al., Regional Extension of Lung Cancer, Int J Rad Onc Biol Phys 6:1013–1020.

than 135,000 platelets) is associated with bone marrow involvement 100% of the time (6 patients) (HIRSCH et al., 1977). DUNNICK et al. (1979) used abdominal CT as an adjunct to staging and found 36% of 145 scans to be abnormal if all patients are scanned. He found 16% with retroperitoneal, 12 patients with liver metastases, and 4 with adrenal metastases.

6.1 Pleural Effusion

Pleural effusion occurs in 12% of patients. It has poor prognosis and causes the tumor to be T_3 whether or not malignant cells are found in the effusion (Fig. 1). If one separates cytologically negative effusions, a small number will be resectable. In one study there were four survivors of 73 patients who had thoracotomy in the presence of pleural effusions (DECKER et al., 1978). The effusion could be due to obstructive pneumonitis or atelectasis, particularly if it is a small amount visible only on CT scan and not on chest x-ray. Measurement of protein in fluid does not correlate with resectability (DECKER et al., 1978).

7 Evaluation for Surgery

Surgery is the patient's best chance for cure, if there is no contraindication. To be eligible for surgery, the tumor needs to be resectable, there can be no extra-thoracic metastases and the patient must be medically operable. Absolute contraindications for surgery are extra-thoracic spread, ipsilateral supraclavicular node involvement, vocal cord paralysis (implying recurrent laryngeal nerve invasion), malignant pleural effusion and usually tumor within 2 cm of the carina. Paraneoplastic syndrome usually signifies metastatic disease, but by itself is not a contraindication, since it can occur with localized disease and can remit after surgery, (VASUDEVAN, et al., 1979; SADOFF and ARONSTAM, 1977) and in oat cell carcinoma, after chemotherapy and irradiation (JENKYN et al., 1980). Invasion of the chest wall is not always a contraindication; this is particularly true for superior sulcus (Pancoast) tumors in which extensive local invasion of bone may occur and not compromise local control or cure. More controversial is mediastinal node involvement. This is usually a contra-indication, but in certain centers, it is treated with mediastinal dissection, particularly if confined to subcarinal nodes. Ipsilateral hilar node involvement is not a contraindication, although if it occurs, the prognosis is jeopardized. In one large series in which stage TINO had a 59% five-year survival, the presence of only a positive hilum decreased it to 52% (MOUNTAIN, 1977).

Age by itself, is not a contraindication. In one review of 80 patients over the age of 70 with lung cancer, a 64% two year survival was found among those who had thoracotomy, compared to a 6% two year survival for those without. Even with an operative mortality of 18%, thoracotomy appeared justified in this group (HARVIEL et al., 1978).

A patient undergoing thoracotomy needs to be medically fit and have adequate pulmonary function to tolerate removal of part or all of his lung. Since smoking is responsible for over 80% of lung cancers and also causes chronic obstructive pulmonary disease, these two are frequently associated. Patients with lung cancer, therefore, frequently have diminished pulmonary tests for reasons besides their cancer. The determination of what is adequate pulmonary function to tolerate surgery varies from asking patients to walk up a flight of stairs in front of the examiner to more objective formal pulmonary function tests and arterial blood gases. KIRSH et al. (1976) used the following set of criteria in elderly patients to eliminate those at high risk from surgery:

1) pCO_2 45 mm Hg at rest or with exercise.
2) pO_2 50 mm at rest or with exercise despite hyperventilation.

3) Forced expiratory volume (FEV_1) 2,000 cc, forced vital capacity (FVC) 2000 cc, or maximum vital capacity (MVC) 50% of predicted in whom pneumonectomy is required.
4) FEV_1 1,500 cc in those requiring lobectomy.
5) Calculated FEV_1 800 cc determined preoperatively by spirometry with a ventilatory perfusion scan.

In older debilitated patients with pulmonary compromise, segmental resection has less morbidity than lobectomy. A 36% five year survival for 31 patients was accomplished by BENNETT and SMITH (1979). HOFFMAN and RANSDELL (1979) found a survival of 85,58, and 26% respectively for one, two and five years for wedge versus 75, 55, and 25% respectively for lobectomy in a review of the Veterans Administration cases. They concluded that patients with peripheral lung cancer can be treated with wedge resection.

In patients in whom the tumor is close to the carina, the sleeve pneumonectomy has been advocated by some. This procedure was first described in 1972 and consists of resection of the right lung and carina and circumferential anastomosis of the left lung to the trachea. Five out of 16 patients in one series were alive 15 months to 7 years after resection (DESLAURIERS et al., 1979).

7.1 Evaluation of Regional Lymph Nodes

Involved ipsilateral supraclavicular nodes is a contraindication for curative surgery. Blind scalene node biopsy can identify non-palpable disease and is worthwhile in selected cases. From a series of 101 patients in whom this procedure was done with an overall incidence of 8.9%, the following conclusions were made (SCHATZLEIN et al., 1981): (1) No patient with a peripheral primary, regardless of the size or histology, was positive. (2) Forty percent (6 out of 15) of centrally located adenocarcinomas were positive. (3) 2.5% (1 out of 40) squamous cell carcinomas were positive. (4) Bilateral biopsies did not increase the yield.

Evaluation of the pulmonary hilum is best done using ipsilateral 55 degree posterior oblique tomography. Interpretation is not difficult; inexplicably, this is used more commonly in Europe and is just getting attention in the United States (JANOWER, 1978).

7.2 Computed Axial Tomography (CT)

This imaging modality has revolutionized radiation therapy treatment planning. It has had less of an impact on staging evaluation and is not sufficiently accurate to replace mediastinoscopy. Table 1 summarizes three studies that investigated the sensitivity (number of positives identified by the test/number of true positives) and the specificity (number of negatives identified by the test/number of true negatives) of CT scanning in detecting mediastinal metastasis.

CT scanning can add other specific information to the staging evaluation but cannot exclude a patient from surgery. For example, for peripheral lesions it can suggest but not prove pleural involvement; pleural effusions can be diagnosed, but benign cannot be separated from malignant; occult lung metastases are rare and a CT search for these is not appropriate. If CT is positive in the mediastinum, then mediastinoscopy needs to be done; if grossly positive, it will have already been seen on a chest x-ray. At this time it is not a major part of the staging evaluation (CENTER, 1981).

7.3 Mediastinal Lymph Nodes

Involvement of the mediastinal lymph nodes by tumor signifies a poor prognosis. In a series of 835 patients, MOUNTAIN et al. (1980) has shown that the five year survival is 8% with mediastinal nodes involved and 48% without. Among patients with squamous cell carcinoma, it is 13% at five years, large cell anaplastic 11%, and adenocarcinoma 2%. On the other hand, in review of 445 patients with mediastinal node metastases, MAR-

Table 1. Ability of CT scanning to detect mediastinal metastases

Author, date	Number of patients	Sensitivity	Specificity	Conclusion
RICHARDSON JV, 1980	65	61%	81%	Added little to staging
UNDERWOOD GA, 1979	18	44%	88%	Added little to staging
FALING LJ, 1981	49	88%	88%	Better than chest x-ray; both had 67% sensitivity for hilar nodes

TINI (1980) found 80 treated with resection and postoperative irradiation. Survival was 49% at three years and adenocarcinoma survival was better than epidermoid (56% versus 44% at three years).

Involvement of the mediastinal nodes in many centers is a sign of inoperability, although this has been challenged by others who do mediastinal node dissection in selected cases. In either case, the identification of mediastinal lymph nodes is important. Selective mediastinoscopy for central tumors will detect involved nodes in about a third of patients, depending on how they are selected. Peripheral tumors less than 2 cm in diameter do not require mediastinoscopy since the yield is so low (WEISSBERG 1977).

Gallium is a radiopharmaceutical used in an attempt to replace mediastinoscopy in detecting lymph node involvement. It is taken up by most lung cancers (ALAZRAKI, 1980), though less frequently by adenocarcinoma than other histologic types consistent with the six-fold difference in intracellular uptake in vitro (THESINGH et al., 1978). The smallest lung cancer that can be identified is 1.5 cm. It has been investigated to replace mediastinoscopy to detect mediastinal lymph nodes involved by cancer. ALAZRAKI (1980) studied 25 patients with uptake of their primary tumors. They had no false negatives and recommended skipping mediastinoscopy if the chest x-ray and gallium scan are negative. RICHARDSON et al. (1980) found a sensitivity of 90% and recommended skipping mediastinoscopy, but he found a 55% specificity and could not rely on negative scan. Gallium scanning at this time has not replaced mediastinoscopy.

8 Irradiation

8.1 Adjunctive Irradiation

Postsurgical irradiation is used when histologic margins are narrow after resection or when mediastinal lymph nodes are involved by tumor. Most patients with T_3, N_1 or N_2 tumors receive adjuvant irradiation. Patients with adenocarcinoma who receive postoperative radiation therapy may have increased one and two year survival (85 versus 51% respectively at one year and 43 versus 8% respectively at five years) (CHOI et al., 1980). Irradiating the mediastinum after adequate surgery in the absence of involved lymph nodes does not affect survival and is not advocated. In fact, in one series, after 6,000 rads to the mediastinum

to T_2N_0 tumors, the survival rate was actually decreased compared to controls (VAN HOUTTE et al., 1980a).

MENDIONDO et al. (1979) treated patients after surgery for Stages I and II non-oat cell cancer with irradiation and found no difference in survival; however, the local recurrence rate was 26.5% versus 8.3% in the irradiated group. Doses ranged from 4,000 to 5,400 rads. COX (1981c) reviewed preoperative irradiation, popularized during the 1960's when it was shown that tumor could be sterilized by the time of surgery. The VA group could not corroborate an increased survival.

In a review of the literature, PEARSON (1980) found that if mediastinal nodes are found at thoracotomy and patients have no postoperative irradiation, the five year survival averaged 11% (0% to 29%); if identified at mediastinoscopy and then resected without adjunctive therapy, the five year survival was 0% in each of three papers; two series indicated a 19% and 35% five year survival when resection was used with postoperative irradiation. He recommends selective resection for N2 cases when they are squamous cell carcinoma and involve the ipsilateral tracheo-bronchial tree, but not the contralateral side or the superior mediastinum.

Interstitial therapy has been popularized by HILARIS and MARTINI (1979) who reported 470 patients treated from 1956–1976 by permanent implant at the time of surgery with radon, ^{198}Au, ^{125}I, or ^{192}Ir seeds. This was supplemented with 3,000–4,000 rads external irradiation. Local control was obtained in 60% of Stage III and 80% of Stages I and II. Seven percent of 340 patients with disease localized to the thorax survived five years.

8.2 Definitive

8.2.1 Treatment Planning

Symptomatic patients with lung cancer can be palliated with irradiation or treated definitively, i.e., with curative intent. Individually shaped lung blocks and computerized axial tomographic treatment planning allows larger doses to be delivered without morbidity, increasing the potential for long term local control. CT evaluation of the extent of tumor has added tremendous accuracy to staging and planning. Pre-radiation evaluation gives a clearer delineation of the tumor three-fourths of the time, changes the assessment of the size of the tumor 43% and can change stage as well (ENAMI et al., 1978b). It is essential for treatment planning in over 50% of cases, in which changes in treatment volume resulted from CT. SEYDEL et al. (1980) reported almost 40% change in treatment volume, causing change in technique.

8.2.2 Dose

The Veterans Administration (PETROVICH 1981) studied 343 patients treated from 1975–1978. They compared 5,000 rads in five weeks to 4,200 rads in three weeks and found no difference in survival, response or control rate. Patients who had a partial or complete response (38%) had a median survival of 50 versus 31 weeks.

CHOI and DOUCETTE (1981) reviewed 169 patients with non-small cell lung cancer treated with high dose external irradiation. Doses were up to 6,400 rads. One hundred and thirty-one patients had T_{2-3}, N_2M_0 stages. All had individual lung blocks; half were reshaped at 2,000 rads. Two year survival was 36% for this group versus 10% for a previous group in lower dose range; at three years it was 28 and 3%. Tumor control increased with dose.

Numerous dose-time fractionation studies have been done comparing varying doses with continuous and split course irradiation. SHAH et al. (1981) compared 5,000 rads in five weeks to 2,000 rads in one week repeated again after a two week rest and 3,000 rads in two weeks was repeated again after a 10 day rest. The two year survival was 33%, 15% and 25%, respectively. The 24 month survival for Stage I, II and III was 85%, 28% and 18%, respectively.

LEE et al. (1976) randomized patients to 2,500 rads in two and a half weeks, repeated after three to four week rest and found no difference in tolerance and survival.

ENAMI et al. (1979) compared 76 patients who received 6,000 rads in six weeks to 24 who received a split course regimen. Local control was achieved in 58.8% continuous and 45.4% split course. Median survival was 12 months. Nineteen percent of the total group survived three years. Stage was not taken into account and small cell cancer was included.

SALAZAR et al. (1976) reviewed 160 patients treated with four different continuous therapy schedules and 59 treated with three different split course regimens. Those in the split course did better with median survival 7.7 months for continous and 11.5 for split course. Split course had higher

response rate, less radiation pneumonitis and decreased incidence of local failure.

HOLSTI and MATTSON (1980) reported 205 patients treated with split course and 158 with continous treatment. The latter received 5,000 rads in five weeks and the former 5,500 rads in seven to eight weeks. They found the split course to be at least as good as continous and better tolerated.

SHANKAR (1980) studied pulmonary function in 15 patients who received split course. Forced vital capacity and forced respiratory volume showed an improvement in half the patients 2–12 months after irradiation compared to before. Adverse effect on lung function was minimal.

The Radiation Therapy Oncology Group (PEREZ et al., 1980) a multi-institutional cooperative group based in the United States, studied 375 patients with non-oat cell primary lung cancer in a prospective randomized fashion. They were divided into one of four treatment arms: (1) 4,000 rads split course (2,000 rads in one week, two week rest, 2,000 rads in one week) or (2) 4,000 rads in four weeks, or (3) 5,000 rads in five weeks, or (4) 6,000 rads in 6 weeks. Overall, there was a 40% one year survival and 10–18% two year survival. Patients treated with split course had the lowest survival (10% at two years), compared with other groups (14–18%). Total response rate was 48% in 4,000 rad groups, 65% in 5,000 rad group and 61% in the 6,000 rad group. The rate of initial intrathoracic recurrence decreased with increasing dose being 38% for 6,000 rads, 45% for 5,000 rads and 51% for 4,000 rads (split) and 64% for 4,100 rads (continuous). Distant metastases were more prevalent in adenocarcinoma or large cell (63%) than in epidermoid (33%). Five thousand or 6,000 rad continous treatment was superior to 4,000 rad continuous or split.

SHERMAN et al. (1981) studied the characteristics of long term survivors of lung cancer after irradiation (greater than 18 months). The local failure rate corresponded to dose: 50% in patients receiving less than 5,000 rads, 22% for 5,000–5,500 rads, 18% for 5,500–5,900 rads and five percent in those receiving greater than 5,900 rads.

One can conclude from the previous studies that: (1) split course is less effective or possibly as effective as continuous for local tumor control, but not more effective. (2) split course is tolerated as well or better as continuous, (3) tumor control increases with dose, (4) CT planning allows a higher dose to be given. It is this author's view that medically inoperable or surgically unresectable Stage I, II or III non-oat cell lung cancer should be treated with high dose continuous radiation therapy to maximize the chance for local control or cure.

9 Small Cell Cancer

Small cell cancer comprises 20–25% of all lung cancer; more than 20,000 people per year contract this disease. It is caused by cigarette smoking and is rare among non-smokers, except for those exposed to whole body irradiation, uranium, and to the chemical chloromethyl ether. Small cell cancers originate from Kulchitsky cells in the bronchial epithelium. These contain enzyme systems for amine precursor uptake and decarboxylation (APUD cells) which account for their high frequency of ectopic polypeptide production, including ACTH, ADH, calcitonin, glucagon, insulin, growth hormone and prolactin (FORBES et al., 1978). Hypercalcemia due to ectopic parathyroid hormone production is more common in squamous cell histology, however.

Small cell cancer is a histologic subtype of primary bronchogenic carcinoma, as defined by the World Health Organization. It consists of oat cell and intermediate cell subtypes (formerly spindle cell and polygonal cell).

Staging of small cell cancer does not utilize the TNM system, but the two broad categories of extensive and limited disease. Extensive means beyond one hemithorax. Limited disease is confined to the ipsilateral hemithorax and includes supraclavicular nodes and pleural effusion (so long as the disease can be included in a radiation portal). Initial work-up may reveal up to 45% of patients having positive marrow biopsy. Only one-third of patients presents with disease limited to the chest (GRECO and OLDHAM, 1979). A subtype of limited disease is the solitary peripheral lesion without spread elsewhere. This may yield up to a 40% five year survival with surgery, with or without additional chemotherapy.

In general, extensive disease is treated with chemotherapy and limited disease with some combination of chemotherapy and radiation.

The average survival of small cell carcinoma without treatment is about three months. With the best of chemotherapy, it is about one year (HARDY et al., 1981). Radiation therapy by itself extends survival. The Medical Research Council of Great Britain (MRC, 1981) compared 121 patients with radiation alone to 115 treated with radiation (3,000 rads in two weeks) followed by three drug chemotherapy in limited disease. Median survival was 25 weeks for radiation therapy and 43 weeks for radiation therapy and chemotherapy. At 36 months, 3% of the radiotherapy and 4% of the radio-chemotherapy group were alive. Recurrence of the primary was in 35% of the x-ray therapy only patients and 32% of the combination. The number of radiation therapy patients alive and free of disease was 8% at 12 months, 2% at 24 months; for the combination, it was 26% at 12 months and 8% at 25 months. Others have found a survival of 5–6 months with the radiation alone, extended to 44 weeks when used as an adjuvant to chemotherapy (BURDON et al., 1978). Giving chemotherapy immediately, rather than waiting for recurrence after radiotherapy, prolongs survival. The Southwest Oncology Group (PEREZ et al., 1981) investigated giving chemotherapy immediately or delaying it after radiation to the chest and brain for limited oat cell cancer. The median survival for x-ray therapy was only 48.4 weeks and 33.6 with the combination.

Stage influences prognosis in small cell cancer with limited disease patients surviving longer than those with extensive disease (CARNEY et al., 1980). Ten to twenty-five percent of patients with limited and three percent of patients with extensive disease may enjoy remissions of two years or longer (WEISENTHAL, 1981). The type of small cell cancer, i.e., oat cell versus intermediate cell type (spindle cell or fusiform) does not affect response rate or survival.

9.1 Role of Radiation Therapy in Small Cell Cancer

Small cell cancer in this context includes the subtypes oat cell and intermediate cell. The latter is included because it behaves clinically more closely to small cell undifferentiated than large cell undifferentiated.

Radiation therapy for small cell cancer can be divided into palliation and adjuvant treatment to chemotherapy, particularly to the chest and brain. Controversy centers about the role of adjuvant treatment to chemotherapy.

9.1.1 Whole Brain Irradiation

Table 2 indicates the effects of prophylactic cranial irradiation on the subsequent development of brain metastases. Irradiation of the whole brain with 3,000 rads in two weeks decreases the fre-

Table 2. Effect of brain-irradiation on survival in small cell lung cancer

Author	Number of patients	Prophylactic brain irradiation	Brain metastases	Median survival
Feld et al (1981)	61 (limited)	No	45%	47 weeks
Moore et al (1978)	152 (extensive)	Yes	3.9%	No effect
SWOG	88 (limited)	Yes	6.8%	No effect
Jackson et al (1977)	29 (limited and extensive)	Yes	0%	No effect
Jackson et al (1977)		No	28%	
Ajaikumar et al (1979)	159	Yes	3-fold decrease in brain mets	No effect
Williams et al (1977)	19	No	32%	No effect
Williams et al (1977)	31	Yes	0%	No effect

quency from up to 45% to 0–6.8%. It does not affect survival. It should be used only in patients who have partial or complete remission.

The case for therapeutic irradiation rather than prophylactic is made by Baglan and Marks (1981). Sixty-four percent of 39 patients had good palliation and were free of neurologic symptoms for the remainder of their lives. Cox et al. (1980), on the other hand, found that 45% of 40 patients with brain metastases died from their brain metastases at the Medical College of Wisconsin and he advocates prophylactic irradiation.

The VA Lung Group has extended prophylactic treatment one step further to non-small cell histologies. The prospectively randomized patients to whole brain irradiation with inoperable lung cancer. Sixteen out of 145 patients who received no brain irradiation developed brain metastases; 7 of 136 who received radiation developed brain metastases (Cox, 1981a).

9.1.2 Chest Irradiation

The indications for treatment of the chest with radiation therapy in small cell cancer are not clear. In extensive disease, there appears to be no rationale for chest irradiation unless bulky disease, there appears to be no rationale for chest irradiation unless bulky disease remains after chemotherapy. Hansen et al. (1980) attempted extensive regional irradiation of chest, adrenals and brain or chest only along with chemotherapy in small cell cancer and found no difference between the two groups.

The high incidence of chest recurrence is illustrated by Byhardt et al. (1981). Of 39 patients, 24 had a complete remission of the primary site with chemotherapy alone, but 20 recurred – most with simultaneous extra-thoracic disease. Chemotherapy alone was insufficient for controlling chest disease.

In limited disease, chest recurrence might be decreased and longevity might be improved by irradiation. Eagan et al. (1981b) reported 30 patients with limited small cell cancer randomized to chemotherapy versus chemotherapy plus whole brain irradiation. There was no pre-planned thoracic irradiation, and 78% failed in the lung (52% solely in the lung) as the first site of treatment failure. The study closed early because the relapse rate was unacceptably high when compared to an 11% failure rate in a preceding study in which median survival was 16 months. None of their patients survived two years without pre-planned thoracic radiation therapy, but with it, greater than 25% two year survival was predicted.

Mira and Livingston (1980) reviewed the site of relapse for small cell cancer. He found in limited disease 9 out of 15 (53%) died of recurrent chest disease. Five of seven patients with chest recurrences had it appear initially outside the radiation volume. Only 2 of 17 had tumor recurrence in the field. Chest irradiation appears to be indicated in patients with limited disease.

Large field investigative irradiation has been tried without success with total body and hemibody irradiation. Eight of eight patients treated with total body irradiation at the onset of their disease, rather than chemotherapy, failed treatment (Byhardt et al., 1979). The Eastern Cooperative Oncology Group did a pilot study of Cytoxan and CCNU plus 2,000 rads to the chest plus 600 rads upper hemi-body radiation therapy. No apparent benefit existed (Salazar et al., 1980).

10 Bronchiolo-Alveolar Carcinoma

This uncommon subtype arises from the periphery of the lung, probably from Type II pneumocytes. Type II pneumocytes are granular ovoid cells which secrete surfactant and proliferate during alveolar injury to replace Type I pneumocyte, a squamoid cell that lines the alveoli. This type of cancer comprises 5 to 6% of all primary lung cancers, and can occur from age 16 to 90 years old. Patients are more frequently females and in their forties (EDGERTON et al., 1981). Twenty percent are asymptomatic at presentation.

It is not uncommon for an asymptomatic patient to have extensive disease on his chest x-ray. Presenting symptoms are cough, dyspnea, chest pain and hemoptysis. Watery expectoration can occur, but frank bronchorrea is rare and when present, signifies advanced disease. Although its analogue in sheep (Jagziekte) is caused by a virus which implies a multi-focal origin, the consensus today is that it is a unifocal disease which spreads through lymphatic and hematologic dissemination (BERKMEN, 1977; EDGARTON et al., 1981; MUNNELL et al., 1978).

X-ray findings show a peripheral nodule with sharp or irregular borders. Nodules do not cavitate; air bronchograms are commonly seen; 50% have psammoma bodies that are not radiologically visible. Pleural effusion occurs in five percent at presentation (BERKMAN, 1977).

There appear to be two clinical syndromes associated with bronchiolo-alveolar carcinoma. The more common type presents as a solitary peripheral lesion, either nodular or infiltrative. It varies from 1 to 10 centimeters.

The second type presents as diffuse changes in both lungs and the patients usually die in three years from respiratory compromise. Aggressive surgery in the diffuse form shortens longevity. But up to 50% of the solitary type are without recurrence at five years after an appropriate surgical procedure (MILLER et al., 1978).

11 Superior Vena Caval Obstruction (SVCO)

SVCO occurs when the superior vena cava is blocked sufficiently that retrograde and collateral flow occur with increased pressure in the venous system that drains the head and neck, upper chest and arms. This results in symptoms of headache, dizziness, dyspnea and blurred vision. On examination there is suffusion and edema of the face, upper chest and eyelids; there may be papilledema; superficial venous collateralization can be found in the anterior chest, cervical veins are dilated in the sitting position.

SVCO is caused by lung cancer 85% of the time, lymphoma 10%, and benign conditions 3–5% (goiter, aortic aneurysm, idiopathic mediastinitis) (PEREZ et al., 1978; LOCHRIDGE et al., 1979). The first reported case of SVCO was due to a syphilitic aneurysm.

Diagnosis of SVCO is confirmed by a ^{99}Tc venogram done through bilateral injections and to identify the lateral extent of the obstruction. Although the location of the obstruction is obtained from this study, intra-luminal thrombus cannot be identified except with a radiographic contrast study. The dye may irritate the intra-luminal surface; however, up to one-third of patients with SVCO have accompanying thrombus and should receive anticoagulant therapy. In this author's opinion, a radiographic contrast study should be reserved for those patients with upper extremity swelling or other evidence of peripheral (subclavian or jugular vein) obstruction. Isolated axillary and subclavian occlusion without SVCO can occur, usually with recurrent lung cancer. This is frequently associated with thrombus and should be treated with anticoagulant, as well as anti-tumor therapy (MASON, 1981).

In recent years, histologic identification of the malignancy has become important because of chemotherapy of small cell cancer. Almost half the patients presenting with SVCO will have small cell cancer. The use of radiation without biopsy until symptoms resolve is allowed, since there is a hazard of bleeding from bulging veins during mediastinoscopy and a poor risk for general anesthesia. Percutaneous biopsy, fiberoptic bronchoscopy and sputa cytology allow diagnosis in most cases prior to treatment.

SVCO has traditionally been considered an emergency; it is one of the few situations for which the radiation therapist will use weekend treatment. Recently, it has been suggested that many cases of SVCO do not require immediate treatment and time can be taken to stage the patient. This may be due to earlier diagnosis and effectiveness of aggressive diuretic therapy.

The treatment of SVCO due to "non-oat cell" lung cancer is irradiation. Large daily fractions of 400 rads calculated mid-plane dose are usually advocated for the first three fractions, followed by 200 rads a day for the rest of the treatment. This provides rapid relief in 60% of patients in one to two days and 86% in three to four days (Scarantino et al., 1979).

Up to a week is required for the majority of patients to clear their edema. Others, however, have used conventional doses of 200 rads a day from the start of treatment without a significant difference in ultimate response (Perez et al., 1978). The prognosis for patients with SVCO is poor, but in most cases no worse than the average patient who has Stage III, inoperable bronchogenic carcinoma. Survivals range from a mean of three to four months (Lochridge et al., 1979) to twelve months (Scarantino et al., 1979). The presence of collateral vein formation on ^{99}Tc scan correlates with poor response to radiation. If 400 rad daily fractions are used and the patient shows no response in 72 h, then his survival is ominous, being three months in one series (Scarantino et al., 1979). Upper airway obstruction, or cerebral edema, are poor signs also leading to survival of less than two months (Lochridge et al., 1979).

There are periodic reports of patients surviving many years, and in one case, 13 years (Percarpio and Gray, 1979) after irradiation for bronchogenic carcinoma causing SVCO. This, along with the palliative effect of radiation, is reason to treat it aggressively.

The use of irradiation for SVCO due to small cell cancer is being replaced by multi-agent systemic chemotherapy. Because small cell cancer is so sensitive to chemotherapy, virtually all patients will have palliative relief whether they have a partial or complete response. Only 20% have no response to aggressive chemotherapy (Kane et al., 1976). Resolution of the syndrome takes about seven days (Dombernowsky and Hansen, 1978). Diuretics, steroids and anticoagulants are used inconstantly. Although chemotherapy is effective in treating SCC-induced SVCO, 30–40% of patients will recur (Dombernowsky and Hansen, 1978). Consolidative irradiation of the chest after several cycles of chemotherapy is probably indicated to control chest disease, especially in limited oat cell cancer and may produce an increase in survival (Eagan et al., 1981 b).

12   Pancoast Tumor

Pancoast tumor is an eponym for a syndrome caused by lung cancer starting in the superior sulcus of either lung, causing shoulder and arm pain with muscular atrophy and Horner's syndrome. It is almost always due to lung cancer. It comprises three percent of lung cancer cases (Canoy, 1976). This group of patients is treated with a combination of surgery and radiation, usually preoperative. Despite extensive local involvement, their survival has been reported as high as 35%, supposedly because most of these are slow-growing squamous cell carcinomas, but survival rates vary among institutions. If these tumors are compared stage for stage though, survival rates are more consistent. For example, if scalene node biopsy, mediastinoscopy and appropriate scans are done preoperatively, the actuarial five year survival is 49.7% (Stanford et al., 1980). In those with nodal involvement, it is 13%, and in those who receive radiation only, 5.5% at four years. Irradiation is effective palliation for pain and is dependent on dose. At least some pain relief was found in all patients receiving over 1,900 rets, but in only half of those receiving less (Morris et al., 1979).

Local control is a predictor for survival. Among 36 patients with Stage III disease, 47% had local control with median survival of 26.5 months versus 6.5 months if there was no local control.

13   Prognosis

Stage I lung cancer has the best prognosis if the histology is not small cell anaplastic. At Memorial Hospital in New York City, 75 out of 81 (93%) patients were alive without disease at one year and 77% at three years (Martini and Beattie, 1977). At the Mayo Clinic, 84% of 495 patients were alive without disease at two years and 69% (actuarial) at five years. If $T_1 N_0$ is separated out from Stage I, it is 80% at five years (Williams et al., 1981). Others have reported lower survivals. Mountain (1977) had a 55% five year survival Stage I which was 59% for $T_1 N_0$ and 49% for $T_2 N_0$. The Veterans Administration Surgical Oncology Group found that for $T_2 N_0$, the five year survival was 40.7%. Lobectomy is the usual surgical procedure for Stage I lung cancer, but segmental resection can give comparatively good results. Fifty-three percent of 168 patients were alive at five years in one study (Jensik et al., 1979).

Stage II disease, a combination of a slightly large tumor (T_2) and positive hilar nodes (N_1), considerably decreases the survival at five years, particularly in adenocarcinoma which was 18% in one series (Mountain, 1981 b). But up to 50% of the solitary type are without recurrence at five years after an appropriate surgical precedure (Miller et al., 1978).

MARTINI et al. (1980) found that of 80 patients with positive mediastinal nodes who underwent resection and postoperative external radiation therapy, the three year survival rate for adenocarcinoma was less than squamous cell carcinoma (56% versus 44%). They found that with patients with peripheral lesions less than 3 cm in diameter, even if they had positive mediastinal nodes, they had a survival rate of three years, similar to T_1N_0 lesions.

SHERMAN et al. (1978) reviewed 49 patients with Stage III lung cancer who received 3,000–4,000 rads preoperatively. They had a 27% cumulative five year survival, higher than experience with x-ray therapy alone.

It is not uncommon for tumor to be present at or near the margin of resection. SOORAE and STEVENSON (1979) reported 64 patients with tumor found microscopically at the margins of resection. There was a 15.6% mortality with four patients dying from bronchopleural fistula. There was no relationship between the length of the resected bronchial stump and survival.

Other than stage, predictors of long term survival are not specific. ASHOI et al. (1975) examined 64 patients surviving ten years or longer after resection. Most had adenocarcinoma of bronchioloalveolar type; none had oat cell. Poor histopathologic signs for survival were blood vessel invasion by tumor and lymph node metastases. Lymphoid infiltrate around the tumor or with blood vessel invasion yielded a longer survival (YOSHIDA et al., 1979). Palliative treatment of metastatic disease, although not curable, has been shown to increase survival (HOLMES et al., 1977). MATTSON and HOLSTI (1980) examined doubling time and found survival longest in slow growing tumors and that doubling time correlated with stage. In a review of 156 of 2,836 patients from the VA who survived over ten years, it was found that the quality of life was better in those who were younger, had less than a pneumonectomy performed and stopped smoking after surgery.

Performance status is an important predictor of response as well as survival (COHEN et al., 1981). Patients who continue to smoke even after the start of treatment for their small cell cancer have a shorter median survival than those who stop (JOHNSTON-EARLY et al., 1980).

Brain metastasis in lung cancer is not immediately lethal and may be curable. Up to 27% of brain metastases in lung cancer patients are solitary. Among 23 patients, 8 had precocious and 15 had metachronous metastases. Five out of 23 lived over two years without neurologic deficit. Three of 23 are alive after 10 years (SALERNO et al., 1978).

14 Chemotherapy for Non-Small Cell Lung Cancer

This provides uniformly poor results. AISNER (1981) listed 28 combination regimens ranging from two to four days and drugs and had partial responses ranging from as high as 30–40%; follow-up studies frequently show response rates of about ten percent. "CAMP" is one popular combination which gave 14 out of 51 partial responses (27%) in one study (LAD et al., 1979).

Chemotherapy added to radiation therapy, either concomitantly or sequentially has not increased longevity, although initial response rates are promising. When cis-platinum and adriamycin are given prior to irradiation to inoperable non-oat cell patients, 37% have a tumor response (EAGAN et al., 1981a). The response increases to 68% after irradiation. A similar response of 46% was present when bleomycin was combined with irradiation, but the median survival was no different than in other series, 13 months (CHAN et al., 1976). Single agent chemotherapy, such as procarbazine (PALMER and KROENING, 1978) or cyclophosphamide (BYAR et al., 1978) when added to irradiation has no effect on survival.

15 Immunotherapy

Immunotherapy at this time has not been shown to be an effective modality for extending survival in lung cancer. C-parvum, BCG and levamisole have been most widely tested (MOUNTAIN et al., 1981a; VAN HOUTTE et al., 1980b).

References

Aisner J, Hansen HH (1981) Commentary: current status of chemotherapy for non-small cell lung cancer, Cancer Treat Rep 65:979–986.

Ajaikumar BS, Barkley HT (1979) The role of radiation therapy in the treatment of small cell undifferentiated bronchogenic cancer, Int J Radiat Oncol Biol Phys 5:977–982.

Alazraki N (1980) Usefulness of gallium imaging in the evaluation of lung cancer, CRC Crit Rev Diagn Imaging 13:249–267.

Aronberg DJ, Sagel SS, LeFrak S, et al (1980) Lung carcinoma associated with bullous lung disease in young men, AJR 134:249–252.

Ashor GL, Kern WH, Meyer BW, et al (1975) Long-term survival in bronchogenic carcinoma, J Thorac Cardiovasc Surg 70:581–589.

Auerbach O, Garfinkel L, Parks VR (1979) Scar cancer of the lung: increase over a 21 year period, Cancer 43:636–642.

Baglan RJ, Marks JE (1981) Comparison of symptomatic and prophylactic irradiation of brain metastases from oat cell carcinoma of the lung, Cancer 47:41–45.

Bennett WF, Smith RA (1979) Segmental resection for bronchogenic carcinoma: a surgical alternative for the compromised patient, Ann Thorac Surg 27:169–172.

Berkmen YM (1977) The many faces of bronchiolo-alveolar carcinoma, Semin Roentgenol 12:207–214.

Burbige EJ, Radigan JJ, Belber JP (1980) Metastatic lung carcinoma involving the gastrointestinal tract, Am J Gastro 74:504–506.

Burdon JGW, Henderson MM, Noon WJ, et al (1978) Combined chemotherapy and radiotherapy for the treatment of small cell carcinoma of the lung, Med J Aust 1:352–355.

Byar D, Kenis Y, Van Andel JG, et al (1978) Results of a EORTC randomized trial of cyclophosphamide and radiotherapy in inoperable lung cancer: prognostic factors and treatment results, Eu J Cancer 14:919–930.

Byhardt RW, Libnoch JA, Cox JD, et al (1981) Local control of intrathoracic disease with chemotherapy and role of prophylactic cranial irradiation in small-cell carcinoma of the lung, Cancer 47:2239–2246.

Canoy NR (1976) Apical lung cancer, Mo Med 73:571–575.

Carney DN, Matthews MJ, Ihde DC, et al (1980) Influence of histologic subtype of small cell carcinoma of the lung on clinical presentation; response to therapy, and survival, JNCI 65:1225–1230.

Center S (1981) Does computed tomography aid in the staging of lung cancer? J Thorac Cardiovasc Surgery 82:334.

Chan PY, Byfield JE, Kagan AR, et al (1976) Unresectable squamous cell carcinoma of the lung and its management by combined bleomycin and radiotherapy; a clinical study of the enhanced results, Cancer 37:2671–2676.

Choi NC, Doucette JA (1981) Improved survival of patients with unresectable non-small-cell bronchogenic carcinoma by an innovated high dose en-bloc radiotherapeutic approach, Cancer 48:101–109.

Choi NC, Grillo C, Gardiello M, et al (1980) Basis for new strategies in postoperative radiotherapy of bronchogenic carcinoma, Int J Radiat Oncol Biol Phys 6:31–35.

Chopra SK, Genouesi UG, Simmons DH, et al (1977) Fiberoptic bronchoscopy in the diagnosis of lung cancer comparison of pre-and post-bronchoscopy sputa, washings, brushings and biopsies, Acta Cytol 21:524–527.

Cohen MH, Makuch R, Johnston-Early A, et al (1981) Laboratory parameters as an alternative to performance status in prognostic stratification of patients with small cell lung cancer, Cancer Treat Rep 65:187–195.

Cox JD, Stanely K, Petrovich Z, et al (1981a) Cranial irradiation in cancer of the lung of all cell types, JAMA 245:469–472.

Cox JD, Yesner RA (1981b) Causes of treatment failure and death in carcinoma of the lung, Yale J Biol Med 54:201–207.

Cox JD, Komaki R, Byhardt RW, et al (1980) Results of whole-brain irradiation for metastases from small cell carcinoma of the lung, Cancer Tret Rep 64:957–961.

Cox JD (1981c) The role of radiation therapy for carcinoma of the lung, Yale J Biol Med 54:195–200.

Davis RS, Flynn MB, Moore C (1977) An unusual presentiation of carcinoma of the lung: 26 patients with cervical node metastases, J Surg Oncol 9:503–507.

Decker DA, Dines DE, Payne WS, et al (1978) The significance of a cytologically negative pleural effusion in bronchogenic carcinoma, Chest 74:640–642.

DeMeester TR, Golomb HM, Kirchner P, et al (1979) The role of gallium-67 scanning in the clinical staging and preoperative evaluation of patients with carcinoma of the lung, Ann Thorac Surg 28:451–464.

Dent PB, McCullouch PB, Wesley-James O, et al (1978) Measurement of carcinoembryonic antigen in patients with bronchogenic carcinoma, Cancer 42:1484–1491.

Deslauriers J, Beaulieu M, Bénazéra A, et al (1979) Sleeve pneumonectomy for bronchogenic carcinoma, Ann Thorac Surg 28:465–474.

Dombernowsky P, Hansen HH (1978) Combination chemotherapy in the management of superior vena caval obstruction in small-cell anaplastic carcinoma of the lung, Acta Med Scand 204:513–516.

Dunnick NR, Ihde DC, Johnston-Early A (1979) Abdominal CT in the evaluation of small carcinoma of the lung, AJR 133:1085–1088.

Eagan RT, Frytak S, Lee RE, et al (1981a) Thoracic radiation therapy and adriamycin/cisplatin-containing chemotherapy for locally advanced non-small-cell lung cancer, Cancer Clin Trials 4:381–388.

Eagan RT, Frytak S, Lee RE, et al (1981b) A case for pre-planned thoracic and prophylactic whole brain irradiation therapy in limited small-cell lung cancer, Cancer Clin Trials 4:261–266.

Edgerton F, Rao U, Takita H, et al (1981) Bronchio-alveolar carcinoma. A clinical overview and bibliography, Oncology 38:269–273.

Emami B, Lee DJ, Munzenrider JE (1978a) The value of supraclavicular area treatment in radiotherapeutic management of lung cancer, Cancer 41:124–129.

Emami B, Melo A, Carter BL, et al (1987b) Value of computed tomography in radiotherapy of lung cancer, AJR 131:63–67.

Emami B, Munzenrider JE, Lee DJ, et al (1979) Radical radiation therapy of advanced lung cancer. Evaluation of prognostic factors and results of continuous and split course treatment, Cancer 44:446–456.

Faling LJ, Pugatch RD, Jung-Legg Y, et al (1981) Computed tomographic scanning of the mediastinum in the staging of bronchogenic carcinoma, Am Rev Respir Dis 124:690–695.

Forbes JT, Greco A, Oldham PK (1978) Immunologic aspects of small cell carcinoma, Semin Oncol 5:263–271.

Ford RM (1978) Primary lung cancer and asthma, Ann Allergy 40:240–242.

Fox RM, Woods RL, Brodie GN, et al (1980) A randomized study: small cell anaplastic lung cancer treated by combination chemotherapy and adjuvant radiotherapy, Int J Radiat Oncol Biol Phys 6:1083–1085.

Fox RM, Woods RL, Tattersall MHN, et al (1979) Undifferentiated carcinoma in young men: the atypical teratoma syndrome, Lancet 1:1316–1318.

Gobien RP, Skucas J, Paris BS (1981) CT-assisted fluoro-scopically guided aspiration biopsy of central hilar and mediastinal masses, Radiology 141:443–447.

Goslin RH, Skarin AT, Zamchek N (1981) Carcinoem-bryonic antigen. A useful monitor of therapy of small cell lung cancer, JAMA 246:2173–2176.

Greco FA, Oldham RK (1979) Current concepts in cancer: small cell lung cancer, N Engl J Med 301:355–358.

Gropp C, Lehmann FG, Bauer HW, et al (1977) Carcino-embryonic antigen, α-fetoprotein, ferritin, and α 2-preg-nancy associated glycoprotein in the serum of lung can-cer patients and its demonstration in lung tumor tissues, Oncology 34:267–272.

Hansen HH, Dombernowsky P, Hirsch FR, et al (1980) Prophylactic irradiation in bronchogenic small cell anap-lastic carcinoma. A comparative trial of localized versus extensive radiotherapy including prophylactic brain irra-diation in patients receiving combination chemotherapy, Cancer 46:279–284.

Hardy JD, Ewing HP, Neely WA, et al (1981) Lung carcino-ma: survey of 2286 cases with emphasis on small cell type, Ann Surg 193:539–548.

Harviel JD, McNamara JJ, Straehley CJ (1978) Surgical treatment of lung cancer in patients over the age of 70 years, J Thorac Cardiovasc Surg 75:802–805.

Hilaris BS, Martini N (1979) Interstitial brachytherapy in cancer of the lung: a 20 year experience, Int J Radiat Oncol Biol Phys 5:1951–1956.

Hillyard CJ, Coombes RC, Greenberg PB, et al (1976) Cal-citonia in breast and lung cancer, Clin Endocrinol 5:1–8.

Hirsch F, Hansen HH, Dombernowsky P, et al (1977) Bone-marrow examination in the staging of small-cell anaplas-tic carcinoma of the lung with special reference to sub-typing. An evaluation of 203 consecutive patients, Can-cer 39:2563–2567.

Hoffman TH, Ransdell HT (1980) Comparison of lobec-tomy and wedge resection for carcinoma of the lung, J Thorac Cardiovasc Surg 79:211–217.

Holmes FF, Olson S, Lasch C, et al (1977) Cancer Data Service: lung carcinoma distantly metastatic at diagno-sis, 1945–1974, J Kans Med Soc 78:292–293.

Holsti LR, Mattson K (1980) A randomized study of split-course radiotheray of lung cancer: long term results, Int J Radiat Oncol Biol Phys 6:977–981.

Hooper RG, Beechler CR, Johnson MC (1978) Radioiso-tope scanning the initial staging of bronchogenic carci-noma, Am Rev Respir Dis 118:279–286.

Horacek J, Pidcek V, Seve J (1977) Histologic types of bron-chogenic cancer in relation to different conditions of radiation exposure, Cancer 40:832–835.

Huhti E, Poukkula A, Uksila E (1980) Serum copper levels in patients with lung cancer, Respiration 40:112–116.

Issell BF, MacFadyen B, Gum ET, et al (1981) Serum zinc levels in lung cancer patients, Cancer 47:1845–1848.

Jacobs L, Kinkel WR, Vincent RG (1977) 'Silent' brain metastasis from lung carcinoma determined by compu-terzed tomography, Arch Neurol 34:690–693.

Janower ML (1978) 55° posterior oblique tomography of the pulmonary hilum, J Can Assoc Radiol 29:158–160.

Jay SJ, Wehr K, Nicholson DP, et al (1980) Diagnostic sen-sitivity and specificity of pulmonary cytology: compari-son of techniques used in conjunction with flexible fiber optic bronchoscopy, Acta Cytol 24:304–312.

Jenkyn LR, Brooks PL, Forcier RJ (1980) Remission of the Lambert-Eaton syndrom and small cell anaplastic

carcinoma of the lung induced by chemotherapy and radiotherapy, Cancer 46:1123–1127.

Jensik RJ, Faber LP, Kittle CF (1979) Segmental resection for bronchogenic carcinoma, Ann Thorac Surg 28:475–583.

Jensik RJ, Faber LP, Kittle CR, et al (1981) Survival follow-ing resection for second primary bronchogenic carcino-ma, J Thorac Cardiovasc Surg 82:658–668.

Johnston-Early A, Cohen MH, Minna JD, et al (1980) Smoking abstinence and small cell lung cancer survival. An association, JAMA 244:2175–2179.

Kallenberg F, Jaqué J (1979) Giant-cell carcinoma of the lung. Clinical and pathological assessment. Comparison with other large-cell anaplastic bronchogenic carcinomas Scand J Thorac Cardiovasc Surg 13:343–346.

Kane RC, Cohen MH, Broder LE, et al (1976) Superior vena caval obstruction due to small cell anaplastic lung carcinoma. Response to chemotherapy, JAMA 235:1717–1718.

Kelly RJ, Cowan RJ, Ferree CB, et al (1979) Efficacy of radionuclide scanning in patients with lung cancer, JAMA 242:2855–2857.

Kharole MU, Gill BS, Grupta PP, et al (1975) Bronchogenic carcinoma in Indian water buffaloes, Vet Pathol 12:462–463.

Kim RY, Perry SR, Levy DS (1979) Metastatic carcinoma to the tongue. A report of two cases and a review of the literature, Cancer 43:386–389.

Kirsh MM, Rotman H, Bore E, et al (1976) Major pulmo-nary resection for bronchogenic carcinoma in the el-derly, An Thorac Surg 22:369–373.

Komaki R, Cox JD, Whitson W (1981) Risk of brain metas-tasis from small cell carcinoma of the lung related to length of survival and prophylactic irradiation, Cancer Treat Rep 65:811–814.

Lad T, Sarma PR, Diekamp U, et al (1979) 'Camp' combi-nation chemotherapy for unresectable non-oat cell bron-chogenic carcinoma, Cancer Clin Trials 2:321–326.

Larsson S, Zettergren L (1976) Histological typing of lung cancer. Application of the World Health Organization classification to 479 cases, Acta Pathol Microbiol Scand 84:529–537.

Lee RE, Carr DT, Childs DS Jr (1976) Comparison of split-course radiation therapy and continuous radiation ther-apy for unresectable bronchogenic carcinoma: 5 year results, AJR 126:116–122.

Libshitz HI, Zornoza J, McLarty JW (1978) Lung cancer in chronic leukemia and lymphoma, Radiology 127:297–300.

Lochridge SK, Knibbe WP, Doty DB (1979) Obstruction of the superior vena cava, Surgery 85:14–24.

Martini N, Flehinger BJ, Zaman HB, et al (1980) Prospec-tive study of 445 lung carcinomas with mediastinal lymph node metastases, J Thorac Cardiovasc Surg 80:390–399.

Martini N, Beattie EJ Jr (1977) Results of surgical treatment in Stage I lung cancer, J Thorac Cardiovasc Surg 74:499–505.

Martini N, Burton GA (1981) Staging and surgical manage-ment of early lung cancer, Bull NY Acad Sci 57:341–348.

Mason BA (1981) Axillary-subclavian vein occlusion in pa-tients with lung neoplasma, Cancer 48:1886–1889.

Mattson K, Holsti LR (1980) Prognostic value of doubling time in lung cancer, Strahlentherapie 156:632–636.

McDonnell L, Long JP (1981) Lung scar cancer – a reappraisal, J Clin Pathol 34:996–999.

Medical Research Council Lung Cancer Working Party (1981) Radiotherapy alone or with chemotherapy in the treatment of small-cell carcinoma of thel ung: the results at 36 months. 2nd report to the medical research council on the 2nd small-cell study, Br J Cancer 44:611–617.

Mendiondo OA, Yoneda J, Maruyama Y, et al (1981) A prospective randomized trial of postoperative irradiation in Stage I and II non-oat cell carcinoma of the lung. A preliminary report, J KY Med Assoc 79:781–788.

Miller WT, Husted J, Freiman D, et al (1978) Bronchioloalveolar carcinoma: two clinical entities with one pathologic diagnosis, AJR 130:905–912.

Mira JG, Livingston RB (1980) Evaluation and radiotherapy implications of chest relapse patterns in small cell lung carcinoma treated with radiotherapy-chemotherapy: study of 34 case and review of the literature, Cancer 46:2557–2565.

Mohsenifar Z, Chopra SK, Simmons DH (1979) Diagnostic value of fiberoptic bronchoscopy in lung cancer presenting as mediastinal mass(es), Cancer 44:1894–1896.

Mok CK, Nandi P, Ong GB (1978) Coexistent bronchogenic carcinoma and active pulmonary tuberculosis, J Thorac Cardiovasc Surg 76:469–472.

Morris RW, Abadir R (1979) Pancoast tumor: the value of high dose radiation therapy, Radiology 132:717–719.

Mountain CF, Gail MH (1981a) Surgical adjuvant intrapleural BCG treatment for stage I non-small cell lung cancer. Preliminary report of the National Cancer Institute Lung Cancer Study Group, J Thorac Cardiovasc Surg 82:649–657.

Mountain CF, McMurtrey MJ, Frazier OH (1980) Regional extension of lung cancer, Int J Radiat Oncol Biol Phys, 6:1013–1020.

Mountain CF (1981b) Staging of lung cancer, Yale J Biol Med 54:161–172.

Mountain CF (1977) Assessment of the role of surgery for control of lung cancer, Ann Thorac Surg 24:365–373.

Munnell ER, Dilling E, Grantham N, et al (1978) Reappraisal of solitary bronchiolar (alveolar cell) carcinoma of the lung, Ann Thorac Surg 25:289–297.

Nugent JL, Bunn PA Jr, Matthews MJ, et al (1979) CNS metastases in small cell bronchogenic carcinoma. Increasing frequency and changing pattern with lengthening survival, Cancer 44:1885–1893.

Palmer RL, Kroening PM (1978) Comparison of low dose radiation therapy alone or combined with procarbazine (NSC-77213) for unresectable epidermoid carcinoma of the lung, stage T3, N1, N2, or M1, Cancer 42:424–428.

Pearson FG (1980) Use of mediastinoscopy in selection of patients for lung cancer operations, Ann Thorac Surg 30:205–207.

Percarpio B, Gray S (1979) Prolonged survival following the superior vena cava syndrome, Chest 75:639–640.

Perez CA, Stanley K, Rubin P, et al (1980) Patterns of tumor recurrence after definitive irradiation for inoperable non-oat cell carcinoma of the lung, Int J Radiat Oncol Biol Phys 6:987–984.

Perez CA, Presant CA, Van Amburg AL III, (1978) Management of superior vena cava syndrome, Semin Oncol 5:123–134.

Perez CA, Krauss S, Bartolucci AA, et al (1981) Thoracic and elective brain irradiation with concomitant or delayed multiagent chemotherapy in the treatment of localized small cell carcinoma of the lung: a randomized prospective study by the Southeastern Cancer Study Group, Cancer 47:2407–2413.

Petrovich Z (1981) Radiotherapy in the management of locally advanced lung cancer of all cell types: final report of randomized trial, Cancer 48:1335–1340.

Quraishi MA, Costanzi JJ, Balachandran S (1981) Iodocholesterol adrenal scanning for the detection of adrenal metastases in lung cancer and its clinical significance, Cancer 48:714–716.

Ramanathan T, Skeme-Smith H, Singh D, et al (1976) Small intestinal perforation due to secondaries from bronchogenic carcinoma, Br J Dis Chest 70:121–124.

Richardson JV, Zenk BA, Rossi NP (1980) Preoperative noninvasive mediastinal staging in bronchogenic carcinoma, Surgery 88:382–385.

Robbins HM, Morrison DA (1979) Biopsy of the main carina. Staging lung cancer with the fiberoptic bronchoscope, Chest 75:484–486.

Sadoff L, Aronstam EM (1977) Operable lung cancer associated with fever, anemia, and hepatomegaly, Arch Intern Med 137:1086–1087.

Salazar OM, Rubin P, Brown JC, et al (1976) The assessment of tumor response to irradiation of lung cancer: continuous versus split-course regimes, Int J Radiat Oncol Biol Phys 1:1107–1118.

Salazar OM, Creech RH, Rubin P, et al (1980) Half-body and local chest irradiation as consolidation following response to standard induction chemotherapy for disseminated small cell lung cancer: an Eastern Cooperative Oncology group pilot report, Int J Radiat Oncol Biol Phys 6:1093–1102.

Salerno T, Munrod D, Little JR (1978) Surgical treatment of bronchogenic carcinoma with a brain metastasis, J Neurosurg 48:350–354.

Scannell JG (1980) 'Bleb' carcinoma of the lung, J Thorac Cardiovasc Surg 80:904–908.

Scarantino C, Salazar OM, Rubin P, et al (1979) The optimum radiation schedule in treatment of superior vena caval obstruction: importance of ^{99m}Tc scintiangiograms, Int J Radiat Oncol Biol Phys 5:1987–1955.

Schatzlein MH, McAuliffe S, Orringer MB, et al (1981) Scalene node biopsy in pulmonary carcinoma: when is it indicated? Ann Thorac Surg 31:322–324.

Seydel HG, Kutcher GJ, Steiner RM, et al (1980) Computer tomography in planning radiation therapy for bronchogenic carcinoma, Int J Radiat Oncol Biol Phys 6:601–606.

Shah K, Olson MH, Ray P, et al ((1981) Comparison of dose-time-fractionation schemes in non-oat cell lung cancer, Cancer 48:1127–1132.

Shankar PS (1981) Laryngeal carcinoma with synchronous or metachronous bronchogenic carcinoma, J Am Geriatr Soc 29:370–372.

Shankar PS (1980) Split-course radiation therapy: effects on pulmonary function in patients with bronchogenic carcinoma, J Am Geriatric Soc 28:547–549.

Shanmugham MS (1976) Metastasis in nose from bronchial carcinoma, J Laryngol Otolog 90:1061–1064.

Sherman DM, Neptune W, Weichselbaum R, et al (1978) An aggressive approach to marginally resectable lung cancer, Cancer 41:2040–2045.

Sherman DM, Weichselbaum R, Hellman S (1981) The characteristics of long-term survivors of lung cancer treated with radiation, Cancer 47:2575–2580.

Shields TW (1979) Multiple primary bronchial carcinomas, Ann Thorac Surg 27:1–2.

Sinner WN, Zailcek J (1976) Implantation metastasis after percutaneous transthoracic needle aspiration biopsy, Acta Radiol Diagn 17:473–480.

Smith HJ (1980) Extrahepatic bile duct obstruction in primary carcinoma of the lung: incidence, diagnosis, and non-operative treatment, J Natl Med Assoc 72:215–220.

Soorae AS, Stevenson HM (1979) Survival with residual tumor on the bronchial margin after resection for bonchogenic carcinoma, J Thorac Cardiovasc Surg 76:175–180.

Standord W, Barnes RP, Tucker AR (1980) Influence of staging in superior sulcus (pancoast) tumors of the lung, Ann Thorac Surg 29:406–409.

Suprun H, Pedio G, Ruttner JR (1980) The diagnostic reliability of cytologic typing in primary lung cancer with a review of the literature, Acta Cytol 24:494–500.

Thesingh CW, Driessen OMJ, Daems WTH, et al (1978) Accumulation and localization of gallium-67 in various types of primary lung carcinoma, J Nucl Med 19:28–30.

Thornbury JR, Burke DP, Naylor B (1981) Transthoracic needle aspiration biopsy: accuracy of cytologic typing of malignant neoplasms, AJR 136:719–724.

Turner P, Haggith JW (1981) Preoperative radionuclide scanning in bronchogenic carcinoma, Br J Dis Chest 75:291–294.

Underwood GH, Jr, Hooper RG, Axelbaum SP, et al (1979) Computed tomographic scanning of the thorax in the staging of bronchogenic carcinoma, N Engl J Med 300:777–778.

Van Houtte P, Rocmans P, Smets P, et al (1980a) Postoperative radiation therapy in lung cancer: a controlled trial after resection of curative design, Int J Radiat Oncol Biol Phys 6:983–986.

Van Houtte P, Bondue H, Rocmans P, et al (1980b) Adjuvant immunotherapy by levamisole in resectable lung cancer: a control study, Eur J Cancer 16:1597–1601.

Van Houtte P, DeJager R, Lustman-Maréchal J, et al (1980c) Prognostic value of the superiro vena cava syndrome as the presenting sign of small cell anaplastic carcinoma of the lung, Eur J Cancer 16:1447–1450.

Vasudevan CP, Suppiah P, Udoshi MB, et al (1981) Reversible autonomic neuropathy and hypertrophic osteoarthropathy in a patient with bronchogenic carcinoma, Chest 79:479–481.

Vincent RG, Chu TM, Fergen TB, et al (1975) Carcinoembryonic antigen in 228 patients with carcinoma of the lung, Cancer 36:2069–2076.

Vincent RG, Dickren JW, Lane WW, et al (1977) The changing histopathology of lung cancer. A review of 1682 cases, Cancer 39:1647–1655.

Wallach SR, Royston I, Taetle R, et al (1981) Plasma calcitonin as a marker of disease activity in patients with small cell carcinoma of the lung, J Clin Endo Metab 53:602–606.

Weisenthal LM (1981) Treatment of small cell lung cancer – 1981, Arch Intern Med 141:1499–1501.

Weissberg D (1977) Mediastinoscopy and anterior mediastinotomy in patients with lung cancer, Isr J Med Sci 13:866–869.

Westcott JL (1981) Percutaneous needle aspiration of hilar and mediastinal masses, Radiology 141:323–329.

Williams DE, Pairoleo PC, Davis CS, et al (1981) Survival of patients surgically treated for stage I lung cancer, J Thorac Cardiovasc Surg 82:70–76.

Winchester DP, Merrill JR, Victor TA, et al (1977) Small bowel perforation secondary to metastatic carcinoma of the lung, Cancer 40:410–415.

Wittes RE, Yeh SDJ (1977) Indications for liver and brain scans. Screening tests for patients with oat cell carcinoma of lung, JAMA 238:506–507.

Yasunami R, Hashimoto Z, Oqura T (1981) Primary lung cancer producing alpha-fetoprotein: a case report, Cancer 47:926–929.

Yoneyama T, Naruke, T, Suemasu K, et al (1976) Bronchial carcinoma in patients with pre-existing unilateral lung disease, Thorax 31:650–651.

Yoshida T, Shirakusa T, Shigematsu N (1979) Histopathological factors predictive for prognosis of lung cancer, Jpn J Surg 9:210–217.

Zimm S, Gardner DF, Waslh JW, et al (1981) Addison's disease as the sole clinical manifestation of recurrent bronchogenic carcinoma, South Med J 74:1016–1018.

Chapter III Lung Cancer: Considerations Related to Gross Anatomy

STEPHEN K. PLUME

CONTENTS

1 Introduction

The objective of this section is to describe anatomic features of particular relevance to the natural history of carcinoma of the lung and to its clinical management. A strict criterion of relevance makes this review highly selective. Readers who wish a comprehensive treatment of thoracic anatomy as such or as a guide to technical aspects of surgical resection or radiation therapy are referred elsewhere.

Critical to an understanding of lung cancer is appreciation of the architecture of the organ in which it occurs. This architecture, including both the internal structure of the lungs and their relationship to adjacent organs, dictates site of development of specific malignancies, patterns of spread, clinical presentation and limitations of local treatment by surgery or radiation.

STEPHEN K. PLUME, M.D.

Department of Surgery, Dartmouth-Hitchcock Medical Center, Hanover, New Hampshire 03755, USA

2 Embryological and Anatomical Considerations

2.1 Lung

Clinical anatomy of the adult lung is best appreciated in the context of at least a brief consideration of embryological development, abstracted here from the works of WEIBEL (1963) and AREY (1965).

The lungs develop from the foregut. At gestational age three weeks the primitive lung bud forms at the caudal end of the laryngotracheal tube. It branches asymmetrically into what will eventually be the right and left mainstem bronchi. By age five weeks these have begun to branch and to invade as yet undifferentiated mesenchyme in the coelomic cavity. They carry with them an investing layer of mesothelium, precursor of the pleura. This layer is reflected upon itself at the (incomplete) fissures between lobes of lung and at the root of the lung where it is continuous with an identical layer lining the inside of the chest wall. A potential space is thus created between the visceral (coating the lungs) and parietal (lining the chest wall) layers of the pleura, a space normally empty except for a few milliliters of fluid thought to serve as lubricant, permitting low friction movement between lungs and chest wall.

2.2 Bronchi

Lobar bronchi are identifiable by age seven weeks. Together with the trachea, they and the next 13 generations of irregularly dichotomously branching lung buds develop into conducting airways, lined by secretory and ciliary epithelium but devoid of respiratory elements. These are the conduits through which bulk gas transport occurs. The ramifying bronchi are the central structures around which pulmonary arteries, bronchial arteries, bronchial veins, and much of the pulmonary lymphatic network differentiate from the surrounding mesenchyme. Blood vessels of the tracheobronchial tree are somewhat variable in origin. Usually there are at least two branches arising directly from the aorta to supply the left lung bronchi, and one or more vessels arising from a systemic artery (which may be an intercostal vessel, subclavian, thryrocervical trunk, or internal mammary artery) to the right side. Congenital or acquired diseases can call forth additional sources of systemic arterial blood to the bronchial network along collateral routes (even from coronary arteries, as seen in patients who have undergone combined heart-lung transplantation) (Jamieson, personal communication, 1983). Systemically derived blood is distributed along bronchi to the level of respiratory bronchioles, where bronchial artery related vessels anastomose with pulmonary parenchymal vascular channels. Beginning at a slightly more proximal level, there are well-defined bronchial veins which drain generally centrally and cephalad along the bronchi into the azygous system, often with contributions from mediastinal veins.

The cellular constituents of the tracheobronchial tree change progressively in the transition from bulk gas flow passages to molecular gas exchange surfaces. The airways become smaller at each branch point (by a factor of 1.4) until bronchioles 0.7 mm in diameter are reached. Beyond this point the airways remain approximately this diameter, although there are several more generations of divisions of the tracheobronchial tree before true alveoli are reached.

The airway is supported by cartilaginous elements from the larynx to the bronchioles. The trachea, 9 to 15 cm long in the adult, maintains its nearly 2-cm diameter with 14 to 16 incomplete rings, open posteriorly. The margins of the horseshoe-shaped cartilaginous rings are connected by the external fibrous membrane. Distal to mainstem bronchi, the larger airways have irregularly shaped, often completely encircling rings. Such elements occur until the airway diameters are down to 1 or 2 mm, beyond which cartilage is not found.

In the larger airways, the epithelium includes goblet cells secreting a product indistinguishable from that of intramural bronchial glands. Goblet cells become less frequent peripherally and disappear altogether by the 13th generation of bronchial divisions. Ciliated cells are found from the trachea to the 10th generation. Clara cells, possibly a source of bronchiolar surfactant, appear in terminal bronchioles.

Although it seems obvious that some combination of airway size, velocity of air flow, size and composition of inhaled particles, and nature of the

Table 1. Nomenclature of pulmonary lobes and bronchopulmonary segments

Right upper lobe	Left upper lobe
anterior	anterior
posterior	apicoposterior
apical	lingula
	superior division
	inferior division
Right middle lobe	
medial	
lateral	
Right lower lobe	Left lower lobe
superior	superior
medial	anteromedial
lateral	lateral
posterior	posterior
anterior	

epithelium at a specific level in the airway creates an environment in which malignant transformation occurs, the range of each of these variables cannot be stated in detail (Ives et al., 1983).

Molecular gas exchange takes place in pulmonary alveoli. Although these occur primarily as the most peripheral element of the tracheobronchial tree, there are alveoli distributed along terminal bronchioles proximal to the true alveolar ducts and sacs. Thus, the terminal bronchioles serve both gas transport and transmembrane gas exchange functions.

Alveoli consist of irregular, polyhedral arrays of air spaces lined by thin Type I alveolar epithelial cells whose basement membranes directly abut those of pulmonary capillary endothelial cells. Molecular gas exchange between alveoli and capillaries occurs here, across a total tissue thickness of 300 to 500 Å. Type I cells are thought to constitute approximately 90% of the surface area of alveoli. Alveolar Type II cells are smaller, thicker, cover a smaller proportion of the alveolar surface area, and are thought to secrete alveolar surfactant (Crapo et al., 1982). At the gross anatomic level, the tracheobronchial tree supplies the two lungs, which are themselves subdivided into lobes and segments – a widely accepted nomenclature which is that of Jackson and Huber (1943) (see Table 1).

Although the total gas exchange surface area is impressively large, perhaps as much as 100 M^2 (Weibel, 1963), it is embedded within an extensive interstitial space occupied by lymphatic vessels, leukocytes, fibroelastic elements, and a dynamic fraction of fluid. Depending on many factors, including state of hydration, presence of inflammation, hydrostatic balance along the pulmonary capillary, and venous or lymphatic obstruction, the interstitium can be a large part of pulmonary parenchymal volume.

2.3 Blood Vessels

Pulmonary parenchymal blood supply, distinct from and much larger than tracheobronchial nutrient flow (comprising as it does the entire cardiac output), is derived embryologically from partition of the truncus arteriosus into the aorta and pulmonary arteries. As mentioned above, the latter accompany the bronchi in the course of embryologic development and, like them, change in structure as a function of size. Proximal portions of pulmonary arteries are thick walled, with definite internal and external elastic laminae. Between diameters of 2,000 and 100 microns the proportion of smooth muscle increases as the walls become thinner and the elastic laminae disappear. Where the vessels lose their continuous muscle coat and have only a single elastic lamina, they become arterioles. At the alveolar level they become true capillaries whose endothelial cells sit on a basement membrane joined to that of adjacent alveolar epithelial cells.

Pulmonary venous drainage does not follow tracheobronchial developmental patterns. Instead, the veins originate as coalescent channels of alveolar capillaries. They follow interalveolar, then interlobular, and finally intersegmental planes as they course centrally toward the heart. On the right side, the upper and middle lobes drain into the right superior pulmonary vein. On the left side, the analog to the middle lobe is the lingula, which does not have a separate investing pleura and which drains with the rest of the upper lobe into the left superior pulmonary vein. The lower lobe on each side drains into its respective inferior pulmonary vein.

2.4 Lymphatics

Lymphatic drainage of the lung is first discernable embryologically during the second month of gestation, thereafter ramifying in richly interconnected networks along the airways, vascular channels, and in loose connective tissue. Lymph vessels are interspersed among all components of the lung except at the tight junction between alveolar Type I and capillary endothelial cells (TOBIN, 1954). In addition to submucosal, intramural, and peribronchial plexuses, adventitial pulmonary artery and vein lymphatics, and interstitial parenchymal lymphatics, there are also extensive subpleural networks. The total number of potential pathways of lymphatic drainage from any specific site within the lung is thus quite large. In general, intrapulmonary lymph channels drain from peripheral to central locations, largely to "hilar" lymph nodes. (Quotation marks are used here because of the notoriously imprecise boundaries of the hilum, an issue addressed below). There are aggregates of lymphoid cells within the lung, most frequently at bronchial bifurcations, but true lymph nodes are infrequent within pulmonary parenchyma (KRAHL, 1964).

In the first few sentences of this chapter it was noted that the lung develops embryologically from the foregut, as a bud off the laryngotracheal tube invading mesenchyme in the coelomic cavity. The branches of the lung bud migrate caudally with their investing layer of pleura, reflected upon itself at the root of the lung where airways and vessels are transmitted. There is no anatomic tissue plane separating proximal and distal respiratory tree. Epithelial linings and lymphatic channels are continuous from trachea to alveoli. The continuity of lymphatic channels along the tracheobronchial tree has great bearing on the spread of lung cancer: just as the tremendous volume of blood through pulmonary vessels accounts for frequent and widespread hematogenous dissemination of malignant tumors (most often to brain, bone, liver, adrenal, and kidney, roughly paralleling distribution of cardiac output at rest), so does the extent of lymphatic drainage in the absence of any sort of proximal barrier or partition imply that lymphatic metastases will occur frequently along tracheobronchial lymph node channels and in lymph nodes which have a shared drainage (ROUVIERE, 1938; BAIRD, 1965). These include groups of lymph nodes which communicate via lymphatics accompanying the large pulmonary vessels, those in mediastinal fat, and those which drain via folds of pleura, notably the inferior pulmonary ligament. The latter put pulmonary lymph in continuity with that in paraesophageal lymphatics and in those related to pericardium.

3 Anatomical Considerations in Staging of Lung Cancer

It is clear that the subsequent behavior of lung cancer is importantly determined by the degree of lymphatic involvement (as well as by other factors discussed below) at the time of diagnosis (Pearson et al., 1982). The absence of limiting membranes at the root of the lung and the imprecise boundaries of the "hilum" (radiographically or surgically) have made it both important and difficult to characterize precisely and to compare subsets of patients who have lung cancer. A major effort led by Mountain resulted in adoption of a clinical lung cancer staging protocol using internationally-accepted TNM (Tumor, Nodal Involvement, Metastasis) criteria (American Joint Committee, 1973, revised 1979). Although much important information has been learned from data gathered in the recommended format (Mountain et al., 1974), a number of factors led to another revision of staging criteria. These factors include evolution of imaging technology (especially computed tomography), increasing familiarity with prethoracotomy invasive staging procedures (mediastinoscopy, parasternal thoroscopy, and needle biopsy), as well as the appreciation that factors other than tumor size, lymph node involvement, and presence of absence of metastases influence the natural history of lung cancer. The central feature of a revision proposed by the American Thoracic Society (Tisi et al., 1983) is the use of specific anatomic landmarks as reference points for locating lymph node stations, because these landmarks can be reliably identified by imaging techniques (Faling et al., 1981), at mediastinoscopy (Pearson et al., 1972), and at thoracotomy.

Briefly, lymph node stations are as follows:
supraclavicular;
high paratracheal (above where the innominate artery crosses the trachea and specified as being to the right or left of the midline);
low paratracheal (extending from innominate artery to azygous vein on the right, or from the level of the top of the aortic arch to the level of carina, medial to the ligamentum arteriosum on the left);
aortopulmonary (lateral to the ligamentum arteriosum and proximal to the first branch of the left pulmonary artery);
anterior mediastinal (anterior to the aorta or innominate artery);
subcarinal (between tracheal bifurcation and right pulmonary artery, but not including nodes attached to the airway);
right tracheobronchial (between azygous vein and right upper lobe bronchus);
left peribronchial (along the left mainstem bronchus, medial to the ligamentum arteriosum);

intrapulmonary (distal to right or left upper lobe bronchus or in the substance of the lung).

(Numbers have been omitted here in favor of descriptive terms to reduce confusion.)

Clinical staging of carcinoma of the lung has been proposed according to the following categories (adapted from the American Joint Committee, 1979, and the American Thoracic Society, Tisi et al., 1983);

Occult Carcinoma
$T_X N_0 M_0$ malignant cytology without detectable mass lesion or metastasis

Stage I
$T_1 N_0 M_0$ primary tumor less than 3 cm in diame-
$T_1 N_1 M_0$ ter surrounded by lung or visceral pleura; not present proximal to a lobar bronchus and *no* adenopathy beyond intrapulmonary nodes
              or
$T_2 N_0 M_0$ tumor greater than 3 cm in diameter or extends to bifurcation of right or left mainstem bronchus (author's approximation of what is usually meant by "hilar")

Stage II
$T_2 N_1 M_0$ T_2 tumors with ipsilateral intrapulmonary nodes

Stage III
T_3 tumor more extensive than T_2 *or* with
N_2 mediastinal *or* distant metastases
M_1

While it is hoped that a refined nomenclature for lymph node mapping will improve the utility of a staging system based on TNM categories, it is also clear that other variables must be taken into account. Clinical outcome is believed to be influenced by cell type (Kirsh et al., 1972; Chung et al., 1982), sex (Kirsh et al., 1972), age (Pemberton et al., 1983), or combinations of these (Rossing and Rossing, 1982). A widely-held belief that small cell carcinoma is not amenable to surgical treatment is being challenged (Shields et al., 1982; Meyer et al., 1982).

Apart from these considerations, one also has to assess apparent anomalies within even a carefully constituted staging system. Some authors argue that extrapulmonary lymph node involvement precludes reasonable expectations of cure by resection (Pearson et al., 1982; Rubinstein et al., 1979); others believe that selected patients with cancer metastatic to mediastinal lymph nodes can benefit from surgery (NARUKE et al., 1978; KIRSH et al., 1971; LEVETT et al., 1982).

A summary statement regarding staging is that specific, precise anatomic criteria most likely will have to be integrated with clinical and biological characteristics of the individual tumor (and perhaps of the individual patient) in order to make it possible to derive gainful information from comparisons of groups of patients and to plan diagnostic and therapeutic interventions for the single patient.

4 Special Anatomical Considerations in Management of Lung Cancer

4.1 Chest Wall

It is also necessary to consider the nonpulmonary anatomy of the chest. Direct extension of a malignancy to adjacent organs is in general a bad but not categorically hopeless finding (PIEHLER et al., 1982). The least gloomy area of involvement is the chest wall. Segmental skeletal support (via the 12 ribs) with generous arterial supply from intercostal arteries originating both posteriorly (directly from the aorta) and anteriorly (from the internal mammary arteries) makes it possible to remove generous sections of chest wall without unduly compromising structural or nutrient support of adjacent tissue. Balanced against this favorable anatomic phenomenon is that intercostal venous drainage from chest wall lesions can infuse malignant cells into the systemic venous circulation via the azygous vein (on the right) or hemiazygous system (on the left) as well as anteriorly through internal mammary veins.

Lymphatic spread from the chest wall can parallel the vessels just mentioned or follow other pathways. The posterior portions of the lower five or six ribs are drained by descending intercostal lymph trunks (WALLS, 1964), running obliquely from lateral and cephalad origins centrally to the cysterna chyli below the diaphragm, from which lymph ascends via the thoracic duct. The latter usually passes into the thorax alongside the aorta, coursing on the anterior surface of the vertebral bodies and eventually emptying into the systemic circulation at the posterolateral junction of the left jugular and subclavian veins. There may be a separate right thoracic duct draining to a comparable location on the right side of the neck. The point to be emphasized is that there is no single or localized pathway from a given point in the chest wall, as there is not from the lung. Multiple potential paths of drainage mandate a careful delineation of the actual extent of disease before embarking upon a putatively curative local procedure for a lesion which has crossed anatomic boundaries which preclude reasonable expectation of success from surgery or radiation.

4.1.1 "Pancoast Tumor"

One specific type of extension of lung cancer to the chest wall which has caused confusion and disagreement is the "Pancoast tumor" or "superior sulcus tumor." PANCOAST described a syndrome reflecting invasion of brachial plexus and sympathetic chain by carcinoma arising in the apex of the upper lobe of the lung (PANCOAST, 1932). He mistakenly attributed malignant potential to "embryonal rest cells" found in the "superior pulmonary sulcus," a term which has no precise anatomic definition. It has variably been used to describe indentation of the upper lobes by innominate and proximal subclavian arteries or referred to as the paravertebral gutter. Since the anatomic boundaries are not clear, and since there is currently thought not to be any unique histologic characteristic of cancer arising in the apex of the lung and invading the chest wall, it is probably best to follow the recommendation that the eponym be dropped (TEIXEIRA, 1983). "Pancoast syndrome" can be used to refer to the symptom complex and physical findings characteristic of pulmonary malignancies with a specific pattern of invasion.

A problem not dealt with by this minor terminological reform is how to explain the surprisingly good later results described by PAULSON and associates for combined surgical and radiation treatment of a group of patients with definite chest wall, brachial plexus, and even vertebral body involvement (SHAW et al., 1961; PAULSON, 1975). Reports of prolonged survival after en bloc resections of lung cancer elsewhere in the chest are essentially anecdotal (NORI et al., 1982; YOSHIMURA et al., 1979).

4.2 Diaphragm

Invasion of the diaphragm usually precludes curative resection, not because the diaphragm cannot be spared or reconstructed, but because extensive venous and lymphatic drainage from the diaphragm almost invariably is associated with disease outside the scope of surgery. There are both subpleural and extraperitoneal lymphatic plexuses on either side of diaphragmatic muscle. Once cancer has crossed both the visceral and parietal layers of pleura into diaphragmatic muscle, there is almost invariably invasion of the liver or metastasis to retroperitoneal lymph nodes. Remarkably, successful resection of adrenal metastases has been described (Twomey et al., 1981), although ordinarily a distant metastasis is taken as an absolute contraindication for pulmonary resection (Clifton, 1966).

5 Specific Resection Procedures

With regard to resection procedures, the thoracic surgeon has several options. *Pneumonectomy* is historically the classic resection performed for lung cancer, but may carry an unacceptable mortality risk in a patient population which typically has reduced cardiovascular and pulmonary reserve (Wilkins et al., 1978). *Lobectomy* will often suffice to remove a tumor and is currently the standard procedure. A patient who cannot afford to lose an entire lobe may benefit from *segmentectomy* (Jensik et al., 1973), a resection designed to remove a segmental bronchus and the pulmonary and vascular tissue associated with it. As there are no pleural linings or even very distinct tissue planes between lobar segments, some surgeons have turned to *wedge resection* (Hoffman and Ransdell, 1980). Segmental anatomy is largely disregarded, and the surgeon concentrates instead on removing the palpable mass with some margin of normal surrounding pulmonary parenchyma. Situations may arise in which a *sleeve resection* is feasible: a bronchus (and, rarely, the vascular structures) can be transected and reimplanted to provide adequate resection margins around some lesions (Bennett and Smith, 1978; Weisel et al., 1979). A special case of this concept is *carinal resection* with reimplantation of a mainstem or lobar bronchus onto the trachea (Grillo, 1978; Pearson, 1981; Jensik et al., 1981).

The nihilist may argue that it has yet to be demonstrated that surgery has a favorable impact on any lung cancer (survival being attributable to case selection rather than to a benefit of resection) (Ball, 1983). In principle, the same challenge can be posed regarding radiation therapy. However, most clinicians believe some lesions can be cured by local measures. The critical issue is to decide what anatomic structures can and should be removed or irradiated in order to provide a reasonable expectation of cure, without killing or crippling the patient in the process.

References

American Joint Committee for Cancer Staging and End Results Reporting (1977) Manual for staging of cancer. American Joint Committee, Chicago, Illinois.

American Joint Committee for Cancer Staging and End Results Reporting Task Force on Carcinoma of the Lung (1973) Clinical staging system for carcinoma of the lung. American Joint Committee, Chicago, Illinois.

American Joint Committee for Cancer Staging and End Results Reporting Task Force on Lung Cancer (1979) Staging of lung cancer. American Joint Committee, Chicago, Illinois.

Arey LB (1965) Developmental anatomy: a textbook and laboratory manual of embryology, 7th edn. Saunders, Philadelphia.

Baird JA (1965) The pathways of lymphatic spread of carcinoma of the lung, Br J Surg 52:868–875.

Ball WC (1983) The effect of surgical treatment on the natural history of lung cancer (editorial). Am Rev Respir Dis 127:1 (see Rossing TH, Rossing RG (1982) Survival in lung cancer: an analysis of the effects of age, resectability, and histopathologic type, Am Rev Respir Dis 126:771–777).

Bennett WF, Smith RA (1978) A twenty-year analysis of the results of sleeve resection for primary bronchogenic carcinoma, J Thorac Cardiovasc Surg 76:840–845.

Chung CK, Zaino R, Stryker JA, et al (1982) Carcinoma of the lung: evaluation of histological grade and factors influencing prognosis, Ann Thorac Surg 33:599–604.

Clifton EE (1966) The criteria for operability and resectability in lung cancer, JAMA 195:1031–1032.

Crapo JD, Barry BE, Gehr P, et al (1982) Cell number and cell characteristics of the normal human lung, Am Rev Respir Dis 126:332–337.

Faling LJ, Pugatch RD, Jung-Legg Y, et al (1981) Computed tomographic scanning of the mediastinum in the staging of bronchogenic carcinoma, Am Rev Respir Dis 124:690–695.

Gordon W (1962) Lymphatic spread in the surgical treatment of lung cancer, Am J Surg 104:866–868.

Grillo HC (1978) Tracheal tumors: surgical management, Ann Thorac Surg 26:112–125.

Hoffman TH, Ransdell HT (1980) Comparison of lobectomy and wedge resection for carcinoma of the lung, J Thorac Cardiovasc Surg 79:211–217.

Ives JC, Buffler PA, Greenberg SD (1983) Environmental association and histopathologic patterns of carcinoma of the lung: the challenge and dilemma in epidemiologic studies, Am Rev Respir Dis 128:195–209.

Jackson CL, Humber JF (1943) Correlated applied anatomy of the bronchial tree and lung with a system of nomenclature, Dis Chest 9:319–326.

Jensik RJ, Faber LP, Milloy FJ, et al (1973) Segmental resection for lung cancer. A fifteen-year experience, J Thorac Cardiovasc Surg 66:563–572.

Jensik RJ, Faber LP, Kittle CF, et al (1982) Survival in patients undergoing tracheal sleeve pneumonoectomy for bronchogenic carcinoma, J Thorac Cardiovasc Surg 84:489–496.

Kirsh MM, Kahn DR, Gago O, et al (1971) Treatment of bronchogenic carcinoma with mediastinal metastases, Ann Thorac Surg 12:11–21.

Kirsh MM, Prior M, Gago O, et al (1972) The effect of histological cell type on the prognosis of patients with bronchogenic carcinoma, Ann Thorac Surg 13:303–310.

Kirsh MM, Tashian J, Sloan H (1982) Carcinoma of the lung in women, Ann Thorac Surg 34:34–39.

Krahl VE (1964) Anatomy of the mammalian lung. In: Fenn WO, Rahn H, (eds) Handbook of physiology, section 3 (Respiration), Vol I, American Physiological Society, Washington, D.C. p 213–284.

Levett JM, Darakjiar HE, DeMeester TR, et al (1982) Bronchogenic carcinoma located in the aortic window. The importance of the primary lesion as a determinant of survival, J Thorac Cardiovasc Surg 83:551–562.

Meyer JA, Comis RL, Ginsberg SJ, et al (1982) Phase II trial of extended indications for resection in small cell carcinoma of the lung, J Thorac Cardiovasc Surg 83:12–19.

Mountain CF, Carr DT, Anderson WAD (1974) A system for the clinical staging of lung cancer, AJR 120:130–138.

Naruke T, Suemasu K, Ishikawa S (1978) Lymph node mapping and curability at various levels of metastasis in resected lung cancer, J Thorac Cardiovasc Surg 76:832–839.

Nori D, Sundaresan N, Bains M, et al (1982) Bronchogenic carcinoma with invasion of the spine. Treatment with combined surgery and perioperative brachytherapy, JAMA 248:2491–2492.

Pancoast HK (1932) Superior pulmonary sulcus tumor. Tumor characterized by pain, Horner's syndrome, destruction of bone and atrophy of hand muscles, JAMA 99:1391–1396.

Paulson DL (1975) Carcinomas in the superior pulmonary sulcus, J Thorac Cardiovasc Surg 70:1095–1104.

Pearson FG, Nelems JM, Henderson RD, et al (1972) The role of mediastinoscopy in the selection of treatment for bronchial carcinoma with involvement of superior mediastinal lymph nodes, J Thorac Cardiovasc Surg 64:382–390.

Pearson FG (1981) Surgery of the trachea. In: Dyde A, Smith RE (eds) The present state of thoracic surgery, The Fifth Coventry Conference. Pitman Medical, London.

Pearson FG, DeLarue NC, Ilves R, et al (1982) Significance of positive superior mediastinal nodes identified at mediastinoscopy in patients with resectable cancer of the lung, J Thorac Cardiovasc Surg 83:1–11.

Pemberton JH, Nagorney DM, Gilmore JC, et al (1983) Bronchogenic carcinoma in patients younger than 40 years. Ann Thorac Surg 36:509–515.

Piehler JM, Pariolero PC, Weiland LH, et al (1982) Bronchogenic carcinoma with chest wall invasion: factors affecting survival following en bloc resection, Ann Thorac Surg 34:684–691.

Rossing TH, Rossing RJ (1982) Survival in lung cancer. An analysis of the effects of age, sex, resectability, and histopathologic type. Am Rev Respir Dis 126:771–777.

Rouviere H (1938) Anatomy of the human lymphatic system (trans Tobias MJ), Edwards, Ann Arbor, Michigan.

Rubinstein I, Baum GL, Kalter Y, et al (1979) The influence of cell type and lymph node metastases on survival of patients with carcinoma of the lung undergoing thoracotomy, Am Rev Respir Dis 119:253–262.

Shaw RR, Paulson DL, Kee KL Jr (1961) Treatment of the superior sulcus tumor by irradiation followed by resection, Ann Surg 154:29–40.

Shields TW, Higgins GA Jr, Matthews MJ, et al (1982) Surgical resection in the management of small cell carcinoma of the lung, J Thorac Cardiovasc Surg 84:481–488.

Teixeira JP (1983) Concerning the Pancoast tumor: what is the superior pulmonary sulcus?, Ann Thorac Surg 35:577–578.

Tisi GM, Friedman PJ, Peters RM, et al (1983) Clinical staging of primary lung cancer, Am Rev Respir Dis 127:659–664.

Tobin CE (1954) Lymphatics of the pulmonary alveoli, Anat Rec 120:625–636.

Twomey P, Montgomery C, Clark O (1982) Successful treatment of adrenal metastases from large-cell carcinoma of the lung, JAMA 248:581–583.

Walls EW (1964) The blood vascular and lymphatic systems. In: Romanes GJ (ed) Cunningham's textbook of anatomy. 12th ed. University Press, Oxford, p 962–963.

Weibel ER (1963) Morphometry of the human lung. Academic Press, New York.

Weisel RD, Cooper JD, Delarue NC, et al (1979) Sleeve lobectomy for carcinoma of the lung, J Thorac Cardiovasc Surg 78:839–849.

Wilkins EW, Scannell JG, Craver JG (1978) Four decades of experience with resections for bronchogenic carcinoma at the Massachusetts General Hospital, J Thorac Cardiovasc Surg 76:364–368.

Yoshimura H, Kazama S, Asari H, et al (1979) Lung cancer involving the superior vena cava: pneumonectomy with concomitant partial resection of superior vena cava, J Thorac Cardiovasc Surg 77:83–86.

Chapter IV Pathologic Aspects of Lung Cancer

CHARLES S. FAULKNER II

CONTENTS

1 Introduction

A rare cancer at the beginning of this century, cancer of the lung has become the leading cause of cancer deaths in males in the United States (RO-DESCU, 1977; SILVERBERG, 1983), and is predicted to become the leading cause of cancer death in females in the United States by 1985 (CARR, 1981). The absolute incidence of lung cancer has almost doubled, decade by decade (RODESCU, 1977; SIL-

CHARLES S. FAULKNER II, M.D., Associate Professor of Clinical Pathology

Dartmouth-Hitchcock Medical Center, Hanover, NH 03756, USA

VERBERG, 1983). It is possible that in the United States we shall see as many as 300,000 new cases annually by 2,000 A.D. (ROSENOW and CARR, 1979).

This pandemic has led to an increasing interest in understanding the pathogenesis, morphogenesis and pathobiology of human lung cancer. Our understanding of this entity is in some ways coming full circle. Lung cancer was originally regarded as an entity. As recently as 1968 WILLIS held that most lung cancers possessed a spectrum of morphologic appearances, and that attempts at subdivision of the entity were "arbitrary" and of "limited" value (WILLIS, 1968). Most clinicans and pathologists, however, tend to regard lung cancer as a variety of different diseases of varying clinical and morphologic characteristics. Nevertheless, recent morphologic studies underline the difficulties in separating these apparent entities, and suggest that there is more interrelationship between the subdivisions than was formerly realized (CARTER and EGGLESTON, 1980). It should not surprise us that lung cancers do not always obey the rules which we have devised for them.

In spite of the validity of this caveat, our current understanding of lung cancer indicates the value of continuing to separate out the various groups as best we can with currently available tools. Important differences in behavior and response to treatment underline the usefulness of this separation.

2 Classification

2.1 General Conditions

As with most efforts at tumor classification, primary neoplasms of the lung are grouped according to our understanding of their origin. According to this belief, the neoplasms derive from the cells which can be found in normal lung, or the precursors of those cells.

Several distinct cell types are recognized in normal human bronchial and bronchiolar epithelium, including basal cells, mucus-producing cells, ciliated cells, neuroendocrine cells and Clara cells (HESS et al., 1981b; MCDOWELL et al., 1978a; CARR, 1981). Over 90% of primary pulmonary neoplasms are included in four major types of carcinoma. The whole basis of the current surgical pathologic classification of these carcinomas depends on relating the histologic appearance of each neoplasm to one of the normal cell types, either directly or indirectly (e.g., via squamous metaplasia). In the majority of cases, this is reproducibly feasible. As we study these neoplasms more closely, for example with the electron microscope, it is becoming apparent that pulmonary carcinomas with features of more than one of the normal cell types are not rare (HESS et al., 1981a; MCDOWELL and TRUMP 1981; AUERBACH et al., 1982; HASHIMOTO et al., 1979; YESNER, 1981), and may even be common (MCDOWELL et al., 1978b; HESS et al., 1981c; GAZDAR et al., 1983; SABA, 1983).

The light microscope is a somewhat limited instrument, and any classification scheme which depends on light microscopic criteria for identifying pulmonary neoplasms will inevitably achieve imperfect success. Nevertheless, for a classification scheme to be useful today, it must be within the reach of pathologists whose morphologic tools do not extend beyond the light microscope, paraffin sections and a small variety of stains. Such a classification should be easily taught and easily learned, should be as scientifically accurate as possible, should be reproducible, and should provide clinically useful information (RAPPAPORT, 1977). These goals are never fully attainable, but are important aiming points for our efforts. New techniques, such as electron microscopy, used appropriately, will add precision to the interpretation of biopsy material (SOBIN, 1983; NASH, 1983).

The World Health Organization (WHO) has devoted major efforts to providing such categorization of human tumors. The first in the long series of published classifications resulting from these efforts was on lung tumors (KREYBERG, 1967). This was widely accepted and employed. Modifications to this classification were proposed in 1973 by the Pathology Panel of the International Workshop for Therapy of Lung Cancer (MATTHEWS, 1973). These changes were also widely accepted, and were subsequently incorporated by the WHO into their formal revision, which was conceived in 1977. Gestation was prolonged, delivery of the completed work not occurring until 1981 (World Health Organization 1981, 1982).

One of the main purposes of the WHO in pro-

Table 1. Histological classification of lung tumours[a]

I. Epithelial tumours

A. Benign
  1. Papillomas
     a) Squamous
     b) "Transitional" papilloma
  2. Adenomas
     a) Pleomorphic adenoma ("mixed" tumour)
     b) Monomorphic adenoma
     c) Others

B. Dysplasia
  Carcinoma in situ

C. Malignant
  1. Squamous cell carcinoma (epidermoid carcinoma)
     Variant:
     a) Spindle cell (squamous) carcinoma
  2. Small cell carcinoma
     a) Oat cell carcinoma
     b) Intermediate cell type
     c) Combined oat cell carcinoma
  3. Adenocarcinoma
     a) Acinar adenocarcinoma
     b) Papillary adenocarcinoma
     c) Bronchiolo-alveolar carcinoma
     d) Solid carcinoma with mucus formation
  4. Large cell carcinoma
     Variants:
     a) Giant cell carcinoma
     b) Clear cell carcinoma
  5. Adenosquamous carcinoma
  6. Carcinoid tumour
  7. Bronchial gland carcinomas
     a) Adenoid cystic carcinoma
     b) Mucoepidermoid carcinoma
     c) Others
  8. Others

II. Soft tissue tumours

III. Mesothelial tumours

A. Benign mesothelioma

B. Malignant mesothelioma
  1. Epithelial
  2. Fibrous (spindle-cell)
  3. Biphasic

IV. Miscellaneous tumours

A. Benign

B. Malignant
  1. Carcinosarcoma
  2. Pulmonary blastoma
  3. Malignant melanoma
  4. Malignant lymphomas
  5. Others

V. Secondary tumours

VI. Unclassified tumours

---

[a] World Health Organization, Histological Typing of Lung Tumours, 3nd edition, Geneva, 1981.

Table 1 (continued)

VII. Tumour-like lesions
  A. Hamartoma
  B. Lymphoproliferative lesions
  C. Tumourlet
  D. Eosinophilic granuloma
  E. "Sclerosing hemangioma"
  F. Inflammatory pseudotumour
  G. Others

mulgating their classifications is to provide a common basis for communication and comparison among interested parties all over the world. In the interests of fulfilling this laudable goal, the following discussion will adhere closely to the WHO groups and criteria. Table 1 lists the different groups identified by the WHO. Our present focus is on the malignant tumors, with emphasis on the numerically predominant groups of carcinoma.

2.2 WHO Classification

2.2.1 Epithelial Tumors

2.2.1.1 Squamous Cell Carcinoma (Syn. Epidermoid Carcinoma). This group comprises 30–45% of lung cancers in most series (MATTHEWS, 1974; PERCY and SOBIN, 1983; CARTER and EGGLESTON, 1980; MATTHEWS et al., 1983), though figures as high at 60% are reported (SPENCER, 1977). Squamous cell carcinoma is defined by the presence in light microscopic sections of keratin and/or intercellular bridges, which correspond to desmosome-tonofilament complexes in the electron microscope. The group consists of a histologic spectrum, ranging from well differentiated tumors, with abundant keratin and numerous intercellular bridges, to poorly differentiated neoplasms, in which one or the other of these elements can be demonstrated only with difficulty. Most of the tumors are between these extremes, in a group best described as moderately differentiated.

These tend to be large, bulky tumors, often centrally located in the lung, usually arising in subsegmental or larger bronchi. They often cause bronchial obstruction. Central necrosis leads to cavity formation in about 10% of the cases (MATTHEWS, 1974; MATTHEWS, 1976; RODESCU, 1977). These neoplasms grow at varying rates (CARTER

et al., 1976), but tend not to metastasize early, perhaps because the cells are more firmly adherent to one another via the relatively numerous desmosomes. As a result, they are more commonly localized to the thorax at the time of diagnosis than the other tumor types (56%) (MATTHEWS, 1974; MATTHEWS et al., 1983). Because of this, squamous cell carcinomas are more often amenable to surgical resection than the other types, and tend to have a longer survival. In one series five-year survival was 22% (IOACHIM, 1978). In another, 18% of patients with resectable squamous cell carcinomas survived ten years (ASHOR et al., 1975).

Squamous cell carcinomas of the bronchi are often preceded by a series of bronchial epithelial changes, starting with squamous metaplasia, and proceeding through dysplasia and carcinoma in situ to frankly invasive carcinoma. This progression is analogous to that seen in the development of squamous cell carcinoma of the uterine cervix. This sequence probably requires a relatively long time, and in some cases the cytologic evidence suggests that even invasive squamous cell carcinoma exists in a prolonged preclinical phase (CARTER et al., 1976; CARTER, 1978). In some studies of pulmonary squamous cell carcinoma, however, it has not been possible to document this series of changes, and at least a few cases appear to arise relatively suddenly in previously normal bronchi (MELAMED and ZAMAN, 1982). Careful study of the bronchial tree in resection specimens often reveals squamous metaplasia and atypical lesions elsewhere (CARTER et al., 1976) and squamous cell carcinomas are more commonly multicentric than the other groups (IOACHIM, 1978; ROSENOW and CARR, 1979; SPENCER, 1977; CARTER and EGGLESTON, 1980; CARTER, 1979; MELAMED and ZAMAN, 1982). These data are consistent with a widespread "field effect", as would be expected with an inhaled agent, such as tobacco smoke.

Cytologic screening efforts in people identified as a high risk population have focussed on squamous cell carcinoma, as the central location and intrabronchial growth yield a higher likelihood of positive cytologic specimens early in the course of the neoplasm (CARTER, 1979; MELAMED and ZAMAN, 1982). At the cost of considerable effort, relatively small numbers of new cancers have been discovered, and some difficulty has been experienced in localizing the lesions responsible for positive cytologic findings (CARTER, 1979). The analogy with carcinoma of the uterine cervix does not seem to extend to screening and sensitive detection of early lesions.

2.2.1.2 Small Cell Carcinoma. Small cell anaplastic carcinoma and small cell undifferentiated carcinoma are terms previously used for this neoplasm. The tumor does possess specific features of differentiation, so the words anaplastic and undifferentiated are inappropriate; accordingly, the WHO no longer uses them. The term oat cell carcinoma is commonly found as a colloquial name for this group. The WHO reserves this term for one specific subgroup of small cell carcinoma, and thus it is not correct to use the term for the whole group.

The histologic features which define this group include the relatively small and uniform size of the cells, and particularly the nuclear detail, which in well-fixed, well-prepared sections is rather characteristic. The nuclei are oval, usually in the range of 2–4 times as large as the nuclei of small lymphocytes, and the chromatin is finely granular and uniformly dispersed. Nucleoli are not prominent. Unfortunately the cells seem fragile, and are fequently severely distorted during biopsy, particularly with small specimens, such as bronchial biopsies. This may render specific diagnosis difficult at times.

The WHO distinguishes two subgroups, on the basis of cytoplasmic differences (World Health Organization 1982). The oat cell type has sparse cytoplasm; the intermediate cell type has more abundant cytoplasm. Intermediate cells are less regular than oat cells. A third type of small cell carcinoma is the combined oat cell type, in which the neoplasm has a component of oat cell type admixed with a squamous and/or an adenocarcinoma component.

Some observers further define small cell carcinoma by requiring ultrastructural demonstration of endosecretory granules (also known as neurosecretory granules, or dense-core vesicles) (COHEN and MATTHEWS, 1978; WHIMSTER, 1983). Other workers feel that some neoplasms in which these structures are not found can still be classified as small cell carcinoma (MATTHEWS and GAZDAR, 1982; GOULD et al., 1983; CARTER, 1983; SABA et al., 1983).

Small cell carcinoma has been the focus of more attention than any of the other pulmonary neoplasms, for a variety of reasons. Its biologic behavior and response to treatment set it apart from the other lung tumors. The neuroendocrine origin of the neoplasm, and the variety of hormones which it can produce have excited the interest of workers from various of the biologic disciplines. Since permanent cell lines derived from these tumors have become available for study (PETTEN-

GILL et al., 1980; GAZDAR et al., 1981 b), it appears that the neoplasm should provide a goldmine of information regarding many aspects of neoplasia, hormone production, gene regulation and so forth.

Small cell carcinoma makes up 20–37% of most series of pulmonary neoplasms (CARR, 1981; IOACHIM, 1978; SPENCER, 1977; PERCY and SOBIN, 1983). These tumors usually arise in central bronchi (CARR, 1981). They tend to grow rapidly, and invade and spread both early and widely. As a result, up to 85% of the cases have spread beyond the thorax at the time of initial diagnosis (MATTHEWS, 1974; CARR, 1981; GRECO and OLDHAM, 1979; RUCKDESCHEL et al., 1979; SHEPHERD et al., 1983). For a number of years oncologists and surgeons have felt that surgery is not a viable treatment for this neoplasm. Recently, however, this uncompromising view has been somewhat softened by more complete understanding of the full spectrum of behavior of these neoplasms. The surgical resectability rate is low, but not nonexistent (RUCKDESCHEL et al., 1979; CARTER, 1983).

Most of these tumors liver up to their reputation for rapid growth. Measurements of tumor doubling times of small numbers of cases have often suggested that these can be among the fastest growing of pulmonary neoplasms (GRECO and OLDHAM, 1979). The labelling index of the tumor cells is often quite high (LIVINGSTON, 1980). In vitro, one permanent cell line has shown a doubling time as short as 24 h (OHARA and OKAMOTO, 1977). Several recent studies, however, underline considerable variation in growth rate from one example to another. Tumor doubling times from 12 to 264 days are reported (BRIGHAM et al., 1978; LENHARD et al., 1981; SHACKNEY et al., 1981). A tumor with a doubling time of less than 30 days is considered a rapidly growing neoplasm; a doubling time of more than 70 days is considered slow growth. Putting this together with the generally high mitotic activity of these neoplasms suggests that rapid cell growth is often accompanied by considerable cell loss. Extensive experience with in vitro tumor growth confirms both the wide spectrum of growth rates and the high rate of cell loss in rapidly growing cell lines (PETTENGILL et al., 1980; GAZDAR et al., 1981 b).

Perhaps relating to the generally rapid mitotic rate, these neoplasms have in the past 10 years proven very responsive to irradiation and chemotherapy. Of all pulmonary malignancies, small cell carcinoma is the most responsive to these modalities (LIVINGSTON, 1980; RUCKDESCHEL, et al., 1979; HIRSCH et al., 1982a; MATTHEWS et al.,

1980; MATTHEWS and HIRSCH, 1981). This fact underlines the importance of correct identification of these neoplasms; fortunately the histopathologic diagnosis of small cell carcinoma has high reproducibility (HIRSCH et al., 1982a; MATTHEWS and HIRSCH, 1981; STANLEY and MATTHEWS, 1981). This has led to a tendency to divide pulmonary carcinoma into small cell and non-small cell, a tendency which may tend to blur the differences between the other types of lung cancer.

Approximately coincidental with the awareness of the full spectrum of growth rates of small cell carcinoma has been the appearance of small but notable groups of long-term survivors in various clinical trials (MATTHEWS et al., 1980; SHACKNEY et al., 1981). Hopes have been raised that it is possible to eradicate the neoplasm. In two series, small numbers of patients treated for small cell carcinoma have died with no evidence of tumor (MATTHEWS and GAZDAR, 1982). Before speaking of real cures, however, we must be sure that we are not dealing with relatively slow-growing examples of this tumor. Therapy which destroys all but a very small number of tumor cells might well be followed by a disease-free interval of 4–5 years (MATTHEWS et al., 1980) or even more.

In studying the spread of small cell carcinoma and the relationship of metastases to prognosis, particular attention has been devoted to the bone marrow and brain. About one-third of the patients present with bone marrow involvement, and these patients have shorter remissions (mean 86 days vs. 182 days) and shorter survivals (mean 149 days vs. 231 days) than patients whose bone marrow biopsies are negative (HIRSCH and HANSEN, 1980). 10–30% of patients present with central nervous system involvement (NUGENT et al., 1979; DOYLE, 1982; HIRSCH et al., 1982b; VANHAZEL et al., 1983). Longer survivals seem to provide more opportunity for central nervous system metastases, with two-year survival being attended by an 80% probability of such involvement (NUGENT et al., 1979). Radiation therapy, however, provides adequate palliation, and the majority of deaths cannot be attributed to central nervous system metastases (NUGENT et al., 1979).

Overall survival in this form of cancer has undergone a considerable improvement with protocols involving radiation therapy and combination chemotherapy. In untreated cases, median survival is 14 weeks for patients with localized disease, and 7 weeks for those with extensive disease. Survival curves with intensive treatment are much better. One is again impressed with the variability of this neoplasm; many respond dramatically to treatment, and some respond very briefly or not at all.

In hopes of finding a way to predict which cases will respond to treatment, many studies have examined the behavior of morphologically defined subgroups of this tumor (KREYBERG, 1967). Experience suggested that the fusiform and polygonal patterns were often found in the same neoplasm, and this led to their combination in the intermediate group (MATTHEWS, 1973; World Health Organization 1982). Many reports in the literature are based on the original four subtypes (BURDON et al., 1979; HIRSCH et al., 1977; NIXON et al., 1979; DOMBERNOWSKY et al., 1979; COHEN and MATTHEWS, 1978; STRAUCHEN et al., 1983), but several recent ones follow the current WHO grouping. These reports are inconsistent in their findings regarding response to therapy and survival. Some find no difference in these variables (GRECO and OLDHAM, 1979; CARNEY et al., 1980; VOLLMER, 1983; TISCHLER, 1978; BUNN et al., 1981; HIRSCH et al., 1983; CARTER and EGGLESTON, 1980), and some find that the oat cell subtype is more amenable to chemotherapy than the intermediate cell subtype (DAVIS and SOBEL, 1981; DAVIS et al., 1981).

Part of this inconsistency can be attributed to difficulties encountered by pathologists in applying criteria for subtyping, and part to the use of different criteria by different pathologists. One study with three pathologists found agreement on the subtype in only 54% of the cases (HIRSCH et al., 1982a). Some observers find admixtures of the two subtypes in many of the cases (DAVIS and SOBEL, 1981; DAVIS et al., 1981; TISCHLER, 1978; CARTER, 1983). Some comment on the difficulties caused by the frequent presence of crush artifact (BURDON et al., 1979; MATTHEWS and HIRSCH, 1981). Some suggest that the features which make the oat cell subtype look different from the intermediate cell subtype could relate more to poor preservation (tumor necrosis and/or autolysis) than to any real differences (HIRSCH et al., 1982a; VOLLMER, 1982). Measurements of cell size show a continuum rather than a biphasic peak (VOLLMER, 1982; KAMEY et al., 1982; CARTER, 1983; CURRIER and FAULKNER, 1983). For all of these reasons, efforts to find morphologic correlates with the different biologic behaviors within the group of small cell carcinoma have so far met with little success. Nor does tumor size appear to correlate with survival (LENHARD, 1981). A study attempting to correlate the rate of growth prior to treatment with the outcome is in progress (LEN-HARD, 1981).

The cell of origin of this neoplasm has been of considerable interest. After this neoplasm was generally accepted as a carcinoma rather than a lymphoma (recognition which occurred within the memory of pathologists whose experience extends back to the early nineteen-fifties), most observers assumed that the cell of origin probably was some sort of primitive reserve or basal cell in the bronchial epithelium (LIEBOW, 1952). Careful ultrastructural studies, however, revealed cells in the bronchial epithelium resembling the Kultschitzky cells of the small intestine. The morphologic features of small cell carcinoma resemble these cells enough to suggest them as the cell of origin (MCDOWELL et al., 1976; BENSCH et al., 1968).

At approximately the same time as these morphologic observations were made, PEARSE was developing and refining his concept of APUD cells (PEARSE, 1966; PEARSE, 1969). The concept dealt with cells which had certain biochemical and morphologic characteristics in common, and which were believed to derive from the neural crest. These cells are widely distributed throughout the body, and serve various neuroendocrine functions. Subsequent work has clearly shown that at least some of the cells included in this APUD group do not migrate from the neural crest, but are locally derived, e.g., in the gastrointestinal mucosa (SIDHU, 1979; MIYAMOTO et al., 1982; VAN-BOGAERT, 1982; GAZDAR et al., 1981a; GOULD et al., 1983; YESNER, 1983; CARTER and EGGLESTON, 1980). PEARSE now states that these cells come from neurally programmed cells, derived fom the same ectoblast from which the entire endoderm evolves (PEARSE, 1977; PEARSE and TAKOR TAKOR, 1979). Most authors now accept that the Kultschitzky-type, or K-type, neuroendocrine cell in the bronchial tree is of endodermal origin. Presumably local microenvironmental factors encourage differentiation towards neuroendocrine form and function (MCDOWELL et al., 1978; SABA et al., 1983; GOULD et al., 1981; MCDOWELL et al., 1981).

The notion that small cell carcinoma is at one end of a spectrum of proliferative lesions related to bronchial Kultschitzky-type cells, first promulgated by BENSCH (BENSCH et al., 1968), is now very widely accepted (GOULD et al., 1983; YESNER, 1983). The spectrum ranges from the small hyperplastic lesions known as tumorlets, through carcinoid tumors and atypical carcinoid tumors, to the small cell carcinoma. The fact that these different proliferative lesions share certain morphologic,

histochemical and biosynthetic features provides solid support for the notion that they are closely related. The impressive epidemiologic differences between carcinoid tumor and small cell carcinoma (see 2.2.1.6) remain unexplained. Perhaps these two neoplasms represent different responses of the same cell to different tumorigenic stimuli (GODWIN and BROWN, 1977). An alternate, but not mutually exclusive hypothesis, is that all pulmonary carcinomas can arise from an "indifferent" epithelial cell, the differentiation of which is controlled by the microenvironment (MCDOWELL et al., 1981).

Such a notion would help explain the observation of foci of glandular and/or squamous differentiation in small cell carcinoma in 1–4% of the cases (EWING et al., 1980; MATTHEWS and GAZDAR 1983). When such differentiation is a prominent feature of the neoplasm, the WHO designates it as a combined type of small cell carcinoma (World Health Organization 1982). No studies have yet assembled sufficient numbers of these variants to determine whether the typical small cell prognosis prevails or is modified.

The presence of small numbers of larger cells is another, more recently recognized variation, occurring in 5–12% of the cases (RADICE et al., 1983; MATTHEWS and GAZDAR 1982; HIRSCH et al., 1983; CARTER, 1983). Where comparisons of response and survival have been possible, the neoplasms with a large cell component behave more aggressively than the "pure" small cell carcinomas (RADICE et al., 1982; HIRSCH et al., 1983; YESNER, 1983; CARTER, 1983; MATTHEWS et al., 1983).

Complete understanding of admixtures of other types of lung cancer in small cell carcinomas is hampered by the fact that some of these neoplasms undergo histologic changes during their course. Such changes have been observed in clinical and autopsy studies (HASHIMOTO et al., 1979; ABELOFF et al., 1979; BRERETON et al., 1978; ABELOFF and EGGLESTON, 1981; MATTHEWS and GAZDAR, 1982). The histologic features of the neoplasm may evolve towards any of the other major types of lung carcinoma. These changes could reflect a change in differentiation of the original tumor, and/or an effect of therapy on the tumor. It seems less likely that they reflect development of a second tumor, as the changed areas are frequently mixed in with the small cell carcinoma.

Morphologic and functional changes have also been observed in some cell lines derived from small cell carcinoma and maintained over long periods of time (GAZDAR et al., 1981b). In other instances, however, the cell lines have remained constant for a number of years (PETTENGILL et al., 1980).

The emergence of morphologic variations may be a reflection of a newly appreciated characteristic of a neoplasm: heterogeneity. We are becoming increasingly aware of this aspect of what we have regarded as monoclonal proliferations. A given neoplasm will show considerable variation from site to site in the patient, and even from cell to cell within a given site. The electron microscope has magnified some of the morphologic variations to the point where they are easy to see. Not only do the numbers of endosecretory granules vary considerably from cell to cell, but variations in differentiation are increasingly frequently found, with bundles of tonofilaments in scattered cells indicating squamous differentiation (SABA et al., 1981; CHURG et al., 1980; SIDHU, 1982), and lumen formation indicating glandular differentiation. The converse also occurs, with non-small cell carcinomas possessing endosecretory granules (McDOWELL et al., 1981; SABA et al., 1983). These newer observations lend support to the notion of commonality of origin of pulmonary carcinomas (McDOWELL et al., 1981; YESNER, 1983). At the biosynthetic level, there are also marked variations in hormone production from cell to cell and from site to site within a given neoplasm (GOULD et al., 1981; RUCKDESCHEL et al., 1979; BAYLIN et al., 1978; BAYLIN and GAZDAR, 1981).

Hormone synthesis by small cell carcinoma has been a particular focus of recent research efforts. The neoplasm has been known for a long time as the most common cause of "ectopic" hormonal syndromes. More recently we have begun to perceive the kaleidoscopic variety of hormones within the repertoire of even a single one of these tumors. A relatively small fraction of patients has a clinical syndrome related to hormone production by the neoplasm (BONDY and GILBY, 1982; LOKICH, 1982; RICHARDSON et al., 1978; GRECO et al., 1981; GOULD et al., 1983), but in vitro cell lines each produce more than one hormone, and a few produce remarkable numbers (SORENSON et al., 1981). Abnormal hormone levels can be measured in the serum of patients, many of whom have no identified syndrome (HANSEN et al., 1980b). Elevated levels are commonly reported for ACTH, ADH and calcitonin.

Hopes have repeatedly been raised that such hormone production may provide a clinical marker for small cell carcinoma, in initial diagnosis and/or for monitoring response to therapy and recurrent (see 4.2).

2.2.1.3 *Adenocarcinoma.* Adenocarcinoma is defined by a tubular, acinar or papillary pattern of growth, and/or by histochemical evidence of mucin production. The WHO defines four subgroups of adenocarcinoma: acinar, papillary, bronchiolo-alveolar and solid with mucin production. Each of the first two groups consists in turn of a spectrum from well differentiated to poorly differentiated. Bronchiolo-alveolar carcinomas are almost always well differentiated, and solid carcinomas with mucin production are poorly differentiated adenocarcinomas.

Adenocarcinomas comprise about 20–40% of pulmonary carcinomas (MATTHEWS, 1974; CARTER and EGGLESTON, 1980; MATTHEWS et al., 1983). They are more often peripheral than central and they tend to be asymptomatic until late in their course (IOACHIM, 1978; ROSENOW and CARR, 1979). They are often relatively slow-growing neoplasms (HAYABUCHI et al., 1983; BRIGHAM et al., 1978; HAINAU et al., 1977), but they tend to metastasize early, perhaps because the junctional complexes binding cell to cell are not strong. Thus, although most appear resectable at the time of diagnosis, many have spread beyond the thorax. In the resectable group ten-year survival is about 20% (ASHOR et al., 1975), while overall five-year survival for adenocarcinoma is only 9% (IOACHIM, 1978).

Adenocarcinoma is the most common type of lung cancer in women, in whom the incidence is rising rapidly (see 2.3.). It is also on the increase in men, and in some series has become the most common lung cancer, surpassing squamous cell carcinoma (COX and YESNER, 1979; VALAITIS et al., 1981; VINCENT et al., 1977).

In their peripheral location, adenocarcinomas arise usually from bronchioles, most commonly from mucus-producing cells or from non-ciliated bronchiolar cells. They are commonly found in association with foci of fibrosis in the lung. Scarring processes often engender proliferation of bronchiolar epithelium in their vicinity, sometimes with considerable cytologic atypia. Continued atypical epithelial proliferation eventually leads to carcinoma in some cases. In recent years the incidence of pulmonary scar carcinoma has increased considerably, to 7–15% of lung tumors (GRAY and O'NEAL, 1980), possibly as a result of increasing length of survival of people with scars in their lung, and/or possibly as a result of increasing numbers of scars in the lung (AUERBACH et al., 1979). A further factor may of course be increasing numbers and amounts of environmental hazards. A scar may disrupt lymphatic drainage in an area of lung, leading to concentration of carcinogens in the area (CARTER and EGGLESTON, 1980, p. 18).

Not all the foci of fibrosis associated with peripheral adenocarcinomas of the lung precede the neoplasms. Adenocarcinomas may bring about foci of central fibrosis (SHIMOSATO et al., 1890; ROSENOW and CARR, 1979; CARTER and EGGLESTON, 1980), and it may be rather difficult to distinguish which came first.

Another point of potential histologic confusion concerns the distinction between primary adenocarcinoma of the lung and metastatic adenocarcinoma of the lung. This determination may in fact be absolutely impossible (IOACHIM, 1978; RODESCU, 1977), and the surgical pathologist faced with adenocarcinoma in the lung may be forced to equivocate. Even a complete autopsy may not provide sufficient data to make this distinction.

Bronchiolo-alveolar cell carcinoma is generally regarded as almost a separate entity within the group of pulmonary adenocarcinoma, although its separateness is challenged by some (CARTER and EGGLESTON, 1980). This neoplasm is defined by its peculiar pattern of growth, in which it uses the existing alveolar septa as its stroma, growing along their surfaces as a neoplastic replacement of the existing alveolar epithelium. Any adenocarcinoma, primary or metastatic, may grow in this fashion at its periphery, and the diagnosis of bronchiolo-alveolar cell carcinoma should be reserved exclusively for those neoplasms which maintain this pattern of growth throughout.

Bronchiolo-alveolar cell carcinomas are almost always well differentiated, with orderly rows of cuboidal to columnar cells (MATTHEWS, 1974; IOACHIM, 1978). Some are mucin-producing, and when they are, they are apt to do so in large quantities. These neoplasms most commonly present as a localized nodule or infiltrate, but may be multiple, or may diffusely involve a large volume of lung (RODESCU, 1977). Such diffusely involved lung, with its solidity, pale color, and admixed anthracotic pigment, has been likened to Roquefort cheese (CARTER and EGGLESTON, 1980).

The prognosis in bronchiolo-alveolar cell carcinoma is quite varied (CARTER and EGGLESTON, 1980; TAO et al., 1978). Those which are surgically resectable tend to have a very high (41% ten-year) survival rate (ASHOR et al., 1975), while those which are not have a low survival rate (CARTER and EGGLESTON, 1980). Metastases occur in about half of the cases (SPENCER, 1977).

The several ultrastructural studies of bronchiolo-alveolar cell carcinoma have produced somewhat different results (SIDHU, 1982). At least the majority of these tumors arise from bronchiolar epithelial cells (GREENBERG et al., 1975; BEDROSSIAN et al., 1975). Some have features of bronchiolar Clara cells (ZOLLIKER and JACQUES, 1981). Some observers find that a few of these neoplasms have ultrastructural characteristics of granular pneumonocytes (type II alveolar epithelial cells) (KIMULA, 1978; BONIKOS et al., 1979; SINGH et al., 1981). A continuous cell line with ultrastructural and biochemical properties consistent with granular pneumonocyst has been derived from a pulmonary adenocarcinoma (LIEBER et al., 1976). Since bronchiolar and alveolar epithelium derive from the same endoderm, it doesn't seem surprising that some fraction of these neoplasms should possess features of alveolar epithelial differentiation (GREENBERG et al., 1975).

2.2.1.4 Large Cell Carcinoma. This category has been described as the wastebasket of pulmonary carcinoma (CARR, 1981; MATTHEWS, 1976; RODESCU, 1977). Those carcinomas in which features of differentiation are too poorly developed to be recognized in the light microscope are classified in this group (World Health Organization 1982). As might be expected, electron microscopic study reveals features of glandular and/or squamous differentiation in many of these neoplasms (AUERBACH et al., 1982; CARTER and EGGLESTON, 1980; CHUNG, 1978; HORIE and OHTA, 1981; SIDHU, 1982; AZAR et al., 1982; TATEISHI and HATTORI, 1982). Although most large cell carcinomas are not further subclassified, the WHO lists two subgroups as variants: the giant cell carinoma and the clear cell carcinoma (World Health Organization 1982).

Large cell carcinomas comprise 7–20% of pulmonary carcinomas (MATTHEWS, 1974; RODESCU, 1977; MITCHELL et al., 1980; MATTHEWS et al., 1983). Many of these neoplasms are peripheral (IOACHIM, 1978). Possibly most of the peripheral ones represent adenocarcinomas which are too poorly differentiated to recognize in the light microscope, and the central ones represent similarly unrecognizable squamous cell carcinomas. They tend to grow as bulky masses, and tend to spread early. In a series of 208 patients (MITCHELL et al., 1980) about half have disseminated disease at the time of diagnosis. 27% underwent resection, with a median survival of 13 months and a five-year survival of 21%. Overall median survival was six months, with a five-year survival of 6%. In this series radiation therapy was ineffective.

The giant cell carcinoma is a variant in which multinucleate giant cells are conspicuous. A few multinucleate tumor cells are seen in many forms of neoplasm. Most observers require that giant cells form a conspicuous component of the neoplasm to justify the term giant cell carcinoma (CARTER and EGGLESTON, 1980). A few set a quantitative threshold (MATTHEWS, 1976). Ultrastructurally, these neoplasms, like the large cell carcinoma, are a blend of poorly differentiated squamous cell carcinoma and poorly differentiated adenocarcinoma (WANG et al., 1976; TATEISHI and HATTORI, 1982). The giant cell carcinoma often is a very aggressive neoplasm (WANG et al., 1976), although there are exceptions to this (CARTER and EGGLESTON, 1980).

The clear cell variant of large cell carcinoma is quite rare (MATTHEWS et al., 1983). Again many carcinomas possess a few cells with clear cytoplasm. To justify the title of clear cell carcinoma, a pulmonary tumor should consist predominantly of clear cells. Such neoplasms may closely resemble metastatic renal cell carcinoma to the lung, and the latter is much more common than primary clear cell carcinoma of the lung (CARTER and EGGLESTON, 1980). These tumors should also be kept distinct from benign clear cells tumors of the lung (so-called "sugar" tumors). At this point there is no evidence to suggest that the presence of a predominantly clear cell appearance has any effect on the outcome of a tumor, and clear cell carcinoma probably should not be regarded as a separate entity (KATZENSTEIN et al., 1980).

2.2.1.5 Adenosquamous Carcinoma. When a tumor possesses features of both squamous cell carcinoma and adenocarcinoma, it is designated as adenosquamous carcinoma (World Health Organization 1982). When strict light microscopic criteria are used, this combination is only 1–2% of pulmonary cancers (CARTER and EGGLESTON, 1980; MATTHEWS et al., 1983). As indicated above, careful study with the electron microscope turns up tumors with mixed adenosquamous features much more frequently (AUERBACH et al., 1982; McDOWELL et al., 1978; SABA et al., 1983). The behavior of these neoplasms is probably closest to that of adenocarcinoma (World Health Organization 1982). It is important to avoid confusing adenosquamous carcinoma with mucoepidermoid carcinoma (see 2.2.1.7).

2.2.1.6 Carcinoid Tumor. Carcinoid tumors have been mentioned briefly in connection with their more malignant relatives, small cell carcinoma. These two types are considered related, based on the current hypothesis of common origin in the bronchial Kultschitzky-type cell (see 2.2.1.2).

Carcinoid tumors are histologically bland neoplasms, consisting of very uniform cells growing in one or more of several characteristic patterns (CARTER and EGGLESTON, 1980; COONEY et al., 1979). Mitoses are usually absent, and there is little or no tumor necrosis. 90% are central neoplasms (SPENCER, 1977; CARTER and EGGLESTON, 1980), tending to grow both intrabronchially as an exophytic lesion, and outside the bronchial wall. The tumor often has a narrow waist where it passes between bronchial cartilage plates, leading to a characteristic dumbbell or collarbutton shape. These neoplasms are only slowly invasive, and metastases occur in only 2–5% of the cases (SPENCER, 1977). Series which have higher numbers with metastases probably include at least some atypical carcinoids (GOODWIN, 1975) (see below).

Although they are histogenetically related to each other, important epidemiologic differences exist between carcinoid tumors and small cell carcinoma:

1. Incidence: carcinoid tumors are much less common than small cell carcinoma, making up 1–2% of lung cancers (SPENCER, 1977; CARTER and EGGLESTON, 1980; CORRIN, 1980).
2. Sex ratio: carcinoid tumors do not show the marked male predominance found in small cell carcinoma (GOODWIN, 1975).
3. Age: the average age of patients with carcinoid tumors is lower (SPENCER, 1977).
4. Inhaled agents: carcinoid tumors appear unrelated to smoking or other known environmental agents (GOODWIN and BROWN, 1977).

These differences have no clear explanation. It is speculated that these two rather distinct neoplasms may represent two different responses of the same bronchial cell to two different carcinogenic stimuli (GOODWIN and BROWN, 1977). An alternate, but not mutually exclusive, hypothesis is that all pulmonary carcinomas can arise from an "indifferent" epithelial cells, the differentiation of which is controlled by the microenvironment. Possibly carcinoid tumors are genetically rather than carcinogenically induced (YESNER, 1983).

The gap between carcinoid tumors and small cell carcinomas is conveniently bridged by neoplasms known as atypical carcinoid tumors, or malignant carcinoid tumors (MILLS et al., 1982; ARRIGONI et al., 1972). Morphologically these are more pleomorphic than carcinoid tumors, with easily discernible mitotic figures, and with areas of necrosis. These neoplasms have a correspondingly intermediate biologic behavior between carcinoid tumors and small cell carcinomas. They have a much more clearcut relationship to smoking than carcinoid tumors, and have the male predominance of other smoking-related lung cancers.

2.2.1.7 Bronchial Gland Carcinomas.

These form a group of neoplasms bearing close resemblances to neoplasms of salivary gland origin (Carter and Eggleston, 1980; Spencer, 1979). They are uncommon, forming less than 1% of pulmonary neoplasms (Carter and Eggleston, 1980; Spencer, 1979). They occur in a very wide age spectrum. While most of them are not very aggressive, important exceptions to this do occur.

Adenoid cystic carcinoma is the most common of the bronchial gland neoplasms. Their growth pattern is infiltrative, with a tendency towards local recurrence. Metastases are rare.

Mucoepidermoid carcinomas are less common than adenoid cystic carcinoma. They are normally composed of admixtures of sheets of cells with little squamous differentiation and glandular elements with mucin production. Depending on the degree of cellular atypia and pleomorphism, these tumors are divided into low-grade and high-grade neoplasms. The latter are much less common than the former, and present some difficulty in histologic differentiation from adenosquamous carcinoma of the lung. The biologic behavior tends to correlate with the histologic appearance, but a case of a neoplasm with low-grade histologic findings and high-grade biologic behavior has recently been reported (Barsky et al., 1983).

Other varieties of salivary-gland-type tumors have been found, with lesser frequencies (Carter and Eggleston, 1980; Spencer, 1979). These include pleomorphic adenoma (formerly known as mixed tumor) and oncocytoma.

2.2.2 Soft Tissue Tumors

Primary mesenchymal tumors of the lung are uncommon, and malignant examples (sarcomas) are particularly rare, occurring in about 1 in 500 cases of pulmonary cancers (Spencer, 1977). The WHO has a separate classification for soft tissue neoplasms (Enzinger et al., 1969), and groups the pulmonary soft tissue tumors according to that scheme. In all categories of sarcoma, metastatic neoplasms from other sites to the lung are much more common than primary lesions in the lung.

Of primary pulmonary sarcomas, leiomyosarcoma and fibrosarcoma are the most common (Carter and Eggleston, 1980; Cameron, 1976; Nascimento et al., 1982). Occasional instances of other types, including liposarcoma, rhabdomyosarcoma, chondrosarcoma, osteogenic sarcoma and others are reported. These neoplasms tend to grow by expansion and local invasion, with relatively little tendency to metastasize (Spencer, 1977). The prognosis tends to relate best to size and involvement of local structures (Nascimento et al., 1982).

2.2.3 Mesothelial Tumors

Tumors of the mesothelial cells lining the pleural surfaces (mesotheliomas) are often included in discussion of pulmonary neoplasms. Once considered a very rare type of tumor, malignant mesotheliomas are becoming common enough that many pathologists have had experience with one or more cases (Suzuki, 1980). This presumably relates to the remarkable increase in use of asbestos during this century, in the manufacture of a bewildering variety of objects found throughout everyday Western life (Craighead and Mossman, 1983; Bhagavan and Koss, 1976). A particular increase in exposure occurred in the shipyard industry in World War II, and at least some of the cases now being seen relate to exposure at that time. The "latent period" between exposure to asbestos and development of malignant mesothelioma is quite variable (Suzuki, 1980; Craighead and Mossman, 1983), and in some series does not appear to be related to the amount or extent of exposure, so that this is unpredictable asbestos-related neoplasm (Craighead and Mossman, 1983; Churg, 1982; Roggli et al., 1982). There probably are cases of malignant mesothelioma in people with little or no previous asbestos experience (Becklake, 1983), but in Western society exposure is so nearly universal (Rosen et al., 1972; Churg and Warnock, 1981; Bhagavan and Koss, 1976; Craighead et al., 1982; Churg, 1982; Roggli et al., 1982) that this is difficult to establish.

These neoplasms tend to grow as coalescing masses along the pleural surfaces, and may encase the lung. They spread locally to involve the chest wall, the diaphragm and the pericardium. The histologic appearances vary from a strong resemblance to adenocarcinoma to a sarcomatous appearance, many examples having some combination of both. Ultrastructural studies reveal that the cells of each of these different-appearing neoplasms form a morphologic continuum (BOLEN and THORNING, 1980; KLIMA and BOSSART, 1983). Evidence is accumulating that differences in biologic behavior correlate with the different morphologic types. Sarcomatous mesotheliomas tend to behave like soft tissue sarcomas, and epithelial mesotheliomas resemble carcinomas in their growth and spread (LAW et al., 1982). Sarcomatous mesotheliomas tend to have shorter survival than epithelial examples (BRENNER et al., 1982; CANTIN et al., 1982; LAW et al., 1982).

Because the clinical and histological features of malignant mesothelioma overlap with those of other neoplasms, the diagnosis may be difficult to establish. In the past, in fact, this has been a diagnosis of exclusion, requiring a complete autopsy to rule out other possible primary sites. This has been particularly true when the patient's exposure to asbestos is thoroughly lost in the murky past of some decades ago. Currently available techniques, however, have allowed the specific diagnosis of mesothelioma on biopsy in some cases (ANTMAN, 1980; KWEE et al., 1982; SUZUKI, 1980). Histochemical studies and electron microscopy each may demonstrate features which can be helpful in making the diagnosis (CARTER and EGGLESTON, 1980; WARHOL et al., 1982; SUZUKI, 1980).

2.2.4   Other Tumors

2.2.4.1 Carcinosarcoma. These are rare lesions, with approximately 33 cases appearing in the literature (CARTER and EGGLESTON, 1980). They are defined by the presence of definitive malignant mesenchymal and epithelial components. Pathologists may have difficulty in differentiating these neoplasms from carcinomas with desmoplasia or with a spindle cell component, and from malignant mesothelioma.

Carcinosarcomas are more frequent in males than females (CARTER and EGGLESTON, 1980; DIACONITA, 1975; EDWARDS et al., 1979). They tend to be bulky neoplasms, and many of them present with polypoid intrabronchial growth (CARTER and EGGLESTON, 1980). They are often thought to be resectable, but five-year survival is no better than that in squamous cell carcinoma of the lung, and may be worse (EDWARDS et al., 1979). Some instances of long survival exist (EDWARDS et al., 1979).

Speculation concerning the origin of these neoplasms is common, and includes simultaneous or collision tumors, malignant change in a hematoma, malignant change in the stroma of a carcinoma, and origin in pluripotential mesenchymal cells (DIACONITA, 1975; EDWARDS et al., 1979).

2.2.4.2 Pulmonary Blastoma. These are malignant tumors of lung with histologic features reminiscent of the pseudoglandular phase of development of the embryonic lung, with a primitive cellular mesenchymal and gland-like spaces (CARTER and EGGLESTON, 1980). Either the mesenchymal or the epithelial elements may undergo some diffferentiation.

These neoplasms make up about 0.5% of primary lung tumors (JACOBSEN and FRANCIS, 1980). They occur over a wide age range, from children to the elderly, with male predominance. They are usually bulky tumors, peripheral in location. Their biologic behavior includes a broad range, with about half the tumors pursuing a benign course (GIBBONS et al., 1981; SCULLY, 1984). Some of the remainder behave in a highly malignant fashion (CARTER and EGGLESTON, 1980). Chemotherapy and radiotherapy are not effective in cases with metastases (GIBBONS et al., 1981).

SPENCER has suggested that pulmonary blastoma may be the pulmonary counterpart of nephroblastoma (SPENCER, 1977). The histologic features bear many resemblances. The distinction of blastoma from carcinosarcoma may also be very difficult, and some cases "transitional" between these two entities have been reported (EDWARDS et al., 1979; ROTH and ELGUEZABAL, 1978).

2.2.4.3 Malignant Melanoma. Rare instances of primary malignant melanoma in the bronchial tree have been reported. Satisfactory proof of primary origin in the lung is often difficult, given the well-known difficulty of locating, or excluding, primary origin in the skin and elsewhere. Generally accepted criteria include absence of a current or previous melanoma elsewhere, involvement of respiratory epithelium in a pattern indicating origin from that epithelium and absence of another primary lesion at autopsy, or long survival following resection of the pulmonary lesion (CARTER and EGGLESTON 1980).

2.2.4.4 Malignant Lymphoma. Malignant lymphomas make up 0.5% of malignancies arising in the lung (SPENCER, 1977). Involvement of the lung as the primary site is much less common than are pulmonary lesions forming part of more widespread disease (KOSS et al., 1983). Any of the spectrum of lymphomas may be seen in the lung, from relatively indolent lymphomas of small lymphocytic origin to the more aggressive large cell lymphomas. The latter, known as "histiocytic" lymphomas in the older Rappaport classification, are generally recognized as the most common of the extranodal lymphomas, particularly in the gastrointestinal tract. No such predominance has been reported in the lung. In the largest series to date, in fact, most of the primary lymphomas were of small lymphoid cells, with relatively low aggressiveness (KOSS et al., 1983). Hodgkin's disease arising in the lung is quite rare, but involvement of the lung by extension from the mediastinum, or as part of more widespread disease, is more common. Distinction of malignant lymphomas from nonmalignant and/or premalignant lymphoid proliferations, such as pseudolymphoma and lymphomatoid granulomatosis, may present considerable difficulty for the pathologist.

2.3 Current Trends

The most obvious trend in lung cancer is the continuing increase, referred to at the beginning of this chapter. As also mentioned above, much of this increase in lung cancer is due to the rapid rise in adenocarcinoma in women. This appears to be at least in part a direct legacy of the marked increase in cigarette consumption by women in the US in the last three decades, an association not mentioned in catchy cigarette advertisements currying favor with trendy youth. The increase in adenocarcinoma is also seen, to a lesser extent, in males, such that even in some Veterans Administration series this type has replaced squamous cell carcinoma as the most common type of lung cancer (COX and YESNER, 1979; VALAITIS et al., 1981; VINCENT et al., 1977). Changes in the criteria for separating the types are another factor in the increase in adenocarcinoma (VINCENT et al., 1977). New and increasing occupational and environmental exposures, aside from smoking, may also be making a contribution (VINCENT et al., 1977). Note must be taken of the rising incidence of lung cancer among nonsmokers (ENSTROM, 1979).

Some variations in incidence of the different types of lung cancer are to be expected, in view of inconsistencies among pathologists in criteria for separating the groups (see 3.1). Part of this difficulty arises from the incompleteness of our understanding of the different pulmonary epithelial cell types, their interrelationships and normal development. More of such knowledge will allow improvements in our classification schemes. Nevertheless it would be optimistic to expect that we can ever devise a set of rules which will predict nature accurately and completely. Neoplasms of the lung, as elsewhere, present a multidimensional continuum, and our efforts to separate out entities from the continuum will always be somewhat arbitrary (HUNTINGTON and HUNTINGTON, 1977; AUERBACH et al., 1982).

The range of survival times in lung cancer remains quite wide, and criteria for predicting prognosis remain very desirable. While the histologic type of the tumor is of value in such prediction, the relationship of disease and host is also important. The extent of the neoplasm (tumor size and stage) and the status of the host (weight loss, Karnofsky performance status) are also factors relating to the eventual outcome (LANZOTTI et al., 1977; STANLEY, 1980).

The overall picture in lung cancer remains grim. 4% of patients survived five years in a prospective study of unselected patients (HUHTI et al., 1981). Obviously any improvement is desirable. A negative side effect of such improvement in survival time will be some increase in the opportunity for development of second primary neoplasms. While some such second primaries occur synchronously with the first, most occur later (MARTINI and MELAMED, 1975; SMITH et al., 1976). Development of a second primary is not yet common, occurring in 0.97% of the patients treated for lung cancer at Memorial from 1955 to 1974 (MARTINI and MELAMED, 1975). It is confined largely to the group of heavy smokers (SMITH et al., 1976), and most of the neoplasms are squamous cell carcinomas (MARTINI and MELAMED, 1975).

3 Diagnosis

3.1 Reproducibility

The principal technique employed in the diagnosis of pulmonary neoplasms remains the biopsy. In view of the problems with and limitations of the light microscopic classification of these neoplasms, an estimate of the reproducibility of this technique is important. Several studies have examined this, from various points of view. In a careful study of interobserver variation (STANLEY and MATTHEWS, 1981), three pathologists of the Working

Party for the Therapy of Lung Cancer found unanimous agreement among themselves in 67% of 476 cases. In 94% of the cases, two of the three pathologists agreed. Not surprisingly, the neoplasms with the most distinctive features (well differentiated neoplasms and small cell carcinoma) were the subject of greatest agreement, while the poorly differentiated carcinomas were the most difficult. Acceptance of the histologic diagnosis rendered by the pathologist at the primary hospital is fraught with some risk. Central review of such material disclosed a 20% disagreement rate in Toronto (JACQUES et al., 1980) and a 13% disagreement rate in Louisiana (ROTHSCHILD et al., 1982).

Of various biopsy sites and routes, rigid bronchoscopy probably provides the least reliable results (LYALL et al., 1980). Needle biopsy of a lung mass may be quite successful (POE and TOBIN, 1980), and, when applicable, lymph node biopsy often provides the best histologic material.

3.2 Cytology

New techniques and better understanding have allowed cytopathologists to assume a greater role in the diagnosis of lung cancer. The assessment of cells obtained from sputum, bronchial washing, bronchial brushing or needle aspiration necessarily has limitations, but in certain circumstances cytology has proven more accurate than biopsy (JOHNSTON and BOSSEN, 1981; YESNER, 1983). This is most often true in the poorly differentiated carcinomas. Cytologic specimens may allow identification of features of differentiation which are obscure in light microscopic study of paraffin sections, but discernible in the electron microscope. In well differentiated neoplasms, cytology may be accurate in up to 100% of the cases (HESS et al., 1981c; KANHOUWA and MATTHEWS, 1976; EVANS and SHELLEY, 1982), and overall accuracy is of the order of 80% or better (PAYNE et al., 1979; HESS et al., 1981c; JAY et al., 1980; LYALL et al., 1980; MATTHEWS et al., 1983). The different techniques of obtaining cytologic specimens have differing sensitivity and specificity, with considerable variation from one series to another (PAYNE et al., 1979; JAY et al., 1980).

3.3 Electron Microscopy

At our present level of understanding, the last word in classification of lung tumors is spoken by the electron microscopist. Ultrastructural studies have contributed notably to our understanding of both normal pulmonary epithelium and neoplasms thereof, and will continue to be very important. Nevertheless, for the forseeable future, electron microscopy will not be available to contribute to the diagnosis of many pulmonary neoplasms, and it remains important to try to refine histologic and cytologic criteria as carefully as possible, so as to allow the practical to move closer to the ideal.

4 Tumor Markers

For a number of years enthuasiasm has waxed for identifying any compound which might be specific for cancer cells in general, or for specific types of cancer in particular. Identification and quantification of such a compound would facilitate diagnosis and treatment of neoplasms. By and large, these hopes have not been completely fulfilled (WOLFE, 1978), although in some circumstances certain substances have been found useful as tumor markers. The search has focussed on antigens associated with neoplasms, on hormones produced by neoplasms, and on certain enzymes. While a diagnostic marker has not yet been found, some tumor products can be used to measure response to treatment (SORENSON et al., 1984; HERBERMAN, 1982).

4.1 Tumor-associated Antigens

No antigen which is truly specific for cancer or any form of cancer has yet been identified (SERROU et al., 1982). As neoplasms develop, they sometimes produce substances associated with fetal growth and differentiation. Prominent among these is carcinoembryonic antigen, considered the prototypic tumor-associated antigen (SORENSON et al., 1984).

Carcinoembryonic antigen may be elevated in 38–80% of patients with any type of pulmonary cancer, and can be increased in various non-neoplastic pulmonary diseases (FORD et al., 1977; PASCAL et al., 1977; VINCENT et al., 1975; MCINTIRE, 1982; GOSLIN et al., 1983). The greatest usefulness lies in monitoring patients following treatment. Persisting elevated values, or the reappearance of elevated values, indicate a poor prognosis.

4.2 Hormones

As discussed above, small cell carcinoma is the type of lung cancer most commonly associated with hormone production. Every cell line derived from small cell carcinoma and evaluated produces at least one hormone, and some produce many (Sorenson et al., 1981). This has led to searches for evidence of in vivo production. Of the hormones evaluated as markers of small cell carcinoma, ACTH, antidiuretic hormone and calcitonin have received the most attention (Sorenson et al., 1984; Ratcliffe, 1982; Hansen et al., 1980a; Wallach et al., 1981). The results of these studies are variable, but do suggest a role for calcitonin in monitoring patients with extensive disease (Ratcliffe, 1982; Wallach et al., 1981). Human neurophysins have been found elevated in 62% of patients with small cell carcinoma (North et al., 1979; North et al., 1980; Maurer et al., 1983). The most recent results indicate no correlation between secretory status of the patient and response to therapy or survival (Maurer et al., 1983).

Hormone production is not confined to small cell carcinoma. In one series, one or more of seven hormones were elevated in 65% of 110 patients with various lung cancers (Gropp et al., 1980). Frequently the elevated level is of a substance immunoreactively similar to a given polypeptide hormone, but with no evidence of clinical hormonal activity. Perhaps the best known such example is ACTH. The "big" form of this hormone is found in elevated quantities in a high proportion of patients with lung cancer of all types (Ayvazian et al., 1975; Bondy, 1981; Gropp et al., 1980; Gewirtz and Yalow, 1974; Hansen et al., 1980b). Clinical evidence of Cushing's disease is not common in any of the non-small cell lung tumors, and is only somewhat more frequently seen in small cell carcinoma (Bondy, 1981; Sorenson et al., 1984; Bondy and Gilby, 1982; Lokich, 1982; Richardson et al., 1978). Unfortunately for its usefulness as a tumor marker, elevated immunoreactive ACTH is also found frequently nonmalignant pulmonary disease (Ayvazian et al., 1975).

Human chorionic gonadotrophin has been evaluated, and is present in the serum in elevated quantities in 4–21% of patients with lung cancer (Broder, 1979; Wilson et al., 1981). Immunohistochemical studies of tumor tissue indicate its presence in most if not all pulmonary tumors (Wilson et al., 1981). It is not clear whether the hormone identified in the tissue is produced but not secreted into the blood, or whether it is secreted in a form which might have a very short half-life. The fact that the hormone is found in the neoplasm with such high frequency has led some to hope that it will be useful as marker. The evidence is not yet in.

Several other hormones have been examined as tumor markers (Bondy, 1981; Gropp et al., 1980; Broder, 1979; Hansen et al., 1980b), but so far none has held much promise. One of the difficulties inherent in this approach is the heterogeneity of individual neoplasms. Hormone production seems to vary from cell to cell in a neoplasm, some having no evidence of such activity, and others producing more than one (Wolfe, 1978; Ruckdeschel et al., 1979; Baylin and Gazcar, 1981). Tumor cells may lose some markers and gain others over time (Wolfe, 1978).

4.3 Enzymes

Of the enzymes which have been considered as markers of pulmonary neoplasms, creatine kinase and neuron-specific enolase seem to have some potential.

The BB iso-enzyme of creatine kinase is present in the serum of 40% of patients with small cell carcinoma of the lung, extensive state (Gazdar et al., 1981b). It is also found in high concentrations in the neoplasms themselves, and in cultures derived from them. In those patients in whom it is present in abnormal levels in the serum, it can be used to monitor response to therapy, and later relapse (Wolfe, 1978).

Neuron-specific enolase is also increased in one study of patients with small cell carcinoma (Carney et al., 1982). Elevated levels are present in 39% of those with limited disease, and 87% of those with extensive disease, and the levels in patients with extensive disease are higher than those with limited disease. In this study, correlation between serum neuron-specific enolase levels and the clinical course was "excellent".

4.4 Other Markers

Modified ribonucleosides, principally the result of metabolism of transfer ribonucleic acid, are secreted in abnormal quantities in the urine of patients with malignant neoplasms. In a study of 29 patients with small cell carcinoma of the lung, five degradation products of transfer ribonucleic acid were analyzed (WAALKES et al., 1982). These products were elevated in the patients more frequently than serum carcinoembryonic antigen. There was 75% agreement between the clinical assessment of response and the urinary ribonucleosides.

Ferritin levels have also been found to be elevated in 65% of 54 patients with lung cancer of various types (URUSHIZAKI and NIITSU, 1982). While the levels did not correlate with the stage of the neoplasm, they did correlate with response to treatment and with recurrence.

4.5 Summary of Marker Studies

Ideal characteristics of tumor markers have been summarized (RICHARDSON et al., 1978). They include production of the marker only by tumor cells; a concentration in the blood or urine reflecting the extent of disease; convenient, inexpensive and accurate assay techniques; and a high frequency of positivity. No marker of lung cancer has yet come close to filling all of these goals. Nevertheless some of the substances assayed can provide useful information in some circumstances, particularly when combined with other available data.

References

Abeloff MD, Eggleston JC (1981) Morphologic changes following therapy. In: Greco FA, Oldham RK, Bunn PA (eds) Small cell lung cancer. Grune and Stratton, New York, pp 235–259.

Abeloff MD, Eggleston JC, Mendelsohn G, et al (1979) Changes in morphologic and biochemical characteristics of small cell carcinoma of the lung, Am J Med 66:757–764.

Antman KH (1980) Current Concepts. Malignant mesothelioma, N Engl J Med 303:200–202.

Arrigoni MG, Woolner LB, Bernatz PE (1972) Atypical carcinoid tumors of the lung, J Thorac Cardiovasc Surg 64:413–421.

Ashor GL, Kern WH, Meyer BW, Lindesmith GG, et al (1975) Long-term survival in bronchogenic carcinoma, J Thorac Cardiovasc Surg 70:581–589.

Auerbach O, Frasca JM, Parks VR, et al (1982) A comparison of world health organization (WHO) classification of lung tumors by light and electron microscopy, Cancer 50:2079–2088.

Auerbach O, Garfinkel L, Parks VR (1979) Scar cancer of the lung. Increase over a 21 year period, Cancer 43:636–642.

Ayvazian LF, Schneider B, Gewirtz G, et al (1975) Ectopic production of big ACTH in carcinoma of the lung, Am Rev Respir Dis 111:279–287.

Azar HA, Espinoza CG, Richman AV, Saba SR, et al (1982) "Undifferentiated" large cell malignancies: an ultra-

structural and immunocytochemical study, Hum Pathol 13:323–333.

Barsky SH, Martin SE, Matthews M, et al (1983) "Low grade" mucoepidermoid carcinoma of the bronchus with "high grade" biologic behavior, Cancer 51:1505–1509.

Baylin SB, Gazdar AF (1981) Endocrine biochemistry in the spectrum of human lung cancer: implications for the cellular origin of small cell carcinoma. In: Greco FA, Oldham RK, Bunn PA (eds) Small cell lung cancer. Grune and Stratton, New York, pp 123–143.

Baylin SB, Weisburger WR, Eggleston JC, et al (1978) Variable content of histaminase, L-DOPA decarboxylase and calcitonin in small-cell carcinoma of the lung, N Engl J Med 299:105–110.

Becklake MR (1982) Exposure to asbestos and human disease, N Engl J Med 306:1480–1482.

Bedrossian CWM, Weilbaecher DG, Bentinck DC, et al (1975) Ultrastructure of human bronchiolo-alveolar cell carcinoma, Cancer 36:1399–1413.

Bensch KG, Corrin B, Pariente R, et al (1968) Oat-cell carcinoma of the lung. Its origin and relationship to bronchial carcinoid, Cancer 22:1163–1172.

Bhagavan BS, Koss LG (1976) Secular trends in prevalence and concentration of pulmonary asbestos bodies – 1940 to 1972, Arch Pathol Lab Med 100:539–541.

van Bogaert L-J (1982) The diffuse endocrine system and derived tumours: histological and histochemical characteristics, Acta Histochem 70:122–129.

Bolen JW, Thorning D (1980) Mesotheliomas. A light- and electron-microscopic study concerning histogenetic relationships between the epithelial and the mesenchymal variants, Am J Surg Pathol 4:451–464.

Bondy PK (1981) The pattern of ectopic hormone production in lung cancer, Yale J Biol Med 54:181–185.

Bondy PK, Gilby ED (1982) Endocrine function in small cell undifferentiated carcinoma of the lung, Cancer 50:2147–2153.

Bonikos DS, Hendrickson M, Bensch KG (1977) Pulmonary alveolar cell carcinoma. Fine structures and in vitro study of a case and critical review of this entity, Am J Surg Pathol 1:93–108.

Brenner J, Sordillo PP, Magill GB, et al (1982) Malignant mesothelioma of the pleura. Review of 123 patients, Cancer 49:2431–2435.

Brereton HD, Mathews MM, Costa J, et al (1978) Mixed anaplastic small-cell and squamous-cell carcinoma of the lung, Ann Intern Med 88:805–806.

Brigham BA, Bunn PA Jr, Minna JD, et al (1978) Growth rates of small cell bronchogenic carcinomas, Cancer 42:2880–2886.

Broder LE (1979) Hormone production by bronchogenic carcinoma: a review. In: Ioachim HL (ed) Pathobiology Annual, Vol 9, Raven, New York, pp 205–224.

Bunn PA Jr, Lichter AS, Glatstein E, et al (1981) Results of recent studies in small cell bronchogenic carcinoma and prospects for future studies. In: Greco FA, Oldham RK, Bunn PA (eds) Small cell lung cancer. Grune and Stratton, New York, pp 413–446.

Burdon JGW, Sinclair RA, Henderson MM (1979) Small cell carcinoma of the lung. Prognosis in relation to histologic subtype, Chest 76:302–304.

Cameron EWJ (1975) Primary sarcoma of the lung, Thorax 30:516–520.

Cantin R, Al-Jabi M, McCaughey WTE (1982) Desmoplastic diffuse mesothelioma, Am J Surg Pathol 6:215–222.

Carney DN, Ihde DC, Cohen MH, et al (1982) Serum neuron-specific enolase: a marker for disease extent and
response to therapy of small-cell lung cancer, Lancet
I:583–585.

Carney DN, Matthews MJ, Ihde DC, et al (1980) Influence
of histologic subtype of small cell carcinoma of the lung
on clinical presentation, response to therapy, and survival, JNCI 65:1225–1230.

Carr DT (1981) Malignant lung disease, Hosp Pract
16(1):97–116.

Carter D (1978) Pathology of early squamous cell carcinoma of the lung. In: Sommers SC, Rosen PP (eds) Pathology Annual, Appleton-Century-Crofts, New York,
Vol 13, Part I, pp 131–147.

Carter, D (1983) Small-cell carcinoma of the lung, Am J
Surg Pathol 7:787–795.

Carter D, Eggleston JC (1980) Tumors of the lower respiratory tract. Fascicle 17, Atlas of tumor pathology, Armed
Forces Institute of Pathology, Washington, D.C.

Carter D, Marsh BR, Baker RR, et al (1976) Relationships
of morphology to clinical presentation in ten cases of
early squamous cell carcinoma of the lung, Cancer
37:1389–1396.

Churg A (1978) The fine structure of large cell undifferentiated carcinoma of the lung. Evidence for its relation
to squamous cell carcinomas and adenocarcinomas,
Hum Pathol 9:143–156.

Churg A (1982) Fiber counting and analysis in the diagnosis
of asbestos-related disease, Hum Pathol 13:381–392.

Churg A, Johnston WH, Stulbarg M (1980) Small cell
squamous and mixed small cell squamous-small cell
anaplastic carcinomas of the lung, Am J Surg Pathol
4:255–263.

Churg AM, Warnock ML (1981) Asbestos and other ferruginous bodies. Their formation and clinical significance,
Am J Pathol 102:447–456.

Cohen MH, Matthews MJ (1978) Small cell bronchogenic
carcinoma: a distinct clinicopathologic entity, Semin
Oncol 5:234–243.

Cooney T, Sweeny EC, Luke D (1979) Pulmonary carcinoid
tumours: a comparative regional study, J Clin Pathol
32:1100–1109.

Corrin B (1980) Lung endocrine tumours, Invest Cell Pathol
3:195–206.

Cox JD, Yesner RA (1979) Adenocarcinoma of the lung:
recent results from the Veterans Administration Lung
Group, Am Rev Respir Dis 120:1025–1029.

Craighead JE, Abraham JL, Churg A, et al (1982) The pathology of asbestos-associated diseases of the lungs and
pleural cavities: diagnostic criteria and proposed grading
shema, Arch Pathol Lab Med 106:544–596.

Craighead JE, Mossman BT (1982) The pathogenesis of
asbestos-associated diseases, N Engl J Med
306:1446–1455.

Currier J, Faulkner CS (1983) unpublished data.

Davis S, Sobel H (1981) Histologic subtypes of small cell
carcinoma of the lung: response to therapy, Eur J Cancer 17:351–354.

Davis S, Stanley KE, Yesner R, et al (1981) Small-cell carcinoma of the lung – survival according to histologic subtype: a Veterans Administration Lung Group Study,
Cancer 47:1863–1866.

Diaconita G (1975) Bronchopulmonary carcinosarcoma,
Thorax 30:682–686.

Dombernowsky P, Hirsch F, Hansen HH, et al (1978) Peritoneoscopy in the staging of 190 patients with small-cell

anaplastic carcinoma of the lung with special reference
to subtyping, Cancer 41:2008–2012.

Doyle TJ (1982) Brain metastasis in the natural history of
small-cell lung cancer, Cancer 50:752–754.

Edwards CW, Saunders AM, Collins F (1979) Mixed malignant tumour of the lung, Thorax 34:629–636.

Enstrom JE (1979) Rising lung cancer mortality among non-
smokers. JNCI 62:755–760.

Enzinger FM, Lattes R, Torloni H (1969) Histological typing of soft tissue tumours. World Health Organization,
Geneva.

Evans DMD, Shelley G (1982) Respiratory cytodiagnosis:
study in observer variation and its relation to quality
of material, Thorax 37:259–263.

Ewing SL, Sumner HW, Ophoven JJ, et al (1980) Small
cell anaplastic carcinoma with differentiation: a report
of 14 cases, Lab Invest 42:115.

Ford CHJ, Newman CE, Lakin J (1977) Role of carcinoembryonic antigen in bronchial carcinoma, Thorax
32:582–588.

Gazdar AF, Carney DN, Guccion JC, et al (1981a) Small
cell carcinoma of the lung: cellular origin and relationship to other pulmonary tumors. In: Greco FA, Oldham
RK, Bunn PA (eds) Small cell lung cancer. Grune and
Stratton, New York, pp 145–175.

Gazdar AF, Carney DN, Minna JD (1981b) In vitro study
of the biology of small cell carcinoma of the lung, Yale
J Biol Med 54:187–193.

Gazdar AF, Carney DN, Minna JD (1983) The biology
of non-small cell lung cancer, Semin Oncol 10:3–19.

Gewirtz G, Yalow RS (1974) Ectopic ACTH production
in carcinoma of the lung, J Clin Invest 53:1022–1032.

Gibbons JRP, McKeown F, Field TW (1981) Pulmonary
blastoma with hilar lymph node metastases: survival for
24 years, Cancer 47:152–155.

Godwin JD II (1975) Carcinoid tumors. An analysis of 2837
cases, Cancer 36:560–569.

Godwin JD II Brown CC (1977) Comparative epidemiology
of carcinoid and oat-cell tumors of the lung, Cancer
40:1671–1673.

Goslin RH, O'Brien MJ, Skarin AT, et al (1983) Immunocytochemical staining for CEA in small cell carcinoma of
lung predicts clinical usefulness of the plasma assay,
Cancer 52:301–306.

Gould VE, Linnoila RI, Memoli VA, et al (1983) Neuroendocrine cells and neuroendocrine neoplasms of the lung.
In: Somers SC, Rosen PP (eds) Pathology Annual, Vol
18, Part I, Appleton-Century-Crofts, Norwalk, pp 287–
330.

Gould VE, Memoli VA, Dardi LE, et al (1981) Neuroendocrine carcinomas with multiple immunoreactive peptides
and melanin production, Ultrastruct Pathol 2:199–217.

Gray RE, O'Neal RM (1980) Multiple pulmonary scar carcinomas in a patient with Hodgkin's disease. Report of
a case and review of the literature, Cancer
46:1868–1872.

Greco FA, Hainsworth J, Sismani A, et al (1981) Hormone
production and paraneoplastic syndromes. In: Greco
FA, Oldham RK, Bunn PA (eds) Small cell lung cancer.
Grune and Stratton, New York, 177–223.

Greco FA, Oldham RK (1979) Current concepts in cancer.
Small-cell lung cancer, N Engl J Med 301:355–358.

Greenberg SD, Smith MN, Spjut HJ (1975) Bronchiolo-
alveolar carcinoma – cell of origin, Am J Clin Pathol
63:153–167.

Gropp C, Havemann K, Scheuer A (1980) Ectopic hormones in lung cancer patients at diagnosis and during therapy, Cancer 46:347–354.

Hainau B, Dombernowsky P, Hansen HH, et al (1977) Cell proliferation and histologic classification of bronchogenic carcinoma, JNCI 59:1113–1118.

Hansen M, Hammer M, Hummer L (1980a) ACTH, ADH and calcitonin concentration as markers of response and relapse in small-cell carcinoma of the lung, Cancer 46:2062–2067.

Hansen M, Hansen HH, Hirsch FR, et al (1980b) Hormonal polypeptides and amine metabolites in small cell carcinoma of the lung, with special reference to stage and subtypes, Cancer 45:1432–1437.

Hashimoto T, Fukuoka M, Nagasawa S, et al (1979) Small cell carcinoma of the lung and its histological origin. Report of a case, Am J Surg Pathol 3:343–351.

Hayabuchi N, Russell WJ, Murakami J (1983) Slow-growing lung cancer in a fixed population sample, radiologic assessment, Cancer 52:1098–1104.

van Hazel GA, Scott M, Eagan RT (1983) The effect of CNS metastases on the survival of patients with small cell carcinoma of the lung, Cancer 51:933–937.

Herberman RB (1982) Tumor markers related to lung cancer: a discussion. In: Colnaghi MI, Buraggi GL, Ghione M (eds) Markers for diagnosis and monitoring of human cancer. Proceedings of the Serono Symposia, Academic Press, New York, Vol 46, pp 123–127.

Hess FG Jr, McDowell EM, Resau JH, et al (1981a) The respiratory epithelium. IX. Validity and reproducibility of revised cytologic criteria for human and hamster respiratory tract tumors, Acta Cytol 25:485–498.

Hess FG Jr, McDowell EM, Trump BF (1981b) The respiratory epithelium. VIII. Interpretation of cytologic criteria for human and hamster respiratory tract tumors, Acta Cytol 25:111–134.

Hess FG Jr, McDowell EM, Trump BF (1981c) Pulmonary cytology. Current status of cytologic typing of respiratory tract tumors, Am J Pathol 103:321–333.

Hirsch FR, Hansen HH (1980) Bone marrow involvement in small cell anaplastic carcinoma of the lung, Cancer 46:206–211.

Hirsch F, Hansen HH, Dombernowsky P, et al (1977) Bone marrow examination in the staging of small-cell anaplastic carcinoma of the lung with special reference to subtyping. An evaluation of 203 consecutive patients, Cancer 39:2563–2567.

Hirsch FR, Matthews MJ, Yesner R (1982a) Histopathologic classification of small cell carcinoma of the lung. Comments based on an interobserver examination, Cancer 50:1360–1366.

Hirsch FR, Osterlind K, Hansen HH (1983) The prognostic significance of histopathologic subtyping of small cell carcinoma of the lung according to the classification of the World Health Organization. A study of 375 consecutive patients, Cancer 52:2144–2150.

Hirsch FR, Paulson OB, Hansen HH, et al (1982b) Intracranial metastases in small cell carcinoma of the lung. Correlation of clinical and autopsy findings, Cancer 50:2433–2437.

Horie A, Ohta M (1981) Ultrastructural features of large cell carcinoma of the lung with reference to the prognosis of patients, Hum Pathol 12:423–432.

Huhti E, Sutinen S, Saloheimo M (1981) Survival among patients with lung cancer. An epidemiologic study, Am Rev Respir Dis 124:13–16.

Huntington RW, Huntington RW III (1977) Classification

of neoplasms: a critical appraisal, Perspect Biol Med 20:215–222.

Ioachim HL (1978) Present trends in lung cancer. In: Thurlbeck WM, Abell MR (eds) The lung: structure, function and disease. Williams and Wilkins, Baltimore, pp 192–214.

Jacobsen M, Francis D (1980) Pulmonary blastoma. A clinico-pathological study of eleven cases, Acta Path Microbiol Scand Sect A 88:151–160.

Jacques J, Hill DP, Shier KJ, et al (1980) Appraisal of the World Health Organization classification of lung tumours, Can Med Assoc J 122:897–901.

Jay SJ, Wehr K, Nicholson DP, et al (1980) Diagnostic sensitivity and specificity of pulmonary cytology. Comparison of techniques used in conjunction with flexible fiber optic bronchoscopy, Acta Cytol 24:304–312.

Johnston WW, Bossen EH (1981) Ten years of respiratory cytopathology at Duke University Medical Center. II. The cytopathologic diagnosis of lung cancer during the years 1970 to 1974, with a comparison between cytopathology and histopathology in the typing of lung cancer, Acta Cytol 25:499–505.

Kameya T, Kodama T, Shimosato Y (1982) Ultrastructure of small-cell carcinoma of the lung (oat and intermediate cell types) in relation to histogenesis and to carcinoid tumor. In: Shimosato Y, Melamed MR, Nettesheim P (eds) Morphogenesis of lung cancer. Vol II CRC Press, Boca Raton, pp 15–43.

Kanhouwa SB, Matthews JM (1976) Reliability of cytologic typing of lung cancer, Acta Cytol 20:229–232.

Katzenstein A-LA, Prioleau PG, Askin FB (1980) The histologic spectrum and significance of clear-cell change in lung carcinoma, Cancer 45:943–947.

Kimula Y (1978) A histochemical and ultrastructural study of adenocarcinoma of the lung, Am J Surg Pathol 2:253–264.

Klima M, Bossart MI (1983) Sarcomatous type of malignant mesothelioma, Ultrastruct Pathol 4:349–358.

Koss MN, Hochholzer L, Nichols PW, Wehunt WD, Lazarus AA (1983) Primary non-Hodgkin's lymphoma and pseudolymphoma of lung, Hum Pathol 14:1024–1038.

Kreyberg L (1967) Histological typing of lung tumours, World Health Organization, Geneva.

Kwee W-S, Veldhuizen RW, Alons CA, et al (1982) Quantitative and qualitative differences between benign and malignant mesothelial cells in pleural fluid, Acta Cytol 26:401–406.

Lanzotti VJ, Thomas DR, Boyle LE, et al (1977) Survival with inoperable lung cancer: an integration of prognostic variables based on simple criteria, Cancer 39:303–313.

Larsson S, Zettergren L (1976) Histological typing of lung cancer. Application of the World Health Organization classification to 479 cases, Acta Pathol Microbiol Scand Sect A 84:529–537.

Law MR, Hodson ME, Heard BE (1982) Malignant mesothelioma of the pleura: relation between histological type and clinical behavior, Thorax 37:810–815.

Lenhard RE Jr, Woo KB, Freund JS, et al (1981) Growth kinetics of small cell carcinoma of the lung, Eur J Cancer Clin Oncol 17:899–904.

Lieber M, Smith B, Szakal A, et al (1976) A continuous tumor-cell line from a human lung carcinoma with properties of type II alveolar epithelial cells, Int J Cancer 17:62–70.

Liebow AA (1952) Tumors of the lower respiratory tract. Armed Forces Institute of Pathology, Washington, Fascicle 17.

Livingston RB (1980) Small cell carcinoma of the lung, Blood 56:575–584.

Lokich JJ (1982) The frequency and clinical biology of the ectopic hormone syndromes of small cell carcinoma, Cancer 50:2111–2114.

Lyall JRW, Summers GD, O'Brien IM, et al (1980) Sequential brush biopsy and conventional biopsy: direct comparison of diagnostic sensitivity in lung malignancy, Thorax 35:929–931.

Martini N, Melamed MR (1975) Multiple primary lung cancers, J Thorac Cardiovasc Surg 70:606–612.

Matthews MJ (1973) Panel Report: morphologic classification of bronchogenic carcinoma, Cancer Chemother Rep, Part 3, 4:299–301.

Matthews MJ (1974) Morphology of lung cancer, Semin Oncol 1:175–182.

Matthews MJ (1976) Problems in morphology and behavior of bronchopulmonary malignant disease. In: Israel L, Chahinian AP (eds) Lung cancer, Natural history, prognosis and therapy. Academic Press, New York, pp 23–62.

Matthews MJ, Gazdar AF (1982) Small-cell carcinoma of the lung – its morphology, behavior and nature. In: Shimosato Y, Melamed MR, Nettesheim P (eds) Morphogenesis of lung cancer. Vol II, CRC Press, Boca Raton, pp 1–14.

Matthews MJ, Hirsch FR (1981) Problems in the diagnosis of small cell carcinoma of the lung. In: Greco FA, Oldham RK, Bunn PA (eds) Small cell lung cancer. Grune and Stratton, New York, 35–50.

Matthews MJ, Mackay B, Lukeman J (1983) The pathology of non-small cell carcinoma of the lung, Semin Oncol 10:34–55.

Matthews MJ, Rozencweig M, Staquet MJ, et al (1980) Long-term survivors with small cell carcinoma of the lung, Eur J Cancer 16:527–531.

Maurer LH, O'Donnell JF, Kennedy S, et al (1983) Human neurophysins in carcinoma of the lung: relation to histology, disease stage, response rate, survival, and syndrome of inappropriate antidiuretic hormone secretion, Cancer Treat Rep 67:971–976.

McDowell EM, Barrett LA, Glavin F, et al (1978a) The respiratory epithelium. I. Human bronchus, JNCI 61:539–549.

McDowell EM, Barrett LA, Trump BF (1976) Observations on small granule cells in adult human bronchial epithelium and in carcinoid and oat cell tumors, Lab Invest 34:202–206.

McDowell EM, McLaughlin JS, Merenyi DK, et al (1978b) The respiratory epithelium. V. Histogenesis of lung carcinomas in the human, JNCI 61:587–606.

McDowell EM, Trump BF (1981) Pulmonary small cell carcinoma showing tripartite differentiation in individual cells, Hum Pathol 12:286–294.

McDowell EM, Wilson TS, Trump BF (1981) Atypical endocrine tumors of the lung, Arch Pathol Lab Med 105:20–28.

McIntire KR (1982) Non-hormone markers of human lung cancer. In: Colnaghi MI, Buraggi GL, Ghione M (eds) Markers for diagnosis and monitoring of human cancer. Proceedings of the Serono Symposia. Academic Press, New York, Vol 46:95–109.

Melamed MR, Zaman MB (1982) Pathogenesis of epidermoid carcinoma of lung. In: Shimosato Y, Melamed MR, Nettesheim P (eds) Morphogenesis of lung cancer, Vol I, CRC Press, Boca Raton, pp 37–64.

Mills SE, Cooper PH, Walker AN, et al (1982) Atypical carcinoid tumor of the lung. A clinicopathologic study of 17 cases, Am J Surg Pathol 6:643–654.

Mitchell DM, Morgan PGM, Ball JB (1980) Prognostic features of large cell anaplastic carcinoma of the bronchus, Thorax 35:118–122.

Miyamoto H, Inoue S, Abe S, et al (1982) Relationship between cytomorphologic features and prognosis in small-cell carcinoma of the lung, Acta Cytol 26:429–433.

Nascimento AG, Unni KK, Bernatz PE (1982) Sarcomas of the lung, Mayo Clin Proc 57:355–359.

Nash G (1983) The diagnosis of lung cancer in the 80 s: will routine light microscopy suffice?, Hum Pathol 14:1021–1023.

Nixon DW, Murphy GF, Sewell CW, et al (1979) Relationship between survival and histologic type in small cell anaplastic carcinoma of the lung, Cancer 44:1045–1049.

North WG, Maurer LH, O'Donnell JF (1979) Human neurophysins (HNPs) and small cell carcinoma (SCC), Clin Res 27:390A.

North WG, Maurer LH, Valtin H, et al (1980) Human neurophysins as potential tumor markers for small cell carcinoma of the lung: application of specific radioimmunoassays, J Clin Endocrinol Metab 51:892–896.

Nugent JL, Bunn PA Jr, Matthews MJ, et al (1979) CNS metastases in small cell bronchogenic carcinoma. Increasing frequency and changing pattern with lengthening survival, Cancer 44:1885–1893.

Ohara H, Okamoto T (1977) A new in vitro cell line established from human oat cell carcinoma of the lung, Cancer Res 37:3088–3095.

Pascal RR, Mesa-Tejada R, Bennett SJ, et al (1977) Carcinoembryonic antigen. Immunohistologic identification in invasive and intraepithelial carcinomas of the lung, Arch Pathol Lab Med 101:568–571.

Payne CR, Stovin PGI, Barker V, et al (1979) Diagnostic accuracy of cytology and biopsy in primary bronchial carcinoma, Thorax 34:294–299.

Pearse AGE (1966) Common cytochemical properties of cells producing polypeptide hormones, with particular reference to calcitonin and the thyroid C cells, Vet Rec 79:587–590.

Pearse AGE (1969) The cytochemistry and ultrastructure of polypeptide hormone-producing cells of the APUD series and the embryologic, physiological and pathologic implications of the concept, J Histochem Cytochem 17:303–313.

Pearse AGE (1977) The diffuse neuroendocrine system and the APUD concept: related "endocrine" peptides in brain, intestine, pituitary, placenta, and anuran cutaneous glands, Med Biol 55:115–125.

Pearse AGE, Takor Takor T (1979) Embryology of the diffuse neuroendocrine system and its relationship to the common peptides, Fed Proc 38:2288–2294.

Percy C, Sobin L (1983) Surveillance, epidemiology and end results: lung cancer data applied to the World Health Organization's classifications of lung tumors, JJNCI 70:663–666.

Pettingill OS, Sorenson GD, Wurster-Hill DH, et al (1980) Isolation and growth characteristics of continuous cell lines from small-cell carcinoma of the lung, Cancer 45:906–918.

Poe RH, Tobin RE (1980) Sensitivity and specificity of needle biopsy in lung malignancy, Am Rev Respir Dis 122:725–729.

Radice PA, Matthews MJ, Ihde DC, et al (1982) The clinical behavior of "mixed" small cell/large cell bronchogenic carcinoma compared to "pure" small cell subtypes, Cancer 50:2894–2902.

Rappaport H (1977) In: Discussion II: Roundtable discussion of histopathologic classification, Cancer Treat Rep 61:1037–1048.

Ratcliffe JG (1982) Hormone markers in lung cancer. In: Colnaghi MI, Buraggi GL, Ghione M (eds) Markers for diagnosis and monitoring of human cancer. Proceedings of the Serono Symposia, Academic Press, New York, Vol 46, pp 85–94.

Richardson RL, Greco FA, Oldham RK, et al (1978) Tumor products and potential markers in small cell lung cancer, Sem Oncol 5:253–262.

Rodescu D (1977) Lung cancer, Med Clin North Am 61:1205–1218.

Roggli VL, McGavran MH, Subach J, et al (1982) Pulmonary asbestos body counts and electron probe analysis of asbestos body cores in patients with mesothelioma, Cancer 50:2423–2432.

Rosen P, Melamed M, Savino A (1972) The "ferruginous body" content of lung tissue: a quantitative study of eighty-six patients, Acta Cytol 16:207–211.

Rosenow EC III, Carr DT (1979) Bronchogenic carcinoma, CA 29:233–245.

Roth JA, Elguezabal A (1978) Pulmonary blastoma evolving into carcinosarcoma: a case study, Am J Surg Pathol 2:407–413.

Rothschild H, Buechner H, Welsh R, et al (1982) Histologic typing of lung cancer in Louisiana, Cancer 49:1874–1877.

Ruckdeschel JC, Caradonna R, Paladine WJ, et al (1979) Small cell anaplastic carcinoma of the lung: changing concepts and emerging problems, CA 29:84–95.

Saba SR, Azar HA, Richman AV, et al (1981) Dual differentiation in small cell carcinoma (oat cell carcinoma) of the lung, Ultrastructural Pathol 2:131–138.

Saba SR, Espinoza CG, Richman AV, et al (1983) Carcinomas of the lung: an ultrastructural and immunocytochemical study, Am J Clin Pathol 80:6–13.

Scully RE (ed) (1984) Case records of the Massachusetts General Hospital Case 3-1984, N Engl J Med 310:178–187.

Serrou B, Cupissol D, Favier F, Favier C (1982) New definitions in the marker approach for diagnosis and monitoring of human cancer: a discussion. In: Colnaghi MI, Buraggi GL, Ghione M (eds) Markers for diagnosis and monitoring of human cancer. Proceedings of the Serono Symposia. Academic Press, New York, Vol; 46, pp 129–134.

Shackney SE, Straus MJ, Bunn PA Jr, (1981) The growth characteristics of small cell carcinoma of the lung. In: Greco FA, Oldham RK, Bunn PA (eds) Small cell lung cancer, Grune and Stratton, London, pp 225–234.

Sheperd FA, Ginsberg RJ, Evans WK, et al (1983) Reduction in local recurrence and improved survival in surgically treated patients with small cell lung cancer, J Thorac Cardiovasc Surg 6:498–506.

Shimosato Y, Hashimoto, T, Kodama T, et al (1980) Prognostic implications of fibrotic focus (scar) in small peripheral lung cancers, Am J Surg Pathol 4:365–373.

Sidhu GS (1979) The endodermal origin of digestive and respiratory tract APUD cells. Histopathologic evidence and a review of the literature, Am J Pathol 96:5–20.

Sidhu GS (1982) The ultrastructure of malignant epithelial neoplasms of the lung. In: Sommers SC, Rosen PP (eds) Pathology Annual, Vol 17, Part I, Appleton-Century-Crofts, Norwalk, pp 235–266.

Silverberg E (1983) Cancer statistics, 1983, CA 33:9–25.

Singh G, Katyal SL, Torikata C (1981) Carcinoma of type II pneumocytes. Immunodiagnosis of a subtype of "bronchiolo-alveolar carcinomas", Am J Pathol 102:195–208.

Smith RA, Nigam BK, Thompson JM (1976) Second primary lung carcinoma, Thorax 31:507–516.

Sobin LH (1983) The histologic classification of lung tumors: the need for a double standard, Hum Pathol 14:1020–1021.

Sorenson GD, Pettingill OS, Brinck-Johnson T, et al (1981) Hormone production by cultures of small-cell carcinoma of the lung, Cancer 47:1289–1296.

Sorenson GD, Pettengill OS, Cate CC, DelPrete SA (1984) Biomarkers in small cell carcinoma of the lung (In Press).

Spencer H (1977) Pathology of the lung, 3rd ed, V1–2, Pergamon, Oxford.

Spencer H (1979) Bronchial mucous gland tumours, Virchows Arch (Path Anat) 383:101–115.

Stanley KE (1980) Prognostic factors for survival in patients with inoperable lung cancer, JNCI 65:25–32.

Stanley KE, Matthews MJ (1981) Analysis of a pathology review of patients with lung tumors, JNCI 66:989–992.

Strauchen JA, Egbert BM, Kosek JC, Mackintosh R, Misfeldt DS (1983) Morphologic and clinical determinants of response to therapy in small cell carcinoma of the lung, Cancer 52:1088–1092.

Suzuki Y (1980) Pathology of human malignant mesothelioma, Semin Oncol 8:268–282.

Tao LC, Delarue NC, Sanders D, et al (1978) Bronchioloalveolar carcinoma. A correlative clinical and cytologic study, Cancer 42:2759–2767.

Tateishi R, Hattori S (1982) Ultrastructure of large-cell and giant-cell carcinoma in the lung in relation to histogenesis. In: Shimosato Y, Melamed MR, Nettesheim P (eds) Morphogenesis of lung cancer. Vol II, CRC Press, Boca Raton, pp 45–66.

Tischler AS (1978) Small cell carcinoma of the lung: cellular origin and relationship to other neoplasms., Semin Oncol 5:244–252.

Urushizaki I, Niitsu Y (1982) Ferritin in diagnosis of lung cancer. In: Colnaghi MI, Buraggi GL, Ghione M (eds) Markers for diagnosis and monitoring of human cancer. Proceedings of the Serono Symposia. Academic Press, New York, Vol. 46, pp 111–121.

Valaitis J, Warren S, Gamble D (1981) Increasing incidence of adenocarcinoma of the lung, Cancer 47:1042–1046.

Vincent RG, Chu TM, Fergen TB, et al (1975) Carcinoembryonic antigen in 228 patients with carcinoma of the lung, Cancer 36:2069–2076.

Vincent RG, Pickren JW, Lane WW, et al (1977) The changing histopathology of lung cancer. A review of 1682 cases, Cancer 39:1647–1655.

Vollmer RT (1982) The effect of cell size on the pathologic diagnosis of small and large cell carcinomas of the lung, Cancer 50:1380–1383.

Waalkes TP, Abeloff MD, Ettinger DS, et al (1982) Biological markers and small cell carcinoma of the lung. A clinical evaluation of urinary ribonucleosides, Cancer 50:2457–2464.

Wallach SR, Royston I, Taetle R, et al (1981) Plasma calcitonin as a marker of disease activity in patients with small cell carcinoma of the lung, J Clin Endocrinol Metab 53:602–606.

Wang N-S, Seemayer TA, Ahmed MN, et al (1976) Giant cell carcinoma of the lung. A light and electron microscopic Hum Pathol 7:3–16.

Warhol MJ, Hickey WF, Corson JM (1982) Malignant mesothelioma. Ultrastructural distinction from adenocarcinoma, Am J Surg Pathol 6:307–314.

Whimster WF (1983) Lung tumours: differentiation and classification. In: Sommers SC, Rosen PP (eds) Pathology Annual, Vol 18, Part I, Appleton-Century-Crofts, pp 121–138.

Willis RA (1967) Pathology of tumours, 4th ed, Butterworth's, London, p 364.

Wilson TS, McDowell EM, McIntire KR, et al (1981) Elaboration of human chorionic gonadotropin by lung tumors. Arch Pathol Lab Med 105:169–173.

Wolfe HJ (1978) Tumor-cell markers: a biologic shell game?, N Engl J Med 299:146–147.

World Health Organization (1981) Histological typing of lung tumours, Tumori 67:253–272.

World Health Organization (1982) The World Health Organization histological typing of lung tumors. Second edition, Am J Clin Pathol 77:123–136.

Yesner R (1981) The dynamic histopathologic spectrum of lung cancer, Yale J Biol Med 54:447–456.

Yesner R (1983) Small cell tumors of the lung, Am J Surg Pathol 7:775–785.

Zolliker AS, Jacques J (1981) Clara cell carcinoma of the lung, Hum Pathol 12:748–750.

Chapter V Diagnostic Workup

FREDERICK RICHARDS and ROBERT H. CHOPLIN

CONTENTS

FREDERICK RICHARDS, II, M.D., Associate Professor of Medicine

ROBERT H. CHOPLIN, M.D., Assistant Professor of Radiology

Bowman Gray School of Medicine of Wake Forest University, 300 South Hawthorne Road, Winston-Salem, NC 27103, USA

1 Diagnostic Workup

Although cough or change in the character of cough is often the first symptom or sign of bronchogenic carcinoma, lung cancer may present in a wide variety of manifestations. An organized approach is necessary for the diagnosis of lung cancer and evaluation of disease extent which is necessary in deciding therapeutic extent. The diagnostic process begins with the posterior-anterior (PA) chest film, and cytological exam of sputum.

1.1 History and Physical

The great majority of patients which lung cancer seek treatment because of symptoms (RICHARDS et al., 1978; ROSENOW and CARR, 1979; COHEN, 1983) (Table 1). Less than five percent of patients are asymptomatic and the tumor discovered on routine chest x-ray. Such symptoms may be related to the primary tumor, to the intrathoracic spread of the tumor, or to distant effects of the tumor. There are no symptoms specific for lung cancer.

Table 1. Clinical symptoms of lung cancer

Bronchopulmonary	Cough, often productive
	Hemoptysis
	Chest pain
	Wheezing, dyspnea, stridor
	Febrile respiratory symptoms
Extrapulmonary intrathoracic	Hoarseness
	Superior vena caval syndrome
	Horner's syndrome
	Dysphagia
	Pleural effusion
	Percarditis
Extrathoracic metastatic	Neurological symptoms
	Bone pain
	Weight loss
	Weakness, anorexia, lassitude, malaise
	Jaundice
	Ascites
	Abdomen, neck, subcutaneous mass

Unfortunately, when cancer of the lung is diagnosed after it causes symptoms, it is usually late in the course and the prognosis is grim.

1.1.1 Symptoms from Primary Tumor

Cough resulting from bronchial irritation is the most common first symptom of lung cancer. Cough may be productive or non-productive and frequently is disregarded by the patient as being a 'cigarette cough'. Production of sputum is of diagnostic significance in that it provides material for cytological examination, but no significance can be attached to its appearance. It may be mucoid, gray, or mucopurulent if there is an associated infection. Voluminous quantities of thin mucoid secretion may be seen in bronchoalveolar carcinoma. Hemoptysis from disruption of the bronchial mucosa occurs in up to 40% of patients. Wheezing or recent increase in shortness of breath is highly suggestive of partial bronchial obstruction. The obstruction may lead to atelectasis with infection of the distal pulmonary parenchyma. The inflammatory process, obstructive pneumonitis, or abscess formation leads to febrile respiration symptoms (WALLACE et al., 1979). Chest pain due to inflammatory involvement of the parietal pleura and chest wall may occur.

1.1.2 Intrathoracic Spread

The first symptoms of a bronchogenic carcinoma may be secondary to invasion of adjacent structures which almost always implies unresectability. Lesions arising in the region of the left hilum, aortic arch, or spread thereof (nodal metastases) may involve the left recurrent laryngeal nerve with resultant left vocal cord paralysis and hoarseness. Diaphragmatic paralysis from phrenic nerve involvement can be diagnosed by means of fluoroscopy with a 'sniff test' (paradoxic motion). Extrinsic compression or direct invasion of the esophagus usually from a primary tumor located in the left main stem bronchus with dysphagia is relatively infrequent. Rarely, a bronchoesophageal fistula with recurrent aspiration pneumonitis may develop. Dysphagia can also be a manifestation of a paralysis of the left recurrent laryngeal nerve. A pharyngoesophageal myotomy may effectively improve swallowing and prevent aspiration (HENDERSON et al., 1974).

External compression or intraluminal invasion

of the vascular wall of the superior vena cava (SVC) from adjacent lymph nodes or direct invasion from a neoplastic growth in the right upper lobe leads to the characteristic SVC syndrome (SALSALI and CLIFFTON, 1968). The SVC syndrome is usually secondary to small cell or squamous cell carcinoma and results in neck vein distention, neck and facial swelling, dyspnea, and diluted venous collaterals over the chest wall and epigastrium. The diagnosis usually can be made on clinical grounds and the chest radiograph. The clinical picture depends on whether the obstruction is proximal or distal to the azygous vein. When diagnosis is in doubt, venography or measurement of venous pressure is confirmatory. Two errors are made in the management of patients with the SVC syndrome: (1) treating without a specific diagnosis; and (2) persuing a diagnosis too vigorously in lieu of treatment. The former probably is more detrimental to the patients as more effective therapy becomes available for specific diagnosis. The major pitfall in the management of SVC syndrome is treatment before a histologic diagnosis is established. Diagnostic tests may be associated with an increased morbidity and should be carefully selected prior to therapy, beginning with the least invasive test and proceeding to mediastinoscopy and thoracotomy if necessary (SHIMM et al., 1981). Radiation therapy has been the conventional form of therapy for tumor related SVC syndrome, but chemotherapy may supplement this modality in certain types of tumor, particularly small cell lung cancer.

Pleural effusions may be caused by extension of cancer to the pleural surface (usually the viceral pleura), by thoracic duct involvement in the mediastinum, or by obstruction of pulmonary lymphatics (LEFF et al., 1978). Thoracentesis and pleural biopsy should be done to establish diagnosis. Pleural effusion from obstructive atelectasis with pneumonitis or pulmonary embolus do not necessarily indicate unresectability. Fluid accumulation in the pleural spaces causes pain and dyspnea from pulmonary embarrassment. Pericardial (most common) or myocardial (less common) involvement from metastases can result in pericardial effusion. This is most commonly seen with poorly differentiated tumors. The onset of a new arrhythmia or electrocardiographic changes and symptoms of congestive heart failure should alert the physician to the possibility of cardiac metastases (STRAUSS et al., 1977).

Extension of tumor to the chest wall with involvement of bone or nerves with resultant pain and restriction of respiratory movement can occur. An unusual type of local spread to the brachial plexus results in Pancoast syndrome (superior sulcus or thoracic inlet tumor) (MILLER et al., 1979). An apical carcinoma invades the chest wall structures and the eighth cervical and first thoracic nerves, producing pain in the shoulder and arm, and may invade the cervical sympathetic nerves producing a Horner's syndrome (unilateral enophthalmos, constricted pupils, and lack of perspiration on the same side of the face and forehead). A 30 to 35% five-year survival is possible when Pancoast's tumor is treated with combined radiation therapy and en bloc resection. Rarely, lung cancer can present as an ipsilateral spontaneous pneumothorax (MAHAJAN et al., 1975).

1.1.3 Metastases and Distant Effects

Systemic effects of lung cancer may result from metastases to various sites that produce effects of mass lesions in the involved viscera and a variety of indirect effects, most common anorexia, weight loss, weakness, and fatigue. Common sites of metastatic spread are lymph nodes, liver, brain, bone, lung, adrenals, and skin. Symptoms arising from the metastases often dominate the clinical picture, complicate the diagnosis, and often make surgery or any other form of therapy futile. The size of the primary tumor does not always govern the extent of spread. Large tumors may not be attended by metastases or conversely small asymptomatic cancer may have widespread metastases.

Peripheral lymphadenopathy from lung cancer may be found on physical exam, most commonly in the ipsilateral supraclavicular region. The chest x-ray may show mediastinal node involvement.

Brain metastases are common, most frequently with small cell lung cancer. Neurologic symptoms from brain metastases may precede pulmonary symptoms. Symptoms include hemiplegia, seizure, personality changes, confusion, speech defects, or only headache. Tumors of the lung usually metastasize to the frontal lobes of the cerebrum, far less frequently to the cerebellum. In 30% of cases, the metastases are solitary. The CT scan is probably more sensitive than the radionucleotide scan. Leptomeningeal involvement with headache and altered mental status, often with focal neurological abnormalities from cranial nerve involvement, is being seen with increased frequency.

Hepatic metastases are frequent in lung cancer. Characteristic symptoms are liver enlargement, pain, hardness, and palpable nodules. Jaundice and ascites are seldom seen. Elevated liver function tests and liver scan are usually sufficient for diagnosis. Rarely is CT scan or ultrasound needed for confirmation. A liver biopsy may be needed for confirmation.

Bone pain and pathologic fracture from metastatic bone involvement may be present on presentation. Most commonly involved are vertebral bodies (70%), pelvic bones (40%), and femur (25%). Paraplegia from fractured vertebra and spinal cord compression may occur. Symptoms include back pain, sensory or motor impairment, or loss of normal bladder or bowel function. Myelography is necessary to localize the lesion. Treatment is decompressive laminectomy and radiation therapy or radiation therapy alone. Other metastatic sites include long bones of the extremities, scapula, sternum, and small bones of wrists and feet. Most are osteolytic lesions, but osteoblastic changes may occur. When bone metastases are present, the skeletal fraction of alkaline phosphatase is often elevated. Roentgenological examination and radionuclide bone scans are usually helpful.

Rarely jaundice, ascites, or an abdominal mass is a major complaint. Neck muscle or subcutaneous tissue masses are present infrequently.

Other metastases including metastases to the remaining lung tissue, opposite lung, pancreas, spleen, heart, thyroid, eye, ovary, kidneys, adrenals, and other internal organs may be observed. Rarely metastases to the skin may occur. There is virtually no organ or tissue to which lung cancer cannot metastasize.

1.1.4 Extrathoracic Nonmetastatic Manifestations

Approximately two percent of patients with bronchogenic carcinoma may manifest symptoms and signs that are not related to the metastatic spread of cancer itself. These paraneoplastic syndromes are usually seen in patients with advanced neoplastic processes but may precede the onset of pulmonary problems related to the malignancy (UMSAWASDI and VALDIVIESO, 1982). The development of these paraneoplastic syndromes have been associated with production of biologically active substances in many cases; while in others the mechanisms remain unknown. Proper recognition and treatment of these syndromes is important because of their potential seriousness. Specific treatment

Table 2. Paraneoplastic syndromes associated with broncho-genic carcinoma

Endocrine	Neurologic
Cushing's syndrome	Cortical degeneration
Hypercalcemia	Subacute cerebellar
Syndrome inappropriate	degeneration
antidiuretic hormone	Progressive multifocal
secretion (SIADH)	leukoencephalopathy
Carcinoid syndrome	Peripheral neuropathy
Hypoglycemia	Polymyositis
Hypercalcitonemia	Transverse myelitis
Gynecomastia	Myasthenic syndrome
Elevated human growth	
hormone	Cardiovascular
Elevated prolactin, follical	Thrombophlebitis
stimulating hormone,	Mirantic endocarditis
leutinizing hormone	
	Cutaneous
Hematologic	Dermatomyositis
Anemia	Acanthosis nigricans
Dysproteinemia	Scleroderma
Dissiminated intravascular	Hyperpigmentation
coagulation	Other dermatoses
Granulocytosis	
Thrombocytosis	Other
Eosinophilia	Nephrotic syndrome
Hypoalbuminemia	Hypouricemia
Pure red cell aplasia	Hypersecretion of
Leukoerythroblastosis	vasoactive intestinal
Plasmacytosis of marrow	peptides, with diarrhea
Thrombocytopenia	Hyperamylasemia
	Anorexia-cachexia
Skeletal	
Clubbing	
Pulmonary hypertrophic	
osteoarthropathy	

is not available for many of these syndromes. Successful treatment of the malignancy may result in amelioration of the syndrome. These manifestations are not specific and may occur in association with malignant lesions other than lung cancer. Table 2 lists these syndromes. The mechanisms of these syndromes are discussed in Section 2.2 – Biochemical Tumor Markers.

1.1.4.1 Endocrine. The secretion of endocrine or endocrine-like substances by the tumor may result in a number of metabolic manifestations. Most of these 'ectopic' hormone syndromes are found in association with small-cell carcinoma.

Cushing's syndrome. This relatively rare manifestation (<1%) of small cell lung carcinoma differs from the classic syndrome. It is characterized by severe hypokalemic alkalosis, progressive weakness, weight loss, muscular wasting, hyper-

glycemia, fewer physical stigmata of typical Cushing's syndrome, and a more rapid fulminating course. An ectopic corticotropin-like (ACTH) substance has been demonstrated in tumor tissue and blood. Although over 70% of patients with lung cancer may have elevated ACTH, less than 2% have the syndrome (WOLFSEN and ODELL, 1979; GROPP et al., 1980). Some cases may be due to secretion of CRF (corticotropin releasing factor). Increased plasma cortisol without diurinal variation which is not suppressed by large doses of dexamethasone. Aminoglutethimide and metyrapone may be helpful in controlling symptoms.

Antidiuretic hormone. Inappropriately increased concentrations of ADH have been reported in 70% of patients with lung cancer, but clinical manifestations are rare (HANSEN et al., 1980). The syndrome of inappropriate anti-diuretic hormone secretion (SIADH), also seen in small cell lung cancer, results in water intoxication with anorexia, nausea, and vomiting accompanied by increasingly severe neurological complications. Provided there is normal renal and adrenal function, the diagnosis is supported by hyponatremia, hyposmolarity of plasma, hyperosmolarity of urine, increased urinary sodium excretion, and elevated ADH (vasopressin) in urine and serum. Occasionally, an associated increase of neurophysin (HNP) is observed. Most respond to fluid restriction but some need hypertonic saline solution and demeclocycline or lithium carbonate. Benign lesions (CNS disorders, pulmonary infections) and chemotherapy (cyclophosphamide/vincristine) may also cause SIADH.

Parathyroid hormone. Hypercalcemia in patients with bronchogenic carcinoma is most often due to bone metastases; however, squamous cell carcinoma of the lung is known to secrete a parathyroid hormone-like (PTH) polypeptide. An accompanying hypophosphatemia is often noted. Prostaglandin E_2 (PGE_2) may also cause hypercalcemia. Clinical symptoms of hypercalcemia include irritability, confusion, lethargy, weakness, anorexia, nausea, constipation, and cardiac arrhythmias. Initial treatment should include vigorous hydration with physiologic saline aided by calciurices diuretics (furosemide or ethacrynic acid). Mithramycin, calcitonin, corticosteroids, prostaglanding inhibitors (aspirin/indomethocin), and/or dichoromethylene diphosphate may be helpful.

The *carcinoid syndrome* is more commonly associated with bronchial carcinoid but has been reported in small cell lung cancer. Clinical features of the syndrome include episodic signs and symptoms related to the release of various vasoactive amines. Many vasoactive substances in addition to serotonin (5-hydroxytryptamine) have been shown to be produced by these tumors: 5-hydroxytryptophan, bradykinin and its precursor enzyme kallikinin, and various catecholamines. Symptoms include flushing or edema, or both, of the face and upper body, tachycardia, wheezing, hyperperistalsis and diarrhea, weight loss, and anorexia. Diagnosis is by 5-hydroxindoleacetic acid in urine.

Ectopic gonadotropin. Rarely bronchogenic carcinoma may produce chorionic gonadotropin (hCG) or placental lactogen (hPL) with tender gynecomastia and testicular atrophy (Fusco and Rosen, 1966). Hypertrophic osteoarthropathy may be been with elevated ectopic growth hormone (hGH) (STEINER et al., 1968). Bombesin may be responsible for weakness, anorexia, and cachexia (MOODY et al., 1983). Some tumors may produce more than one hormone with overlapping effects.

A variety of nonendocrinological manifestations may occur with cancer. These include neuromuscular disorders, dermatologic disorders, and hematologic disorders.

1.1.4.2 Neuromuscular Disorders.

Carcinomatous neuromyopathies are the most frequent extrathoracic, non-metastatic manifestation of lung cancer. In one review, 56% had small cell lung cancer, 22% squamous cell carcinoma, 16% large cell carcinoma, and 5% adenocarcinoma (MORTON et al., 1966).

Subacute cortical cerebellar degeneration with severe dysarthria, vertigo, and predominant ataxia of the upper extremities may occur. Nystagmus is uncommon. Bilateral and symmetric abnormalities and normal cerebrospinal fluid are keys to diagnosis. A cerebral encephalomyelopathy characterized by progressive dementia, psychosis, or organic brain syndrome may occur. Moderate spinal fluid pleocytosis and a characteristic slow electroencephalograph are characteristic (JOYNT, 1974). There is no therapy for these conditions.

A polyneuropathy predominantly affecting the lower extremities of a sensorimotor type that may respond to corticosteroids can occur. Pure sensory neuropathy is rare.

A polymyositis with progressive proximal muscle weakness that usually involves extensor muscles of the arm intially usually without muscle wasting, hypoflexia is common. Androgens or corticosteroids may help. A Myasthenic (Eaton-Lambert) syndrome with proximal muscle weakness without ocular and bulbar involvement that may respond to Guanidine hydrochloride or calcium is rare (CHERINGTON, 1976). Electromyogram in both is characteristic. As mentioned earlier, alteration in mental status may be secondary to ectopic hormone production (i.e. hypercalcemia, hyponatremia).

1.1.4.3 Dermatologic.

A number of dermatological conditions may be associated with lung cancer including acanthosis nigricans, pruritis, tylosis, urticaria, herpes zoster, scleroderma, acquired ichthyosis, hyperpigmentation, and an exfoliative dermatitis. Dermatomyositis is more common with adenocarcinoma and presents with symmetrical proximal muscle weakness (pelvic girdle greater than shoulder muscles) and a violaceous facial rash in a butterfly distribution. Corticosteroids may improve the symptoms. Useful diagnostic laboratory tests include electromyography, muscle biopsy, and evaluation of serum enzymes including SGOT, SGPT, and aldolase.

1.1.4.4 Skeletal.

Hypertrophic pulmonary osteoarthropathy (HPO) (Bamberger-Marie Disease) characterized by clubbing of fingers and toes, painful and symmetric arthropathy of ankles, wrists, and knees, and a proliferative periostitis of long bones may be seen in up to five percent of patients with lung cancer (SCHUMACHER, 1976). Bone x-rays and radionuclide bone scans may be helpful for diagnosis. HPO occurs only rarely, if ever, in small cell lung tumors. Its occurrence is distributed equally among the other three major cell types. The etiology of this syndrome is unknown, although estrogens, growth hormone, and neurologic innervation have been suggested.

1.1.4.5 Vascular Manifestations.

Recurrent or migratory thrombophlebitis often resistant to anticoagulation may be the first indication of the presence of lung cancer (BYRD et al., 1967). Non-bacterial verrucal, marantic endocarditis, characterized by the deposition of sterile fibrin plaques on the heart valves and resultant arterial embolization may occur (CROWTHER and BATEMAN, 1972). The mechanisms of these complications are unknown.

1.1.4.6 Hematologic.

Normocytic, normochromic anemia, red cell aplasia, fibrinolytic purpura, erythrocytosis, thrombocytosis, eosinophilia, and non specific leukocytosis have been reported in patients with lung cancer.

2 Laboratory Data

2.1 Hematologic

Hematological disturbances are frequent with lung cancer (Moody et al., 1983). They usually occur late in the course when there is widespread or recurrent tumor. These abnormalities may include anemia, granulocytosis, leukoerythroblastosis, thrombocytosis, leukopenia, or disturbances in blood coagulation.

2.1.1 Red Blood Cell Abnormalities

Anemia commonly develops in lung cancer. Simple investigations after pertinent history and physical examination will often reveal the cause. Most commonly this is due to dyserythropoiesis in which there is decreased utilization of iron. This is due to the non-specific toxic effects of the lung cancer with associated block of reticulo-endothelial iron release. The red blood cells are usually normocytic and normochromic but hypochromic and microcytic cells are also present (dimorphic anemia). Characteristically, the anemia is mild with reduced serum iron and total iron binding capacity and increased iron in the bone marrow. Rarely, a sideroblastic anemia occurs with raised serum iron and increased saturation of iron binding protein. It is characterized by a dimorphic peripheral smear and 'ring' sideroblasts. Leukoerythroblastic anemia results from infiltration of the bone marrow and is characterized by the occurrence of immature white and red cells in the peripheral blood. Infrequently, anemia may be due to hemorrhage, deficiency of iron, folate, or vitamin B-12. Hemolytic anemia has been rarely described with lung cancer (Horne and McAnally, 1978). Anemia is frequent after cytotoxic therapy.

Secondary erythrocytosis has been infrequently associated with lung cancer (Hammond and Winnick, 1974). It is usually mild and requires no treatment.

2.1.2 White Cell Abnormalities

A peripheral blood leukocytosis (or leukemoid reaction) which resembles leukemia may occur in bronchogenic cancer. A granulocytic leukemoid reaction is most common and is characterized by elevation of the white blood cell with a shift to the left (Dalal et al., 1980). The leukemoid reaction differs from leukemia in that the cell count is usually below $50 - 10^9/L$, splenomegaly is absent, other hemopoietic elements are often normal, and the leukocyte alkaline phosphatase is usually high. Bone marrow metastases may be a contributing factor in some cases. Monocytic leukemoid reactions and lymphocytic leukemoid reactions are rare. Eosinophilic reactions have also been associated with lung cancer (Varindani et al., 1982). There does not appear to be a relationship between survival and granulocyte count, monocyte count, and lymphocyte count (Markman, 1982).

A leukoerythroblastic blood picture consisting of myeloblasts, neutrophilic myelocytes, or erythroblasts in the circulating blood is indicative of malignant infiltration of the bone marrow (Ihde et al., 1979). A mild anemia and/or thrombocytopenia are common. The white blood cell count may be increased, decreased, or within normal limits. Only about 25 to 35% of patients with bone marrow involvement have leucoerythroblastic anemia. The bone marrow frequently has osteoblastic changes and fibrotic reactions and the serum alkaline phosphatase is elevated. Leukopenia is usually the result of cytotoxic chemotherapy or radiotherapy.

2.1.3 Platelet Abnormalities

Thrombocytosis is frequent (60%) with lung carcinoma and thrombocytopenia is relatively rare (2.6%) at presentation with lung cancer (Silvis et al., 1970). Thrombocytosis may also occur after administration of drugs, particularly steroids and vincristine. Thrombocytopenia as a result of therapy is associated with a hypoplastic marrow; spontaneous bleeding can occur with counts below $20-30 \times 10^9/L$.

2.1.4 Coagulation Disorders

Bronchogenic carcinoma is often associated with thrombotic disturbances, variously ascribed to the release of thromboplastic substances, alterations in coagulation factors, thrombocytosis, increased platelet adhesiveness, increased fibrinogen deposition, and decreased fibrinolysis. Probably the most important mechanism is DIC (disseminated intravascular coagulation) from release of thromboplastic and proteolytic substances. Patients may have migrating thrombophlebitis (Trousseau's syndrome), arterial embolism (with or without thrombotic non-bacterial endocarditis), and hemorrhage phenomena, depending on the degree of coagulopathy (SACK et al., 1977).

2.1.5 Disturbances from Cytotoxic Drug Therapy

Neutropenia and thrombocytopenia from chemotherapy are common. Anemia is also frequent. The bone marrow is generally hypoplastic. The changes are usually brief and temporary but may be prolonged.

2.2 Biochemical Tumor Cell Markers

Many biological products or marker substances are produced by lung cancer or found in association with lung cancer (VINCENT, 1982; BRODER and PRIMACK, 1983). These products may be categorized as follows: tumor-associated hormones, both fetal and tumor-associated antigens, enzymes, and others (Table III). A large number of these substances have been evaluated as potential markers of the presence of lung cancer (MERRILL and BONDY, 1982). It is felt that these biological markers of tumor growth may reflect change in total body tumor burden.

A wide variety of 'ectopic' hormones have been found to be associated with lung cancer. Among the many hormones that may be produced are the corticotropic hormones, antidiuretic hormone, calcitonin, growth hormone, glycoprotein hormones, prolactin, gastrin, etc. Hormonal production may be associated with various paraneoplastic syndromes, however, in most instances the secreted polypeptide or glycopolypeptide materials may be immunologically similar but biochemically nonfunctional.

The exact mechanism of production of these markers is as yet unknown. Two general theories have been proposed to explain 'ectopic' hormones. The first and most widely held view is that there is a derepression or other dysregulation of genetic information leading to the expression of 'inappropriate' portions of the cellular genome. However, there is evidence that specific gene depression is not the cause of ectopic hormone production and that failure to control the intracellular abundance of messenger RNA coding for a specific hormone rather than new synthesis from previously inactive genes is responsible (SHIELDS, 1978). A second popular theory suggests that cells of neuroectodermal crest origin migrate to various

Table 3. Tumor cell markers in carcinoma of the lung

Hormone production	Adrenocorticotropin hormone (ACTH)
	Melanocyte-stimulating hormone (MSH)
	Human chorionic gonadotropin (hCG)
	Human placental lactogen (hPL)
	Human growth hormone (hGH)
	Parathyroid hormone (PTH)
	Calcitonin (hCT)
	Antidiuretic hormone (ADH)
	Prolactin
	Bombesin
	5-Hydroxytryptophan (serotonin)
	Estradiol
	Hypoglycemic factor
	Renin
	Erythropoietin
	Glucagon
Fetoproteins	Alpha fetoprotein (AFP)
	Carcinoembryonic antigen (CEA)
Enzymes	Placental alkaline phosphatase (PAP)
	Histaminase
	L-dopadecarboxylase
Antigens	
Polyamines	
Chromosomal abnormalities	

body sites during development. These neural crest cells subsequently undergo malignant transformations and secrete 'ectopic' hormones (LOKICH, 1978).

For example, the large polypeptide "big" ACTH or pro-ACTH is found in all histological types of lung cancer – not merely small cell which sometimes manifests abnormalities in adrenocortical control – and it was present in 74% of a series of 74 patients (WOLFSEN and O'DELL, 1979). All 26 patients with benign abnormalities had normal plasma ACTH reactivity. A more recent report casts doubt on the use of this marker for lung cancer (TORSTENSSON et al., 1980).

A number of nonhormonal substances may be produced in excess in patients with bronchogenic carcinoma and are found in higher concentrations in serum or plasma of patients with bronchogenic cancer than in that of normal subjects. None of these tumor markers studies so far have been proven exclusively tumor specific; serial elevation of markers in body fluids can occur in non-neoplastic conditions, and some cancers fail to produce the marker under the study (WOLFE, 1978). The use of these markers for estimation of tumor response and survival is under investigation; preliminary results are encouraging.

Probably the best known of these substances is carcinoembryonic antigen (CEA), whose relationship to bronchogenic carcinoma is being increasingly appreciated (DENT et al., 1978). Elevated serum levels of CEA may occur in 60 to 85% of patients with bronchogenic carcinoma, particularly adenocarcinoma and small cell carcinoma. Unfortunately measurements of CEA have little clinical utility because elevated levels may be found in benign conditions. There are also false negatives. Post-operative CEA levels seem to correlate with extent of disease and survival whether or not the patient is rendered disease free and rising CEA levels may help in the differential diagnosis of recurrent disease in lung cancer patients. Serial determination of serum carbohydrates (fucose, mannose, and galactose) with CEA can be of aid in the assessment of tumor status with small cell lung cancer (WAALKES et al., 1983). In addition, determination of marker substances in body fluids (i.e. effusion fluid, bronchial washings, cerebrospinal fluid) may be of aid in the diagnosis and the detection of metastatic or primary disease.

The recent development of radioactive antitumor antibodies directed against such markers may produce potential application for cancer associated antigens as diagnostic and therapeutic tools (RITTGERS et al., 1978). A 131 I-labelled IgG to CEA localized with enough selectivity in metastatic colon cancer to be of useful diagnostic and perhaps useful therapeutic agent (GOLDENBERG et al., 1978).

2.3 Blood Chemistry and Urine Studies

Lung cancer has been associated with a number of biochemical abnormalities. While none of these laboratory abnormalities is specific for bronchogenic carcinoma, the recognition is of importance in the management of bronchogenic carcinoma.

Serum electrolyte and other metabolic abnormalities (hypokalemic alkalosis, hyponatremia, hypercalcemia, etc) secondary to ectopic hormone production and their management have been previously discussed under the paraneoplastic syndromes. These abnormalities may also be seen with organ dysfunction secondary to tumor metastases (i.e. bone, adrenal, renal, and liver involvement). Prompt recognition is of importance.

Elevation of liver chemistries such as serum glutamic-oxaloacetic transaminase (S-GOT), S-GPT, serum prothrombin time, and serum lactic dehydrogenase (S-LDH) are useful in the detection of liver metastases. It should be remembered, however, that positive biochemical tests may be caused by the presence of non-malignant hepatic disorders, such as cirrhosis of fatty degeneration of the liver which occurs with a high incidence in patients with lung cancer. Despite suspicion of metastases raised by positive scans and enzymes, proof still rests on the liver biopsy (MARGOLIS et al., 1974). Lactic acidosis has been reported with extensive liver metastases (SPECHLER et al., 1978).

Increase in serum alkaline phosphatase occurs with bone metastases in addition to liver metastases. Hypercalcemia or hypocalcemia is seen with bone metastases. Increased urinary excretion or increased serum hydroxyproline occurs with bone metastases.

Neoplastic diseases may be associated with a nonspecific disturbance of serum proteins which is characterized by hypoalbuminemia and increased concentrations of α 1, 2-globulins (SUNDERMAN, 1964). Plasmacytic dyscrasia with elaboration of a monoclonal protein may occur in lung cancer (ISOBE and OSSERMAN, 1971). A nephrotic syndrome with mild to moderate proteinuria may be seen (VINCENT, 1978; RUDMAN et al., 1979). Possible causes of this complication include immune complex glomerulonephropathy, renal amyloidosis, or renal vein thrombosis.

Depression of plasma zinc is frequent in lung cancer but of little diagnostic significance (DAVIES et al., 1968). Ferritin, or iron binding protein, may be elevated in bronchogenic carcinoma (GROPP et al., 1970).

2.4 Chromosome Abnormalities

A variety of chromosomal abnormalities in lung cancer have been described (GAZDAR et al., 1983). A specific acquired chromosome defect, depletion 3p (14–23) appears to be specific for small cell lung cancer (WHANG-PENG et al., 1982).

3 Radiographic (Imaging) Evaluation in Patients with Lung Cancer

When evaluating patients with lung cancer, the diagnostic radiologist must identify the carcinoma, help determine the stage of the disease, and sometimes evaluate regional lung function for preoperative assessment of the patient's pulmonary reserve. While certain radiographic patterns usually represent tumor, it must be remembered that currently used methods are histologically nonspecific and pathological confirmation of tumor as well as determination of cell type is important for selection of the proper treatment. Indeed, a major thrust of imaging for staging purposes should be to identify those areas most likely to be positive on biopsy as well as the safest access route to those sites.

3.1 Identifying the Carcinoma

The radiographic patterns produced by the primary tumor or its secondary effects may be grouped as central or peripheral masses; infiltrates; segmental, lobar, or lung collapse; and pleural effusions. Several excellent discussions of these radiographic patterns and their histological correlates are available (HEITZMAN et al., 1982; FRASER et al., 1978; THEROS, 1977). While most cancers are visible on the plain chest radiograph, occasionally fluoroscopy or tomography is necessary to identify its presence. Use of the chest radiograph as a tool for cancer screening is discussed elsewhere.

The discovery of a solitary pulmonary nodule presents a particular problem in differential diagnosis. Documented stability over at least a two year period of time is the most reliable indicator that a nodule is benign. However, in patients for whom no previous examination is available; central, lamellar, or diffuse calcification usually indicates a benign lesion. It was suggested in 1980 that the extraordinary ability of computed tomography to discriminate densities could be used to detect calcification in a nodule which was not otherwise demonstrated on plain films or conventional tomography (SIEGELMAN et al., 1980). In a series of 88 patients without clearly calcified nodules, 20 had relatively high density lesions and were spared a diagnostic thoracotomy. These lesions had all remained stable on follow up out to 18 months. While other investigators initially had difficulty in duplicating this work, recent modifications of the technique have been made to broaden its applicability and the original work has now been confirmed (PROTO 1983). The lower limit of

density will vary from scanner to scanner but will generally be in the range of 160–200 Hounsfield units. Lesions with densities below this level should be considered indeterminate for benign vs malignant and should be removed.

3.2 Determining the Stage of Disease

Proper staging of patients with lung cancer is important to identify those suitable for resectional surgery, as an aid in determining prognosis, and for proper reporting of end results. About 50% of patients can be assigned to Stage III by physical examination and a simple chest radiograph at the time of presentation (MINTZ et al., 1979). While imaging procedures may be required to confirm distant metastatic disease, few of these patients will prove to be candidates for surgery.

Imaging studies performed on the remaining patients attempt to define the extent of disease both regionally and at distant sites. While controversy exists about the most optimal use of these imaging studies; conventional tomography, computed tomography and radionuclide scanning have all demonstrated some benefit in properly staging patients. Clear cut guidelines are not present be-

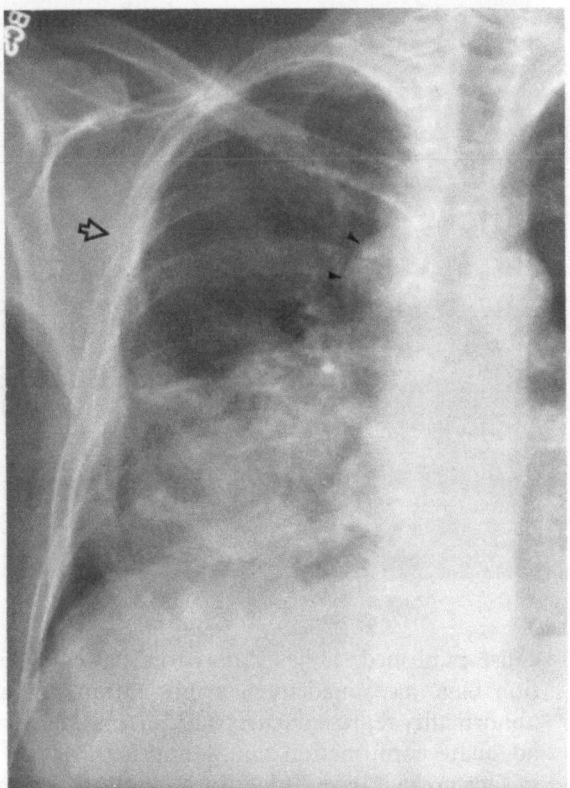

Fig. 1. Plain film evidence of mediastinal and skeletal metastasis. Chest radiograph of a man with poorly differentiated lung cancer demonstrates a mass at the inferior right hilum and consolidation of the middle lobe. Enlargement of the azygous lymph node region (*arrowhead*) and paratracheal widening almost always indicates mediastinal metastasis as in this patient. A metastasis to the right lateral fourth rib is also noted (*open arrow*)

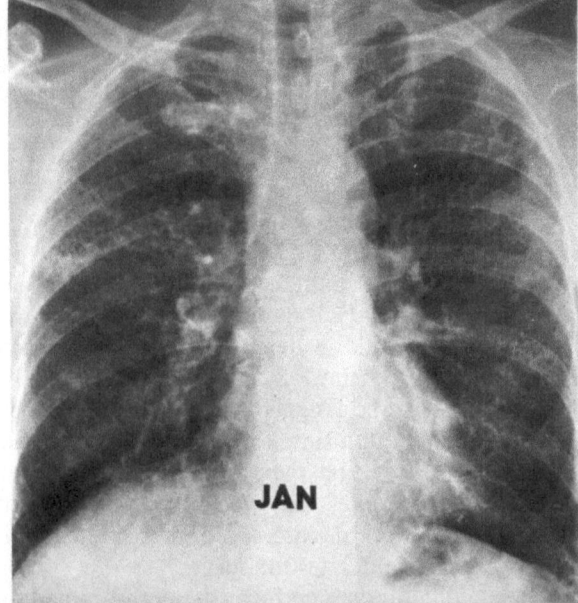

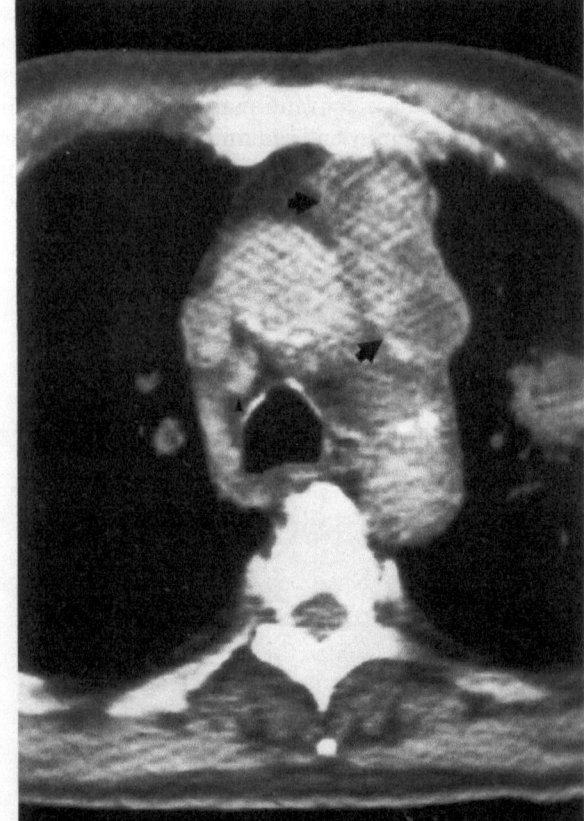

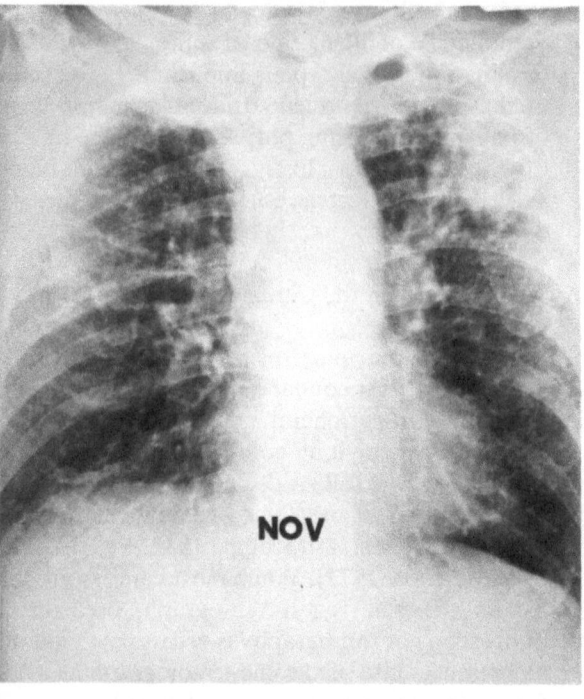

Fig. 2a–c. Preaortic and pretracheal lymphnode enlargement. A 61 year old man developed infiltrate in the left upper lobe in November which was diagnosed as squamous cell carcinoma. While the mediastinal contours appear similar to a previous examination in January and were thought to be normal, computed tomographic evaluation demonstrates a $2^1/_2$ by 5 cm mass of matted lymph nodes in the preaortic mediastinum (*arrows*). Additional note is made of a lymph node in the retrocaval pretracheal space (*arrowhead*). Lymph nodes in this location must usually be greater than 2 cm in size to be visualized on the plain chest radiograph

nary estimates of clinical staging, and use different techniques and equipment to obtain the images. Because of these limitations, it has been suggested that large multi-institutional national trials be conducted to help resolve these questions (LIBSHITZ, 1983).

3.2.1 Identifying Regional Extent of Disease

Radiographic procedures utilized in evaluation of regional extent of disease include the plain chest radiograph, conventional tomography, computed tomography and nuclear scanning with tumor seeking radiopharmaceuticals. Methods currently undergoing active research include nuclear magnetic resonance imaging and imaging with radiolabelled monoclonal antibodies. It is hoped that the latter two technologies will not only be able to

cause published studies suffer from patient selection bias, have inadequate confirmation that an abnormality represents metastatic disease, have inadequate confirmation that a "normal" study is in fact normal, give little information on prelimi-

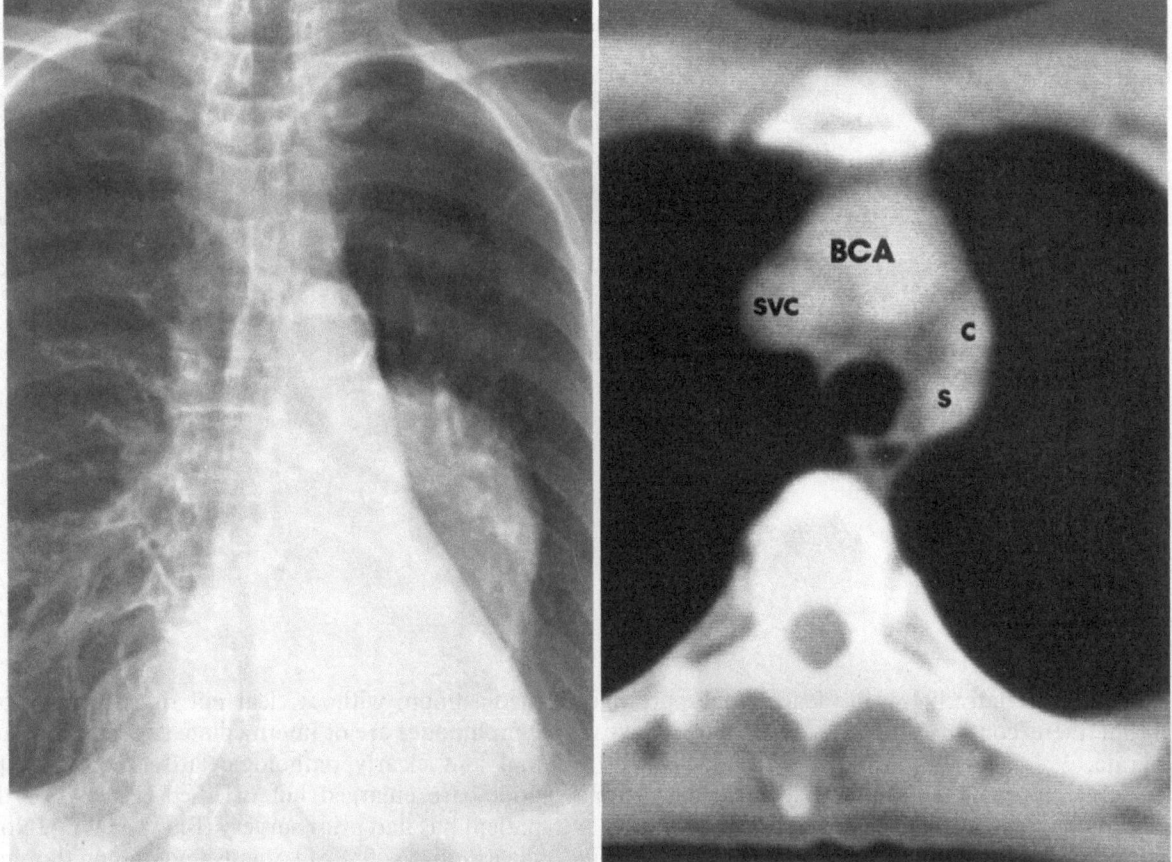

identify areas of abnormality but also contribute information as to their histological character.

The plain chest radiograph continues to be the quickest and least expensive method of imaging the primary tumor, hilum, and mediastinum. While hilar or paratracheal lymph node enlargement (Fig. 1) may be readily identified; the position of the subcarinal, pretracheal and preaortic lymph nodes is such that they will not usually be detected until of considerable size (Fig. 2). Moreover tortuous blood vessels or mediastinal fat deposition may result in water density shadows which may be interpreted as hilar or mediastinal metastases (Fig. 3). While a positive plain radiograph correctly predicts the presence of mediastinal metastasis in 85–100% of patients, the predictive value of a negative test is only about 55% (OSBORNE et al., 1982). Because of this high proportion of false negatives, additional evaluation by conventional or computed tomography has been performed for a majority of patients.

Conventional tomography identifies mediastinal involvement in 40–90% of patients subsequently demonstrated to have mediastinal metas-

Fig. 3a, b. Widened superior mediastinum from a tortuous brachiocephalic artery. This 60 year old woman has a large carcinomatous mass in the left lower lobe. The upper mediastinum is widened and could possibly represent metastatic disease. Computed tomographic scan just above the level of the aortic arch shows an enlarged brachiocephalic artery (*BCA*), which accounts for the apparent widening. There was no evidence of metastasis to the mediastinum at this level. Left common carotid artery (*C*), left subclavian artery (*S*), and superior vena cava (*SVC*)

tasis (OSBORNE et al., 1982; SHEVLAND et al., 1978; MINTZER et al., 1979). Since conventional tomography relies on detecting soft tissue contour abnormalities of the hilum or mediastinum, its limitations are similar to plain film evaluation. The pretracheal, preaortic and subcarinal lymph node groups must be considerably enlarged before abnormality is identified although the enlargement may be less than that required for detection by plain film. Finally, conventional tomography cannot reliably identify mediastinal invasion from a contiguous tumor, vascular encasement, mediastinal lipomatosis or simple vascular tortuosity. The

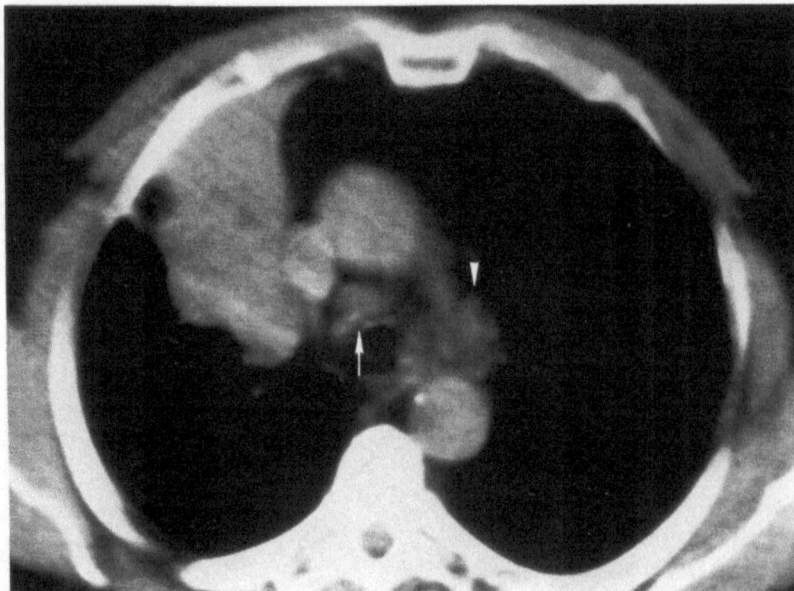

Fig. 4. Approach to biopsy of mediastinal lymph nodes. Computed tomographic scan of a patient with a right upper lobe carcinoma taken just above the pulmonary artery. A pretracheal retrocaval lymph node is enlarged (*arrow*). Lymph nodes in this location are most easily biopsied by transcervical mediastinoscopy. In addition, there is an enlarged lymph node just anterior to the descending aorta (*arrowhead*). Biopsy of lymph nodes in this location is most easily accomplished by a parasternal mediastinotomy

test has a relatively low incidence of false positives but there continues to be a 20% false negative rate.

Computed body tomography has been used as a method of evaluating the mediastinum in patients with lung cancer since it was introduced in 1975. Initial reports using machines with long scanning times were unable to demonstrate clear cut advantage over conventional tomography (UNDERWOOD et al., 1979; MOAK et al., 1982). More recent studies utilizing sub-5 second scanners have demonstrated a sensitivity of 80–94% and specificity of 62–100% (OSBORNE et al., 1982; FALING et al., 1981; REA et al., 1981; BARON et al., 1982). A compilation of data covering 265 patients from five studies demonstrates a sensitivity of 89%, specificity of 89% and accuracy of 89% (BREYER et al.). Because of the low incidence of false negative examinations, surgeons have been able to eliminate mediastinoscopy with its attendant costs and morbidity in patients with a normal mediastinum by CT. In others, computed tomography has been helpful in deciding whether transcervical mediastinoscopy or parasternal mediastinotomy is the most appropriate approach by which to biopsy a mediastinal abnormality (Fig. 4). A few patients with metastatic disease in normal sized mediastinal lymph nodes will remain undetected by CT and undergo thoracotomy.

In about 18% of patients undergoing CT, the examination will be indeterminate because the mass is contiguous with but inseparable from the mediastinum without clear cut signs of invasion, lymph nodes are of intermediate size between normal and clearly pathologic (1.0–1.5 cm), lymph nodes are enlarged but calcified (Fig. 5), or the patient has had prior surgery (BREYER et al.). Nontheless, up to 90% of patients undergoing thoracotomy after CT evaluation have proven to have resectable disease which compares to 76% after mediastinoscopy alone (BARON et al., 1982).

A final advantage of computed tomography over conventional tomography is the ability to demonstrate direct mediastinal or chest wall invasion from contiguous tumor. A confident diagnosis of invasion depends on demonstration of interdigitation of the mass into the mediastinum or chest wall or encasement of a vessel or bronchus (Fig. 6). Mere obliteration of fat planes between tumor and mediastinum/chest wall may occur from mass effect alone and these patients should be considered indeterminate for invasion. The ability to distinguish vascular structures by administration of contrast is a major advantage of computed tomography over conventional tomography.

Nuclear scanning with tumor seeking radiopharmaceuticals is the only other approach to intrathoracic staging for which considerable experience is available. ^{67}Ga-citrate and [57]Co-bleomycin are the two agents with extensive use although a relatively large number of radiopharmaceuticals have been tried. While approximately 90% of primary lung tumors, irrespective of cell type, demonstrate uptake with ^{67}Ga, the ability to predict me-

diastinal metastases has been quite variable and
the accuracy of the study ranges from 50–90%
(ALAZRAKI, 1980; NIEWEG et al., 1983; PANNIER
et al., 1982). Moreover, radionuclide scanning is
unable to assess mediastinal invasion by a contiguous tumor. In view of these limitations, staging
with tumor seeking radiopharmaceuticals has not
received wide acceptance.

Scanning with radiopharmaceutical tagged
monoclonal anti-lung tumor antibodies is a research technique with potential applicability for
staging patients with lung cancer (CUTTITTA et al.,
1981). Most likely these radiopharmaceuticals will
be used in conjunction with emission computed
tomography scanners which are also in the research stage of development. To date, no large
clinical trials evaluating this technique are available.

Nuclear magnetic resonance imaging is another research procedure which holds promise for
accurately staging patients with lung carcinoma.
While reports of its usefulness have been anecdotal
to date, technological improvements are developing at a rapid place and the images available are
continually improving (COHEN et al., 1983; GAMSU
et al., 1983). The known advantages of NMR imaging are that no ionizing radiation is used, flow-
ing blood provides a natural contrast medium to
outline the vessels of the mediastinum and hilum
(Fig. 7), and the tomographic section may be oriented in any plane. A hoped for advantage is the
ability to distinguish benign from malignant

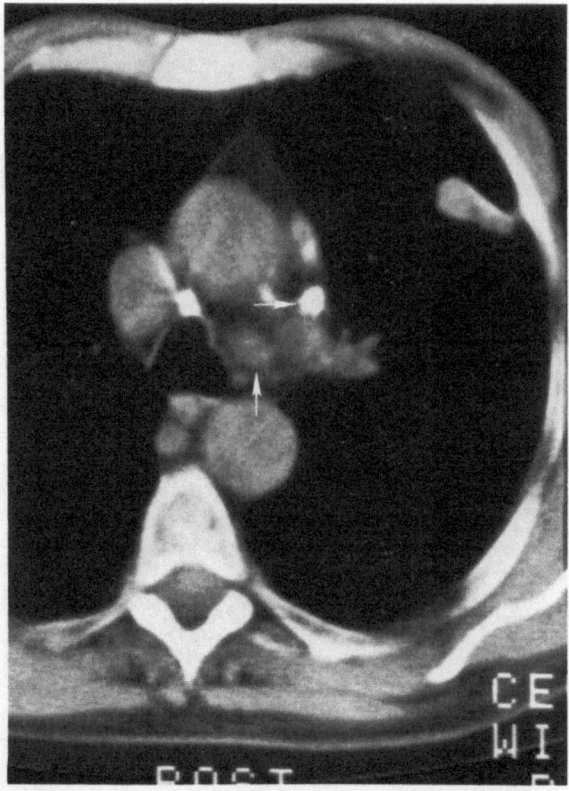

Fig. 5. Lymph nodes indeterminate for metastatic disease.
A carcinoma of the left upper lobe and enlarged mediastinal
lymph nodes (*arrows*) are demonstrated at the level of the
aorticopulmonary window. Some of these lymph nodes are
calcified so that either granulomatous disease or carcinoma
could account for the lymphadenopathy. Carcinoma was
present in the non-calcified lymph nodes

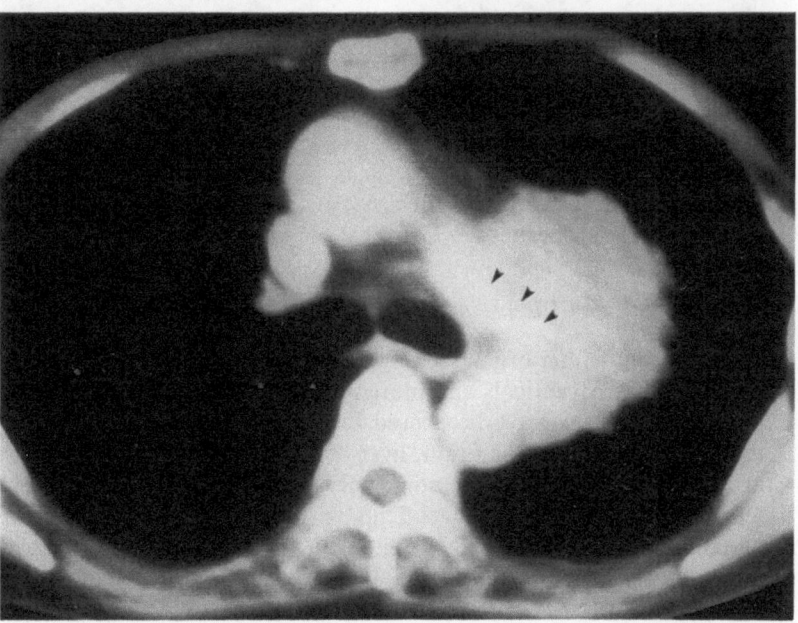

Fig. 6. Encasement of the left
pulmonary artery by tumor.
Computed tomography with
contrast infusion demonstrates
complete encasement of the
pulmonary artery (*arrowheads*) by
a carcinoma at the superior left
hilum

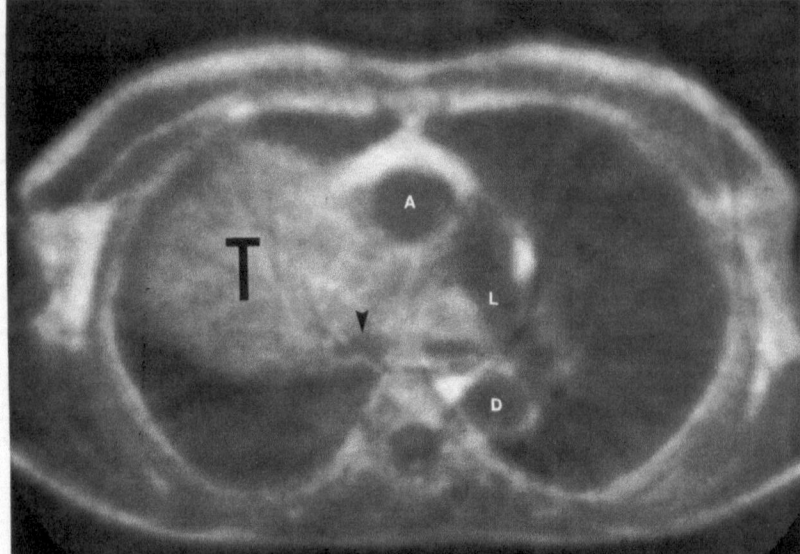

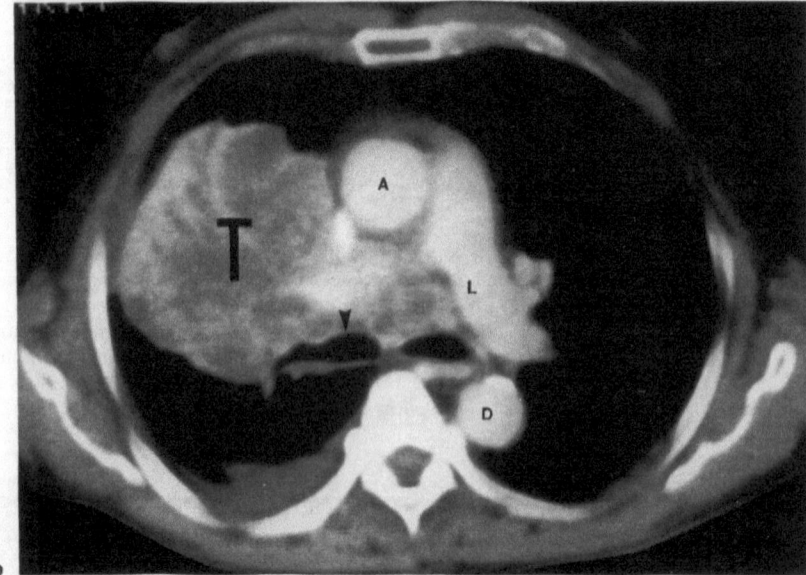

Fig. 7a, b. Nuclear magnetic resonance image of the mediastinum. (**a**) Nuclear magnetic resonance image taken at the level of the carina demonstrates a large cell carcinoma of the right upper lobe. The tumor completely crosses the mediastinum and abuts the left pulmonary artery. Areas of high signal intensity such as fat appear white in the image. Areas of low signal intensity such as the lungs, mediastinal vessels, bronchi, and thoracic musculature appear black. (**b**) The computed tomographic image at the same level shows similar findings to the magnetic resonance image. Although the necrotic nature of the tumor is better appreciated on post contrast infusion computed tomography, advances in nuclear magnetic resonance imaging may change this discrepancy.
A ascending aorta, *D* descending aorta, *L* left pulmonary artery, *T* tumor, *arrowhead* right main stem bronchus

lymph nodes irrespective of their size by analysis of their NMR properties.

3.2.2 Identifying Disease at Distant Sites

Scanning with either organ seeking or tumor seeking radiopharmaceuticals and more recently computed tomography have been used for identification of metastases to the brain, liver and skeleton in patients with lung carcinoma. Radionuclide scans are usually positive in patients with clinical or laboratory evidence suggesting organ involvement (GUTIERREZ et al., 1975; DONATO et al.,

1979; RAMSDELL et al., 1977). However, positive examinations have been reported to be present in 18–37% of patients who are asymptomatic and have normal laboratory values (KELLY et al., 1979). This wide range of positivity has given rise to controversy over the cost effectiveness of these tests in this setting. As previously stated, results are difficult to compare because of different patient selection procedures and methods of performing the examinations.

While most studies evaluate separate multiorgan imaging, whole-body gallium imaging may occasionally demonstrate metastases not found by

Fig. 8. Upper abdominal computed tomographic scan. A patient with small cell carcinoma has enlargement of the left adrenal gland (*arrowhead*), multiple low density areas in the liver and an enlarged retrocrural lymph node (*black arrow*) all representing metastatic disease

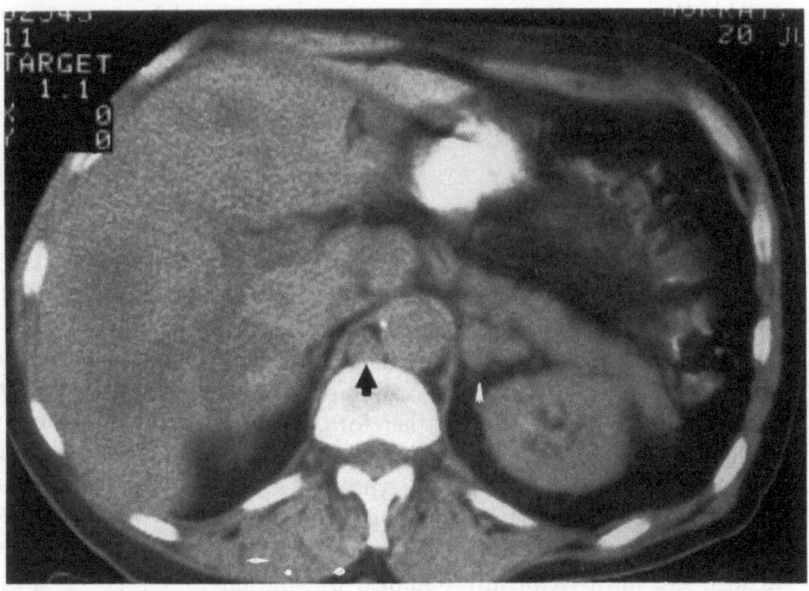

the other procedures (MINTZ et al., 1979). In patients with small cell carcinoma, gallium scanning may be useful in defining the tumor, hilar and mediastinal lymph nodes, and liver metastases in a single test. It is less useful in detecting brain and bone metastases (BITRAN et al., 1981).

Computed tomography has been used to detect metastatic disease in the brain, liver and adrenal. Since brain computed tomography is able to identify small lesions than the radionuclide brain scan, it has generally supplanted it in patient evaluation (MINTZ et al., 1979; LUSINS et al., 1980). The use of brain CT in asymptomatic patients is controversial with regard to cost effectiveness, but it may demonstrate metastatic disease in up to 6% of these patients (JACOBS et al., 1977).

Both computed tomography and liver scintigraphy have a sensitivity for detection of liver metastases of about 90% in patients with a wide variety of neoplasms (SNOW et al., 1979). However, in patients with lung cancer, it has been suggested that the radionuclide scan may be less sensitive than computed tomography (KNOPF et al., 1982). Moreover, upper abdominal computed tomography may detect unsuspected metastatic disease in the lung bases, the upper abdominal lymph nodes or the adrenal glands none of which can be detected by liver spleen scanning. Upper abdominal computed tomography may be particularly beneficial in patients with small cell carcinoma in whom 16–25% will show evidence of liver metastases and a smaller percentage will have other areas involved

(Fig. 8) (DUNNICK et al., 1979). Whether or not computed tomography is the imaging procedure of choice for the upper abdomen depends, in part, on its availability (POON et al., 1982).

Finally, CT has been advocated for routine preoperative evaluation of the adrenal gland in patients with bronchogenic carcinoma (CHAPMAN et al., 1982; SANDLER et al., 1982). Approximately 15% of patients at presentation will be found to have adrenal metastases and in some this may be the only site of metastatic disease. It should be noted that asymptomatic adrenal adenomas are relatively common and histopathological confirmation of metastasis is important.

3.3 Evaluating Regional Pulmonary Function

While the majority of patients with lung cancer may undergo resectional surgery without difficulty, chronic obstructive pulmonary disease is of sufficient severity in about 10–20% of patients to influence the decision regarding surgery (OLSEN et al., 1974). Patients with marginal pulmonary reserve have mortality rates up to 18% and are at risk of becoming respiratory cripples if a pneumonectomy is required (OLSEN et al., 1975). While routine pulmonary physiologic tests may detect decreases in pulmonary function, they do not define the regional distribution of the abnormality. Quantitative nuclear medicine techniques have been developed to evaluate regional ventilation and perfusion as well as predict the postoperative

FEV$_1$ (Wernly 1980). Patients with predicted postoperative FEV$_1$ less than 800 cc are at high risk for developing postoperative respiratory failure and are usually considered non-surgical candidates.

4 Definitive Diagnostic Procedures

Major factors which influence treatment with lung cancer are the histological cell type and the stage of disease. The different types are associated with differences in their natural history and response to treatment. It is not adequate, therefore, to make a diagnosis of lung cancer without knowledge of the cell type as the histological type will affect management. Histological or cytological type will affect management. Histological or cytological diagnosis are most frequently obtained by sputum cytology, cytological examinations of bronchoscopic brush specimens, biopsy at bronchoscopy, or percutaneous needle aspiration.

4.1 Sputum Cytology

Sputum cytology examination can be rewarding in verifying the diagnosis of lung cancer; however, bronchoscopic examination may also be necessary. Postbronchoscopy sputum during the first two hours or the following morning is frequently of value. Early morning sputum represents the best specimen for deep sampling of the lung; induction methods may be used to increase diagnostic yield. Meticulous instruction in coughing and expectorating to secure lower respiratory tract mucous without food contamination is essential, as are prompt fixation and experienced and careful microscopic interpretation. In one study of patients with primary lung cancer, one or two sputum samples yielded a positive result in 59 percent, three sputum in 69%, and four sputa in 85% (Oswald et al., 1971). False positive incidence may vary but is probably less than two the three percent. The diagnostic yield is greater with central (75%) lesions than with peripheral (45%) lesions. Bronchial washings via bronchial catheter under fluoroscopic image-intensifier guidance system and during fibroptic bronchoscopic examination are usually necessary for peripherally located lesions. Sputum cytology correlates very favorably with bronchial brush specimens and with biopsies (Payne et al., 1979).

Cell type as determined correlates with final histology in about 85 to 95% of patients.

4.2 Bronchoscopy and Transthoracic (Percutaneous) Fine Needle Aspiration Biopsy

4.2.1 Bronchoscopy

Most patients suspected of having bronchogenic carcinoma should have endoscopic examination of the tracheobronchial tree (Zavala, 1975; Marsh and Wang, 1983). At present, two types of endoscopes are used widely: the rigid bronchoscope and the flexible fiberoptic bronchoscope. In most instances, the flexible fiberoptic bronchoscope is preferred because it is better tolerated by patients and permits improved visualization of the tracheobronchial tree. It has a high efficiency (80 to 90%) in confirming a diagnosis when transbronchial biopsy, brush specimens, and cytological study of bronchial secretions are used along with directed biopsy of suspected lesions. Bronchoscopy is a minor, safe procedure that is usually performed on an out-patient basis. The rigid bronchoscope is still used particularly for lesions of the proximal bronchial tree and for occasional preoperative assessment of resectability.

In addition to confirming lung cancer, bronchoscopy helps determine resectability and extent of disease (Robbins et al., 1981). The length of normal bronchi proximal to the tumor and the status of the carina may be determined. The presence or absence of immobility and rigidity of either main stem bronchus, as well as the bronchus intermedius on the right may be assessed. Rigidity and fixation of this area and widening of the carina imply unresectability. Finding bilateral tumors, vocal cord paralysis, or small cell carcinoma would indicate incurability.

Transbronchial lung biopsy consists of inserting biopsy forceps or a needle via the instrumentation channel of the fiberoptic bronchoscope, through the bronchial wall to the target lesion site under x-ray television monitoring (Anderson, 1978; Wang et al., 1978; Herf et al., 1977). It is a relatively safe procedure with a diagnostic rate of 60 to 80% in diffuse pulmonary disease or peripheral nodules. The complication rate is about 5 to 15%. Pneumothorax occurs in about five percent, most heal spontaneously, others require a tube thoracostomy. Bleeding is frequent with bloody sputum or hemoptysis.

4.2.2 Percutaneous (Transthoracic) Needle Biopsy

Material from peripherally located lung lesions that cannot be reached by bronchoscope may be obtained by percutaneous needle aspiration under fluoroscopic control (SINNER, 1979; SMITH et al., 1974). The success rate may be as high as 80 to 90% with lesions of 1.5 cm or larger. This is a valuable procedure not only for coin lesions but in other pulmonary lesions where one wants histologic confirmation short of thoracotomy. The technique is applicable to suspected malignancy in surgical poor risk patients or those with obvious bone or brain metastases in whom sputum cytology and bronchoscopic washings have failed to provide diagnosis. If the lesion is large and close to the chest wall, this technique is safe and productive. If the lesion is small and lies deep in the lung, pneumothorax, intrapulmonary hemorrhage, and hemoptysis may be significant complications. Rare complications include air embolism, massive hemorrhage, or implantation of the needle tract with malignant cells.

4.3 Mediastinoscopy and Mediastinotomy

Mediastinoscopy and mediastinotomy have a major role in bronchogenic carcinoma (SARIN and NOHL-OSER, 1969; GOLDBERG et al., 1983; CARLENS, 1959; MCNEIL and CHAMBERLAIN, 1966; LARSSON, 1973; PEARSON, 1968; PAGE et al., 1980; JOLLY et al., 1980). In some cases, these procedures lead to a histological diagnosis when other diagnostic methods have failed. However, these examinations are essentially a staging procedure. The results of these examinations will separate resectable cases with considerable accuracy. The low morbidity and negligible mortality of these procedures makes them an excellent means to predict who will benefit from thoracotomy and resection.

4.3.1 Mediastinoscopy

Mediastinoscopy consists of making a small incision in the supra-sternal notch with blunt dissection to the tracheal carina and inserting the mediastinoscope into the upper mediastinum. Lymph nodes in the area are then biopsied. In lung cancer, the degree of lymphatic spread to the mediastinum determines survival rate after surgical treatment. The presence of lymph node enlargement in the mediastinum does not always indicate metastases and conversely about one-third of patients with apparently normal mediastinum on x-rays will have microscopic spread to the nodes.

Mediastinoscopy is generally a safe procedure with a very low morbidity rate and a mortality

rate of less than 0.5%. However, complications can arise such as hemorrhage, pneumothorax, mediastinal emphysema, mediastinitis, implantation metastases, perforation of the esophagus, or injury to the recurrent laryngeal nerve.

4.3.2 Anterior Mediastinotomy

Anterior mediastinotomy may be employed for evaluation of surgical resectability and diagnosis. This consists of resection of the second or third intercostal cartilage to expose the lung root. It may be advantageous for left upper lobe and left hilar lesion to detect spread to subaortic and anterior mediastinal lymph nodes and for diagnosis in cases of superior cava obstruction (MCNEIL and CHAMBERLAIN, 1966; PAGE et al., 1980; JOLLY et al., 1980). Complications are similar to mediastinoscopy.

4.4 Biopsy of Distant Metastatic Focus

The biopsy of a distant metastatic site (i.e. lymph node, skin nodule, pleura, liver, bone marrow) precludes successful resection. Scalene lymph nodes are often the first extrathoracic manifestation of lung cancer and when a node is palpable in this area, even though it is less than 1 cm in diameter, in a patient with known lung cancer, it is likely to contain metastases; only about 3 to 4% of non-palpable scalene nodes contain metastases (DANIELS, 1949). Likewise, metastases in other lymph nodes, subcutaneous nodules, liver, bone marrow, or pleura are readily biopsied so that the diagnosis may be made easily from such lesions.

Bone marrow involvement is particularly common with small cell lung cancer and bilateral bone marrow aspirate and biopsy has a high diagnostic yield even when peripheral blood values are normal. The presence of anemia, leukopenia, leukocytosis, thrombocytopenia, and thrombocytosis is often associated with marrow involvement. A leukoerythroblastic peripheral blood picture is indicative of bone marrow involvement (IHDE et al., 1979).

Abnormalities in liver function tests when correlated with liver scan are suggestive of metastatic involvement. Liver biopsy may be performed percutaneously or at laparoscopic examination.

Lung cancer sometimes first presents clinically as involvement of the pleural (more commonly) or pericardium (less commonly) by direct or lymphatic extension. Thoracentesis or pericardiocentesis fluid cytology may yield a diagnosis in 40 to 50% of cases. Multiple specimens increase the diagnostic yield. A combination of cytology and closed needle biopsy of pleura may provide the diagnosis in up to 80 to 90% of cases (Salyer et al., 1975; Winkelman and Pfitzer, 1981).

4.5 Exploratory Thoracotomy

It is rarely necessary to resort to thoracotomy to establish a diagnosis. One should understand that this is a major operative intervention that is not well tolerated by older patients with associated chronic obstructive pulmonary disease and heart disease. The operative mortality rate ranges between two and ten percent depending on patient selection and surgeon skill (Bryer et al., 1981; Nagasaki et al., 1982).

Possible exception is the patient with the solitary pulmonary nodule that is uncalcified and is either unstable (doubling time less than two years) or of unknown stability (no previous chest x-ray to permit calculation of growth rate). Resection of solitary malignant nodule results in a five-year cure rate of 30 to 50% (Jackman et al., 1969).

References

Alazraki N (1980) Usefulness of gallium imaging in the evaluation of lung cancer, CRC Critical Reviews in Diagnostic Imaging 13:249–267.

Anderson HA (1978) Transbronchoscopic lung biopsy for diffuse pulmonary diseases, Chest 73:734–736.

Baron RL, Levitt RG, Sagel SS, et al (1982) Computed tomography in the preoperative evaluation of bronchogenic carcinoma, Radiology 145:727–732.

Bitran JD, Bekerman C, Pinski S (1981) Sequential scintigraphic staging of small cell carcinoma, Cancer 47:1971–1975.

Breyer RH, Karstaedt N, Mills SA, Johnston FR, Choplin RH, Wolfman NT, Hudspeth AS, Cordell AR. Computed tomography for evaluation of mediastinal lymph nodes in lung cancer: correlation with surgical staging, Annals of Thoracic Surgery (To be published)

Breyer RH, Zippe C, Pharr WF, et al (1981) Thoracotomy in patients over age seventy years, ten-year experience, J Thorac Cardiovasc Surg 81:187–193.

Broder LE, Primack A (1983) Marker substances in bronchogenic carcinoma: a review. In: Strauss MJ (ed) Lung cancer – clinical diagnosis and treatment. Grune and Stratton, New York, pp. 37–61.

Byrd RB, Divertie MB, Spittell JA (1967) Bronchogenic carcinoma and thromboembolic disease, JAMA 202:1019–1022.

Carlens E (1959) Mediastinoscopy: a method for ispection and tissue biopsy of the superior mediastinum, Dis Chest 36:343–352.

Chapman GS, Kumar D, Redmond J IV, et al (1982) Upper

abdominal CT scanning in staging non-oat-cell lung carcinoma, J Engl J Med 307:189.

Cherington M (1976) Guanidine and germine in Eaton-Lambert syndrome, Neurology 26:944–946.

Cohen AM, Creviston S, LiPuma JP, et al (1983) NMR evaluation of hilar and mediastinal lymphadenopathy, Radiology 148:739–742.

Cohen MH (1983) Signs and symptoms of bronchogenic carcinoma. In: Strauss MJ (ed) Lung cancer – clinical diagnosis and treatment. Grune and Stratton, New York, pp. 97–111.

Crowther D, Bateman CJT (1972) Malignant disease, Clin Hematol 1:447–473.

Cuttitta F, Rosen S, Gazdar AF et al (1981) Monoclonal antibodies that demonstrate specificity for several types of human lung cancer, Proc Nat Acad Sci USA 78:4591–4595.

Dalal PR, Rosenthal R, Sarkar TK (1980) Leukemoid reaction in pulmonary carcinoma, J Natl Med Assoc 72:683–686.

Daniels AC (1949) A method of biopsy useful in diagnosing certain intrathoracic diseases, Dis Chest 16:360–367.

Davies IJT, Musa M, Dormandy TL (1968) Measurements of plasma zinc. Part I: In health and disease, Part II: In malignant disease, J Clin Pathol 21:359–365.

Dent PB, McCulloch PB, Wesley-James O, et al (1978) Measurement of carcinoembryonic antigen in patients with bronchogenic carcinoma, Cancer 42:1484–1491.

Donato AT, Ammerman EG, Sullesta O (1979) Bone scanning in the evaluation of patients with lung cancer, Ann Thorac Surg 27:300–304.

Dunnick NR, Ihde DC, Johnston-Early A (1979) Abdominal CT in the evaluation of small cell carcinoma of the lung, AJR 133:1085–1088.

Faling LJ, Pugatch RD, Jung-Legg Y, et al (1981) Computed tomographic scanning of the mediastinum in the staging of bronchogenic carcinoma, Am Rev Respir Dis 124:690–695.

Fraser RG, Pare JAP (1978) Diagnosis of diseases of the chest, 2nd ed. WB Saunders, Philadelphia, pp. 1002–1073.

Fusco FD, Rosen SW (1966) Gonadotropin-producing anaplastic large-cell carcinomas of the lung, N Engl J Med 275:507–515.

Gamsu G, Webb WR, Sheldon P, et al (1983) Nuclear Magnetic resonance imaging of the thorax, Radiology 147:473–480.

Gazdar AF, Carney DN, Minna JD (1983) The biology of non-small cell lung cancer, Semin Oncol 10:3–19.

Goldenberg DM, Deland F, Kin E, et al (1978) Use of radiolabeled antibodies to carcinoembryonic antigen for the detection and localization of diverse cancers by external photoscanning, N Engl J Med 298:1384–1388.

Goldberg EM, Goldberg MC, Bekerman C (1983) Mediastinoscopy in assessment of lung cancer. In: Strauss MJ (ed) Lung cancer – clinical diagnosis and treatment. Grune and Stratton, New York, pp. 135–155.

Gropp C, Havemann K. Lehmann FG (1978) Carcinoembryonic antigen and ferratin in patients with lung cancer before and during therapy, Cancer 42:2802–2808.

Gropp C, Havemann K, Scheuer A (1980) Ectopic hormones in lung cancer patients at diagnosis and during therapy, Cancer 46:347–354.

Gutierrez AC, Vincent RG, Bakshi S et al (1975) Radioisotope scans in the evaluation of metastatic bronchogenic carcinoma, J Thorac Cardiovasc Surg 69:934–941.

Hammond D, Winnick S (1974) Paraneoplastic erythrocytosis and ectopic erythropoietins, Ann NY Acad Sci 230:219–227.

Hansen M, Hammer M, Hummer L (1980) ACTH, ADH, and calcitonin as markers of response and relapse in small cell lung cancer, Cancer 46:2062–2067.

Heitzman ER, Markarian B, Raasch BN, et al (1982) Pathways of tumor spread through the lung: radiologic correlations with anatomy and pathology, Radiology 144:3–14.

Henderson RD, Bosko A, van Nostrand AWP (1974) Pharyngoesophageal dysphagia and recurrent laryngeal nerve palsey, J Thorac Cardiovasc Surg 68:507–512.

Herf SM, Suratt PM, Arora NS (1977) Deaths and complications associated with transbronchial lung biopsy, Am Rev Respir Dis 115:708–711.

Horne McK III, McAnally TP (1978) Hemolytic anemia with lung carcinoma: case reports, Milit Med 143:188–189.

Ihde DC, Simms EB, Matthews MJ, et al (1979) Bone marrow metastases in small cell carcinoma of the lung: frequency, distribution, and influence on chemotherapeutic toxicity and prognosis, Blood 53:677–686.

Isobe T, Osserman EF (1971) Pathologic conditions associated with plasma cell dyscrasias: a study of 806 cases, Ann NY Acad Sci 190:507–518.

Jackman RJ, Good CA, Clagett OT, et al (1969) Survival rates in peripheral bronchogenic carcinomas up to four centimeters in diameter presenting as solitary pulmonary nodules, J Thorac Cardiovas Surg 57:1–8.

Jacobs L, Kinkel WR, Vincent RG (1977) 'Silent' brain metastases from lung carcinoma determined by computerized tomography, Arch Neurol 34:690–693.

Jolly PC, Weil L, Anderson RP (1980) Anterior and cervical mediastinoscopy for determining operability and predicting resectability in lung cancer, J Thorac Cardiovasc Surg 79:366–371.

Joynt RJ (1974) The brain's uneasy peace with tumors, Ann NY Acad Sci 230:342–347.

Kelly RJ, Cowan RJ, Ferree CB, et al (1979) Efficacy of radionuclide scanning in patients with lung cancer, JAMA 242:2855–2857.

Knopf DR, Torres WE, Fajman WJ, et al (1982) Liver lesions: comparative accuracy of scintigraphy and computed tomography, AJR 138:623–627.

Larsson S (1973) Pretreatment classification and staging of bronchogenic carcinoma, Scand J Thorac Cardiovasc Surg 7 (Suppl 10):1–147.

Leff A, Hopewell PC, Costello J (1978) Pleural effusion from malignancy, Ann Intern Med 88:532–537.

Libshitz HI (1983) CT of mediastinal lymph nodes in lung cancer: is there a "State of the Art"?, AJR 141:1081–1085.

Lokich JJ (1978) Tumor markers: hormones, antigens, and enzymes in malignant disease, Oncology 35:54–57.

Lusins JO, Chayes Z, Nakagawa H (1980) Computed tomography and radionuclide brain scanning, NY State J Med 80:185–189.

Mahajan V, Kupferer CF, Van Ordstrand HS (1975) Pneumothorax: a rare manifestation of primary lung cancer, Chest 68:730–732.

Margolis R, Hansen HH, Muggia FM, et al (1974) Diagnosis of liver metastases in bronchogenic carcinoma: a comparative study of liver scans, function tests and peritoneoscopy with liver biopsy in 111 patients, Cancer 34:1825–1829.

Markman M (1982) Pretreatment peripheral blood counts in small-cell carcinoma of the lung, JAMA 248:550.

Marsh BR, Wang KP (1983) Bronchoscopy. In: Strauss MJ (ed) Lung cancer – clinical diagnosis and treatment, Grune and Stratton, New York, pp. 127–133.

McNeil TM, Chamberlin JM (1966) Diagnostic anterior mediastinotomy, Ann Thorac Surg 2:532–539.

Merrill WW, Bondy PK (1982) Production of biochemical marker substances by bronchogenic carcinomas, In: Matthay RA (ed) Clin Chest Med 3(2):307–320.

Miller JI, Mansour KA, Hatcher CR (1979) Carcinoma of the superior pulmonary sulcus, Ann Thorac Surg 28:4–47.

Mintz U, DeMeester TR, Golomb HM, et al (1979) Sequential staging in bronchogenic carcinoma, Chest 76:653–657.

Mintzer RA, Malave SR, Neiman HL, et al (1979) Computed vs conventional tomography in evaluation of primary and secondary pulmonary neoplasms, Radiology 132:653–659.

Moak GD, Cockerill EM, Farber MO, et al (1982) Computed tomography vs standard radiology in the evaluation of mediastinal adenopathy, Chest 82:69–75.

Moody TW, Russell EK, O'Donohue TL, et al (1983) Bombesin-like peptides in small cell lung cancer: biochemical characterization and secretion from a cell line, Life Sci 32:487–493.

Morton DL, Itabashi HH, Grimes OF (1966) Nonmetastatic neurological complications of bronchogenic carcinoma: the carcinomatous neuromyopathies, J Thorac Cardiovasc Surg 51:14–29.

Nagasaki F, Flehinger BJ, Martini N (1982) Complications of surgery in the treatment of carcinoma of the lung, Chest 82:25–29.

Nieweg OE, Beekhuis H, Piers DA, et al (1983) [57]Co-bleomycin and ^{67}Ga-citrate in detecting and staging lung cancer, Thorax 38:16–21.

Olsen GN, Block AJ, Tobias JA (1974) Prediction of post pneumoonectomy pulmonary function using quantitative macroaggregate lung scanning, Chest 66:13–16.

Olsen GN, Block AJ, Swenson ED, et al (1975) Pulmonary function evaluation of the lung resection candidate: a prospective study, Am Rev Respir Dis 111:379–387.

Osborne DR, Korobkin M, Ravin CE, et al (1982) Comparison of plain radiography, conventional tomography, and computed tomography in detecting intrathoracic lymph node metastases from lung carcinoma, Radiology 142:157–161.

Oswald NC, Hinson KFW, Canti G, et al (1971) The diagnosis of primary lung cancer with special reference to sputum cytology, Thorax 26:623–631.

Pagé A, Mercier C, Verdant A, et al (1980) Parasternal mediastinoscopy in bronchial carcinoma of the left upper lobe, Can J Surg 23:171–172.

Pannier R, Verlinde I, Puspowidjono I, et al (1982) The role of gallium-67 thoracic scintigraphy in the diagnosis and staging of patients suspected of bronchial carcinoma, Thorax 37:264–269.

Payne CR, Stovin PGI, Barker V, et al (1979) Diagnostic accuracy of cytology and biopsy in primary bronchial carcinoma, Thorax 34:294–299.

Pearson FG (1968) An evaluation of mediastinoscopy in the management of presumably operable bronchial carcinoma, J Thorac Cardiovasc Surg 55:617–625.

Poon PY, Feld R, Evans WK et al (1982) Computed tomography of the brain, liver, and upper abdomen in the staging of small cell carcinoma of the lung, J Comput Assist Tomogr 6:963–965.

Proto A (1983) CT analysis of the pulmonary nodule, Radiology 149(P):42.

Ramsdell JW, Peters RM, Taylor AT Jr, et al (1977) Multiorgan scans for staging lung cancer. Correlation with clinical evaluation, J Thorac Cardiovasc Surg 73:653–659.

Rea HH, Shevland JE, House AJS (1981) Accuracy of computed tomographic scanning in assessment of the mediastinum in bronchial carcinoma, J Thorac Cardiovasc Surg 81:825–829.

Richards F II, Muss HB, White DR, et al (1978) Current concepts: management of lung cancer, NC Med J 39:535–540.

Rittgers RA, Loewenstein MS, Feinerman AE, et al (1978) Carcinoembryonic antigen levels in benign and malignant pleural effusions, Ann Intern Med 88:631–636.

Robbins HM, Sweet ME, Jefferson SE, et al (1981) The determination of resectability of lung cancer by fiberoptic bronchoscopy, Arch Intern Med 141:649–650.

Rosenow EC III, Carr DT (1979) Bronchogenic carcinoma, CA 29:233–245.

Rudman D, Chawla RK, Nixon DW, et al (1979) Proteinuria with disseminated neoplastic disease, Cancer Res 39:699–703.

Sack GH Jr, Levin J, Bell WR (1977) Trousseau's syndrome and other manifestations of chronic disseminated coagulopathy in patients with neoplasms: clinical pathophysiologic, and therapeutic features, Medicine 56:1–37.

Salsali M, Cliffton EE (1968) Superior vena caval obstruction with lung cancer, Ann Thorac Surg 6:437–42.

Salyer WR, Eggleston JC, Erozan YS (1975) Efficacy of pleural needle biopsy and pleural fluid cytopathology in the diagnosis of malignant neoplasm involving the pleura, Chest 67:536–539.

Sandler MA, Pearlberg JL, Madrazo BL, et al (1982) Computed tomographic evaluation of the adrenal gland in the preoperative assessment of bronchogenic carcinoma, Radiology 145:733–736.

Sarin CL, Nohl-Oser HC (1969) Mediastinoscopy: a clinical evaluation of 400 consecutive cases, Thorax 24:585–588.

Schumacher HR Jr, (1976) Articular manifestation of hypertrophic pulmonary osteoarthropathy in bronchogenic carcinoma, Arthritis Rheum 19:629–636.

Shevland JE, Chiu LC, Schapior RL, et al (1978) The role of conventional tomography and computed tomography in assessing the resectability of primary lung cancer: a preliminary report, CT 2:1–19.

Shields R (1978) Ectopic hormone production by tumours, Nature 272:494.

Shimm DS, Logue GL, Rigsby LC (1981) Evaluating the superior vena cava syndrome, JAMA 245:951–953.

Siegelman SS, Zerhouni EA, Leo FP, et al (1980) CT of the solitary pulmonary nodule, AJR 135:1–13.

Silvis SE, Turkbas N, Doscherholmen A (1970) Thrombocytosis in patients with lung cancer, JAMA 211:1852–1853.

Sinner WN (1979) Pulmonary neoplasms diagnosed with transthoracic needle biopsy, Cancer 43:1533–1540.

Smith J, McSweeney JJ, Melamed MR, et al (1974) Percutaneous needle aspiration lung biopsy, Clin Bull 4:63–68.

Snow JH Jr, Goldstein HM, Wallace S (1979) Comparison of scintigraphy, sonography, and computed tomography in the evaluation of hepatic neoplasm, AJR 132:915–918.

Spechler SJ, Esposito AL, Koff RS, et al (1978) Lactic acidosis in oat cell carcinoma with extensive hepatic metastases, Arch Intern Med 138:1663–1664.

Steiner H, Dahlbäck O, Waldenström J (1968) Ectopic growth-hormone production and osteoarthropathy in carcinoma of the bronchus, Lancet 1:783–785.

Strauss BL, Matthews MJ, Cohen MH, et al (1977) Cardiac metastases in lung cancer, Chest 71:607–611.

Sunderman FW Jr (1964) Studies of the serum proteins. VI. Recent advances in clinical interpretation of electrophoretic fractionations, Am J Clin Pathol 42:1–21.

Theros EG (1977) Varying manifestations of peripheral pulmonary neoplasms: a radiology-pathologic correlative study, AJR 128:893–914.

Torstensson S, Thorén M, Hall K (1980) Plasma ACTH in patients with bronchogenic carcinoma, Acta Med Scand 207:353–357.

Umsawasdi T, Valdivieso M (1982) Paraneoplastic syndromes in lung cancer, Semin Resp Med 3:200–209.

Underwood GH Jr, Hooper RG, Axelbaum SP, et al (1979) Computed tomographic scanning of the thorax in the staging of bronchogenic carcinoma, New Engl J Med 300:777–778.

Varindani MK, Ptichumoni CS, Lucariello RJ (1982) Eosinophilic leukemoid reaction in pulmonary carcinoma, NY State J Med 82:347–348.

Vincent FM (1978) Paraneoplastic CNS and renal syndromes, JAMA 240:862–863.

Vincent RG (1982) Biologic markers in lung cancer, Semin Respir Med 3:184–193.

Waalkes TP, Abeloff MD, Ettinger DS, et al (1983) Serum protein-bound carbohydrates and small cell carcinoma of the lung, Cancer 52:131–139.

Wallace RJ, Cohen A, Awe RJ, et al (1979) Carcinomatous lung abscess: diagnosis by bronchoscopy and cytopathology, JAMA 242:521–522.

Wang KP, Terry P, Marsh B (1978) Bronchoscopic needle aspiration biopsy of paratracheal tumor, Am Rev Respir Dis 118:17–21.

Wernly JA, DeMeester TR, Kirchner PT, et al (1980) Clinical value of quantitative ventilation-perfusion lung scans in the surgical management of bronchogenic carcinoma, J Thorac Cardiovasc Surg 80:535–543.

Whank-Peng J, Kao-Shan CS, Lee EC (1982) Specific chromosomal defect associated with human small cell lung cancer: deletion 3p(14–23), Science 215:181–189.

Winkelmann M, Pfitzer P (1981) Blind pleural biopsy in combination with cytology of pleural effusions, Acta Cytol 25:373–376.

Wolfe HJ (1978) Tumor-cell markers: a biological shell game?, N Engl J Med 299:146–147.

Wolfsen AR, Odell WD (1979) Pro ACTH: use for early detection of lung cancer, Am J Med 66:765–772.

Zavala DC (1975) Diagnostic fiberoptic bronchoscopy: techniques and results of biopsy in 600 patients, Chest 68:12–19.

Chapter VI Radiation Therapy in Cancer of the Lung

Thomas O'Connor

CONTENTS

1 Introduction

Technique in any discipline is the acting out of the thinking process. It does not exist isolated from the stream of the general care of a patient with lung cancer; it is not an end in itself. It is a means to an end, either the creation of conditions that will allow for a cure of the patient or the palliation of his symptoms if cure is precluded by the extent of his disease.

Lung cancer is not a new disease. The review of the 19th Century literature by MILTON ROSEN-

Thomas O'Connor, M.D., Chief of Radiation Therapy Community Hospitals, 1500 North Ritter Avenue, Indianapolis, IN 46219, USA

BLATT illustrates that quite adequately (ROSEN-BLATT, 1964). While there is general consensus that the incidence of lung cancer has increased since the beginning of the 20th Century, it was known to our predecessors in all of its lethal manifestations of locally extensive disease, superior vena caval obstruction, bone metastases, brain metastases, spinal cord compression, as well as the increasing incidence at autopsy. Even a scheme of pathogenesis was known or hypothesized with the speculated sites of origin being the bronchial mucosa, the bronchial mucous gland and the alveolus. However, the major distinction came to be the distinction made between cancer of the lung and tuberculosis, however, the importance of this distinction became consequential only after the successful chemotherapy for tuberculosis.

According to American Cancer Society statistics of 1983, cancer of the lung will be the site of 22% of all male cancers and 9% of all female cancers in the U.S.A. (SILVERBERG, 1983). It will be the first cause of death in 35% of all male cancers and in 17% of all female cancers, the second most frequent cause of death after carcinoma of the breast. 10,124 men between 35–54 will die as will 46,049 men from 55–74. Tragically, the incidence continues to rise in both men and women. The total number of patients involved is 135,000 (94,000 men and 41,000 women). 117,000 of these will die (83,000 men and 34,000 women). The 5-year survival of patients with lung cancer has risen by 2% from 1960–63 to 1970–73. It rose from 8% to 10% for whites and 5% to 7% for blacks.

Successful treatment of cancer of the lung is dictated by the extent of disease at the time of diagnosis. This sad reality is demonstrated by the consistent 25% survivability of patients with cancer of the lung who are resected (SELAWRY et al., 1973). Simply, this means that after curative resection 75% of the patients with cancer of the lung will die of their disease. Those with small cell carcinoma will behave as though they already have metastatic disease, and non-small cell cancers of the lung will behave according to the extent of their disease at the time of diagnosis (Mountain et al., 1974).

The forces of mortality in cancer of the lung are associated with the histological cell type of the tumor, the extent of the primary tumor designated as the T Compartment, the presence or absence of metastatic events within regional nodes designated the N Compartment, and the presence or absence of distant metastases designated the M Compartment.

Histological classification of the primary tumor indicates that the prognosis for squamous cell carcinoma has a superior prognosis versus the adenocarcinoma or undifferentiated large cell carcinoma which have the same survival curve. Patients with undifferentiated small cell carcinoma of the lung have a tragic course with virtually no hope of rescue by loco-regional therapy (Mountain et al., 1974). The hope for small cell cancer is based upon systemic treatment which is predominantly chemotherapy plus adjuvant radiotherapy in some ill-defined role. There have been some successes in this effort, but thus far there is little to celebrate since true success, i.e. cure of the patient with tolerable toxicity, is still elusive (Einhorn, 1983).

Primary cancers of the lung begin in the bronchial mucosa as a consequence of some carcinogenic events. The tumor will grow according to rules that are dictated by its biology and anatomical environment. It will also change in its cellular characteristics so that the tumor that is clinically apparent is a polyclonal system with multiple phenotypes demonstrating remarkable biological diversity (Fidler et al., 1982). This phenotypic diversity, which allows selected variants to develop from the primary tumor, means not only that primary tumor and metastases differ in their responses to treatment, but also that individual metastases differ from one another. Also, the forces of evolution acting on a tumor usually cause the metastatic lesion to become more malignant with more rapid growth and metastatic potential. Although the possibility of evolution to a less malignant form can occur, it probably does so with small frequency. However, this process could explain the phenomenon of spontaneous regression of tumor as well as the very large metastases with either small or undiagnosable primary tumors.

Prognostic factors associated with the primary tumor, T Compartment, are related to its size, its location, external margination, complications such as atelectasis, obstructive pneumonitis, pleural effusion or some evidence of local extension such as hoarseness, chest pain or dysphagia. There is

a reciprocal correlation between the increasing anatomical extent of the primary tumor and survivability (Mountain et al., 1974). T_1 squamous cell carcinoma will have a 5-year survival of 48% versus 29% for T_2 versus less than 10% for T_3. Adenocarcinoma, T_1, has a 5-year survival of 32% with a fall to 14% for T_2 to less than 5% for T_3. Undifferentiated large cell carcinoma has a 18% 5-year survival for T_1 lesions, 18% for T_2 lesions and a nonexistent 5-year survival for T_3 lesions (Mountain et al., 1974).

The influence of the regional node compartment on survival is consequential in that a new event has occured, i.e. metastases, and metastases are different in their behavior from the primary tumor in their growth and response to treatment (Fidler et al., 1982). This difference in biological behavior and presence of lymph nodal metastases at the hilum, as well as in the mediastinum, is reflected in survival.

Squamous cell carcinoma with no nodes involved (N_0) has a 5-year survival of 30% versus 18% for adenocarcinoma versus 20% for undifferentiated squamous cell carcinoma. However, progression of N_1 status, i.e. ipsilateral hilar nodal involvement, produces a 5-year survival of 16% for large cell carcinoma, 8% for adenocarcinoma and 6% for large cell carcinoma. An N_2 status, mediastinal adenopathy, produces a catastrophically low 5% 5-year survival for squamous cell carcinoma, 2% for adenocarcinoma and less than 2% for large cell carcinoma. It can be seen that the presence of a metastatic event N_0 to N_1 or N_2 has serious prognostic consequences.

Evidence of disease in the metastatic compartment, M_1, produces a fall in 5-year survival from the M_0 state of 38% to zero for squamous cell carcinoma, 19% to nearly zero for the adenocarcinoma and 17% to nearly zero for the large cell carcinoma. Included in the M_1 state are the scalene/cervical lymph nodes, as well as the contralateral hilum and distant organs (Mountain et al., 1974).

The causes of death in lung cancer are predominantly related to extensive local tumor and associated complications or distant metastases. In 271/633 cases the cause of death was pulmonary infection, 147/633 widespread metastases and 102/633 due to heart and pericardial involvement by tumor (Luomanen and Watson, 1968).

Given an overall survival rate of about 5%, is it feasible that improved local control will produce an increase in survival? Are there sufficiently large numbers of patients with T_+ N_+ M_0 disease to warrant increased efforts at local control given the present state of the patients at the time of diagnosis? We know that the American Cancer Society no longer recommends routine chest x-ray looking for neoplastic disease, since the control group and the study group had the same numbers of deaths (American Cancer Society, 1980).

In an autopsy series from 1935 of 69 cases, 11% of patients with squamous cell carcinoma had only the primary tumor and 18% had only the primary and regional nodes at the time of death. Twelve percent of patients with adenocarcinoma had only the primary tumor and 6% more had extended into the regional nodes. Undifferentiated carcinoma had no patient without at least evidence of nodal metastases, and only 5% of the total had no distant metastases (OLSEN, 1935). At least in the non-intervened, there exists a quantity of patients who are either $T_+ N_0 M_0$ or $T_+ N_+ M_0$ that exceeds the present 5-year survival rate who potentially could benefit from improved loco-regional control of their lung cancer.

2 Patient Selection

The military metaphor is frequently used in reference to cancer with terms like crusade, aggressive treatment, war on cancer, etc. (SONTAG, 1979). However, the use of triage is used only in terms of trauma in medicine. It is applicable to the Radiation Oncologist in his evaluation of the patient with lung cancer. The Radiation Oncologists divide the patient population into three divisions (Triage): (1) those patients who are potentially curable, i.e. $T_+ N_0 M_0$ or $T_+ N_+ M_0$; (2) those who are not curable, M_+, but are symptomatic from their lung cancer; (3) those who are not curable, but are asymptomatic from their cancer. The method of triage is primarily the elimination by history, physical, radiological and laboratory means of evidence for metastatic disease. The sites of metastases are independent of the cell types of lung cancer, but the frequency is related to cell type with undifferentiated cancers being most frequent, adenocarcinoma intermediate and the squamous cell carcinoma being least frequent.

The sites of metastases via the lymphatic system are most frequent into the hilar nodes 502/676, mediastinal nodes 420/676 and 129/676 into the supraclavicular nodes. Sites of hematogenous metastases are 296/676 in the adrenal glands, 289/676 in the liver, 234/676 in the bone and 130/676 in the brain (LUOMANEN and WATSON, 1968).

In this entire series there were only 83/676 single metastatic sites, 16/676 to the other lung, 16/676 to the bone, 15/676 to the liver, 13/676 to the brain, 12/676 to the heart and 11/676 to the adrenals (LUOMANEN and WATSON, 1968).

The metastatic pattern of cancer of the lung therefore dictates the evaluation to eliminate patients from the potentially curable group and place them into the palliative group. Evaluation of the patient who is non-resectable is already placed into the T_3 or $T_{1-2} N_2$ group with an associated poor survival of 5% or less. In these patients evaluation of the retroperitoneum with CT to investigate the liver, adrenal glands and para-aortic nodes is appropriate with useful results present in 4/16 patients with non-oat cell cancers of the lung, i.e. adrenal metastases (CHAPMAN et al., 1982).

In a larger series CT evaluation of biopsy proven non-oat cell cancers of the lung showed adrenal masses in 21.4% of the patients (NEILSEN et al., 1982). Another series, 110 patients by SANDLER, showed a 10% positive rate in the adrenal glands (SANDLER et al., 1982). In small cell carcinoma of the lung where metastases are known to be more frequent from autopsy studies, the CT of the upper abdomen was positive in 16/45 (36%) patients with the most common site being the liver in 27% of the patients (DUNNICK et al., 1979).

Evaluation of the patient's brain without symptoms by CT has produced a pre-operative positivity of 6% (JACOBS et al., 1977). These patients otherwise would have been subjected to attempted resection. This same frequency, 5%, of silent brain metastases was shown by BUTLER et al. (1979). It seems, therefore, that the use of the CT scan to evaluate the upper abdomen can uncover metastatic diseases with a useful frequency of 10–25%, while CT scans of the brain will uncover metastases at about a 5% rate. The detection of disease outside of the chest is sufficient to change the patient from one with curative potential to an individual who may need no treatment at the present, or to one who needs an intervention to a site other than the primary site.

History, the most important part of the examination, along with physical examination indicates evidence for poor prognostic factors or suggests lines of inquiry to develop evidence for poor prognostic factors. The poor prognostic factors are acute pneumonia dyspnea, loss of weight, anorexia, asthenia more so than cough, chest pain, fever, atelectasis or recurrent pneumonia. Patients with acute pneumonia, weight loss, anorexia and asthenia had a median survival of 3 months. Those with fever survived 5 months. Patients with proximal metastases as evidenced by supraclavicular nodes, hoarseness, dysphagia, superior vena caval obstruction, pleural effusion or pericardial involvement survived 3 months. Any patients with metastases to the brain, bone, spinal cord, abdomen and high cervical or axillary nodes survived for 2 months (GREEN et al., 1971).

An attempt was made by FEINSTEIN to develop a staging system based upon the clinical findings of patients with cancer of the lung. The outcome for patients with cancer of the lung in his series is a function of their clinical (function) anatomical (form) state (FEINSTEIN, 1967a, b).

This functional criterion is now recognized as a most important semi-quantative clinical prognostic feature and is incorporated as the performance status.

On the basis of performance evaluation of 0–100 with 0 being dead and 100 being free of any sign of disease, patients in the series by PETROVICH with a performance greater than 80 survived 44 weeks while those less than 80 survived 34 weeks (PETROVICH et al., 1981). In an analysis of 65 lung cancer patients by PATER and LOEB, it was found that weight loss and performance status significantly affected patients' outcome independent of stage, histology and treatment (PATER and LOEB, 1982).

3 Review of Curative Efforts with Radiation Therapy

Surgery has come to be the treatment of choice for localized non-small cell cancers of the lung. Since 1933 when GRAHAM did the first successful pneumonectomy for a Stage (T_1 N_0 M_0) squamous cell carcinoma with a Radon seed implant around the bronchial stump (GRAHAM and SINGER, 1933), the cure rate has progressed to 25% overall 5-year survival for resected lesions (SELAWRY et al., 1973). Attempts to show that radiation therapy has a place in the primary treatment of cancer of the lung was shown to have some hope as early as 1940 when LEDDY and MOERSCH showed that there were no survivors at 1 year in untreated patients but a 20%, 12% and 4% survival at 1 year, $1^1/_2$ years and 5 years when treated with radiotherapy (LEDDY and MOERSCH, 1940). SMART, in highly selected group of 40 potentially operable patients, showed a 5-year survival of 22.5% (SMART, 1966). Since none of these patients were further triaged

by attempted surgery, or treated by supervoltage equipment, the outcome is even more impressive.

In patients who undergo "curative" surgical resection, there is evidence of failure to control the tumor in 75%. This failure to control the tumor is a consequence of undiagnosed metastases and unresected local disease. MATTHEWS demonstrated in a combined autopsy series on patients dying within 30 days of surgery that 44/131 (33%) of patients with epidermoid carcinoma had persistent disease with 22/44 (50%) of the residual being local and the remainder being distant metastases. For patients with adenocarcinoma the rate was 13/30 (43%) with 1/13 being local and 12/13 being distant. In large cell carcinoma 3/22 (14%) had distant metastases only. In small cell carcinoma, as one might expect, 13/19 (70%) had persistent disease with 1/13 being local and the remaining 12/13 being distant (MATTHEWS et al., 1973). This is a local accuracy of 88% and a distant metastatic evaluation accuracy of 76%.

Pre-operative radiation therapy has the attractiveness of treating a tumor with surgically undisturbed anatomy with an intact vasculature and unperturbed tumor kinetics to a moderate dose so as to make an unresectable tumor resectable and reduce any surgical dissemination of clonogenic cells either locally or distantly. It has the disadvantage of adding radiation injury to the soon to be operated surgical field producing the possibility of exaggerated complications. The mechanism of potential injury is through the fibrosis caused by radiation destroying the important tissue planes necessary for the good surgical dissection if surgery is delayed for months. If surgery is undertaken at shorter intervals after radiation, then the trauma may precipitate latent radiation injury in the slowly proliferating deep tissues and unexpected bad results may be obtained often expressed by excessive bleeding (DEELEY, 1967).

In the 1967 review by DEELEY, he concluded that at that time there was some improvement in the ability to "technically" resect otherwise unresectable tumors that did not translate into increased survivability. He felt that a controlled clinical trial examining both survival and morbidity was necessary to answer the question (DEELEY, 1967). In a review published in 1982, KJAER concluded that on the basis of the four randomized studies of pre-operative radiation therapy that none of the studies showed any benefit for pre-operative irradiation. While the doses used of 4000–5000 rads produced a 25% sterilization rate, this did not translate into improved survival. The cost of complications was high and he could not exclude an adverse effect on survival (KJAER, 1982).

If pre-operative irradiation does not prove to be useful, then would post-operative irradiation prove to be useful in producing prolonged survival? This presupposes that the further triage of the patients via surgery will define those who are still potentially curable in spite of local metastases. A glance back at the data of MOUNTAIN et al. shows that the rate of mortality for patients with T_3 disease is 95% at 5 years and 97% with N_2 disease at 5 years (MOUNTAIN et al., 1974). It follows that the size of the T_+ N_2 compartment available to be rescued by enhanced local control is small indeed. In fact, another glance at the autopsy data of MATTHEWS suggests that it is only those with squamous cell carcinoma that have any chance of being benefitted, since it is only they who had a prominence of local disease (MATTHEWS et al., 1973).

One could also speculate in a very general way on the likelihood of a given series being adequate to show a difference between a control group and a treated group in the correct direction by referral to BOAG et al. (1971). To obtain a 75% chance of detecting a 10% difference in the appropriate direction, a trial would require 200 to 300 patients in each arm. It is unlikely that a sufficient number of patients will be counted to produce the group that is necessary. In general, in patients without the presence of N_1 or N_2 nodes, post-operative radiation is not indicated (CHUNG et al., 1982; KIRSH et al., 1981; VANHOUTTE et al., 1980). Whether there is some utility in irradiating N_1 or N_2 patients is undetermined at this juncture. In an editorial by CHOI, he expresses implicitly there is utility in post-operative radiation and that this can be brought out by increasing the dose to 5,400–5,600 rads (CHOI, 1982). This is consistent with his paper that showed local failures in squamous cell carcinoma up to 5,000 rads post-operatively (CHOI, 1980). PEREZ in an editorial (PEREZ, 1982) while agreeing there is no "statistically sound evidence to demonstrate this …. it is possible that this group of patients may benefit from post-operative radiotherapy". KJAER in his review expresses the view that no effect of post-operative irradiation after adequate surgery has been demonstrated. He is careful to note that the number of patients in the randomized trials is small (KJAER, 1982).

4 Radiotherapy in Inoperable Cancer of the Lung

4.1 Background

A review of survival data at 5-years in patients treated with radiotherapy for inoperable cancer of the lung show a range from about 3% to 10% who are, in fact, alive (GUTTMAN, 1966; JOHNSON et al., 1973; SHERMAN et al., 1981; COY et al., 1980). This sad state of affairs is further made dismal by studies by DURRANT et al. that showed it made no difference whether the patient was treated immediately with radiotherapy or just as his symptoms arose (DURRANT et al., 1971). This study later was supported by BERRY et al. in the second Oxford trial suggesting that radiotherapy has no routine place in the treatment of inoperable cancer of the lung except in the treatment of small cell lesions or nearly operable lesions. They felt that radiotherapy was only of value in patients who were overtly symptomatic from their cancer (BERRY et al., 1977). However, there is some light in the dismay of the radiotherapy of lung cancer in that if the intrathoracic tumor is controlled in a patient with a high performance status, that the 5-year survival was 22% as reported by COX et al. (1980). It is therefore possible to use radiotherapy in patients who do not demonstrate disease outside of the chest, whose clinical status is good with some hope of providing a survival advantage.

The intent and goal of the radiotherapist is to cure a patient of his cancer. Cure means for the individual that he will become free of the risk of dying from this cancer. This is not able to be known in a clinical situation. A cure for a population of such patients is the time when their rate of demise is parallel to that of a normal control group not afflicted with cancer of the lung (DEELEY, 1967; McBRIDE et al., 1983; EASSON, 1967). This event arises in the third to fourth year after the diagnosis.

In an effort to give patients the opportunity for cure one must first obtain a complete remission. There must be no diagnosable disease after the completion of radiotherapy. The loco-regional causes of mortality must be controlled if the patients who are free of distant metastases are to show themselves simply by surviving in contrast to those who are doomed to die as a consequence of the development of metastases over the next 3 years (DEELEY, 1967).

4.2   Dose

The parameters of dose, volume and to a lesser degree fractionation are consequential to the radiotherapist since he can only control these once he has selected a patient for a curative attempt. If one reviews FLETCHER's textbook regarding possible doses and by analogy takes the information from head and neck cancer and applies it to the cancer of the lung, doses of 6,000 rads are recommended for superficial lesions of the glottis with progression to 7,000 rads for bulky lesions. These are T_1–T_2 lesions of the vocal cords (JESSE et al., 1980).

For patients who are freed of gross metastatic disease after a neck dissection, a minimum dose of 5,500 rads in $5^1/_2$ weeks is recommended. In patients with strongly suspected residual disease after a neck dissection then 6,000 rads is recommended (JESSE et al., 1980). A review of the literature of the treatment of cancer of the lung shows that the doses used have been lower. In fact, a study by DEELEY showed that patients who received 3,000 rads did better than those receiving 4,000 rads (DEELEY, 1966). This study suggested that the cause of mortality was due to increased lung fibrosis. However, if one looks at the field distribution shown in DEELEY's review, then one can appreciate that efforts made to spare the spinal cord were done so at the expense of lung tissue and that no dose correction was made for the increase in lung transmission (DEELEY, 1967).

As early as 1963 Peresligin showed a response curve to the effects of radiation. There was an increase in response rate up to 6,650 rads with a fall-off on either side. At 3,800 rads there was a 10% response, at 4,750 rads a 29% response, at 5,700 rads a 75% response and a 92% response at 6,650 rads (SELAWRY et al., 1973).

One needs to recall that we are looking for a dose to treat a variety of different histological types of non-oat cell cancer of the lung, and we know that to some degree histology determines the outcome (COX et al., 1979). We know that squamous cell carcinoma will more frequently cause death and complications locally than will large cell carcinoma or adenocarcinoma which are more likely to cause problems distantly. We seek a dose without any knowledge of the kinetics of the tumor, yet we know that the doubling time is related to survival, i.e. those with slower growth rates have a superior prognosis (MEYER, 1973). We know that in some degree the growth characteristics of the primary and the metastases differs

(FIDLER and HART, 1982; STRAUS, 1974), and very likely that this accounts for the increase in sterilization rate in lymph nodes in contrast to the primary tumors in pre-operative series, e.g. BLOEDORN with 35% sterilization of the primary and 77% of the regional nodes (BLOEDORN et al., 1961; BLOEDORN et al., 1964).

With all of the unknowables, exploration for a dose undertaken by the Radiation Therapy Oncology Group was presented by PEREZ et al. (1980). They showed that there was a complete response of 8%, 18%, 21% and 21% for 4,000 rads split, 4,000 rads continuous, 5,000 rads continuous and 6,000 rads continuous indicating a distinct dose response curve as manifested by the complete response, partial response and chest recurrence with the 5,000 and 6,000 rads being equivalent. There was also a greater frequency of complete and partial response for smaller tumors than larger tumors, i.e. 82% for T_1 67% for T_2 and 46–56% for T_3. Histology played an important role in response, in that squamous cell carcinoma had a higher local control at 5,000 rads than 4,000 rads. The other histologies did not. The recommended dose from this study is in the order of 5,000 to 6,000 rads. The patients with a complete remission have a longer survival than those who do not attain a complete remission (COX et al., 1978). COX also demonstrated that control of the local disease is highly correlated with survival. They were able to obtain a complete response of 3% with a total response of 34% (PETROVICH et al., 1981).

4.3   Volume

W.T. MURPHY's Rule of Radiotherapy is "Put the Radiation Where the Cancer Is!" (unpublished). The treatment volume to encompass all of the tumor in all of the patients would be a field to cover the entire body. This clearly is impractical although efforts have been suggested and made to treat half the body with large single fractions without dramatic improvement, albeit modest toxicity (SALAZAR et al., 1980). A more temperate approach is to treat the causes of mortality that are found within the thorax, i.e. the primary and the metastases in the nodes of the hilum and the mediastinum. While one recognizes that progress from a T_1 to T_3 seriously decreases survivability as well as progression from N_0 to N_1 to N_2, there still exists the evidence previously mentioned that survivability is related to tumor control locally.

Therefore, the minimum tumor volume is the primary tumor with a margin around the opacity visualized on chest x-ray. Certainly the adjacent hilum and the entire mediastinum needs to be included. Supraclavicular nodes are not a force of mortality, and if they are involved they indicate dissemination of the cancer. If they are not clinically involved they have a local failure rate of 4.3% if they are not irradiated (EISERT et al., 1976). Since it is simple enough to do, and associated with no excess morbidity over the usual radiation fields, then they ought to be included particularly in those with small cell carcinoma and those with demonstrated mediastinal involvement. It goes without saying that all tissues that do not need to be treated are shielded. The normal lung is shielded out. The spinal cord is protected from very high dose with a small risk by a posterior shield or with a boosting technique of oblique radiation fields. CHOI in his editorial expresses the belief that radiation complications in the lung are related to the increased volume of the lung treated by three fields, or rotational fields in contrast to the simpler parallel opposed fields with careful shielding (CHOI, 1982).

4.4 Fractionation

Fractionation other than the rather standard daily fractions of about 200 rads per day are enigmatic at this point. However, there are two characteristics that make split course radiation attractive according to KJAER (1982). Firstly, the total time required to treat a patient with a short life expectancy is significantly reduced. Secondly, it is possible to exclude patients from the second course of treatment who have shown progression locally or evidence of metastases distantly. Also, split course therapy allows modification of the radiation fields if the patient has had a significant response to the irradiation. Even if the patient demonstrates new demonstrations of his disease, he will likely have already received a high enough dose of radiation to control his symptoms.

Outcomes for split course radiotherapy waxed in an early study by ABRAMSON and CAVANAUGH comparing 6,000 rads in 30 fractions versus 2,000 rads for 5 days followed by a repetition after a 3 week rest. At 1 year the split course group had 43% alive versus the 14% for continuous irradiation. They also recorded few complications and fewer failing to complete treatment (ABRAMSON and CAVANAUGH, 1970). JOHNSON et al. in 1973

failed to show any difference in survival or symptom relief if the patients were treated with 4,800 rads in 20 fractions over 4 weeks with Co60; or with 2,800 rads in four 700-rad fractions with a 35 MEV. They all had 30% 1-year survival and 6% 6-year survival (JOHNSON et al., 1973). In 1979 EMAMI et al. showed that patients treated with 6,000 rads in 30 fractions in 6 weeks had superior survival over split course technique of 2,500 rads in 10 fractions repeated after a 2-week hiatus. This result was independent of favorable or nonfavorable prognostic factors (EMAMI et al., 1979).

In 1980 PEREZ, representing the Radiation Therapy Oncology Group, showed a lower complete response rate for the 4,000-rad split course group of 8% versus 18–21% for the remaining arms including 4,000 rads continuous irradiation. There was also a high local recurrence rate of 51% versus 45% for 5,000 rads and 38% for 6,000 rads. Patients treated in the split course group had the lowest survival of 10% versus 16–18% for the other groups. Complication rates were not different among the various aims for the study (PEREZ et al., 1980).

In 1982 SEALY et al. showed that there was no overall difference in survival between two split courses of radiotherapy (SEALY et al., 1982). There was, however, the expected much improved survival with a complete response. The complete response was found in 6% of the short course which was 2,000 rads in 5 fractions in 5 days followed by 3 weeks rest and then repetition. The long course was 3,000 rads in 15 fractions, 2 weeks rest and a further 2,000 rads in 10 fractions in 2 weeks. In 1981, SHAH reported that he was able to attain a 24-month survival of 33% with 5,000 rads, but only 15% with 4,000 rads split dose and 25% with a 6,000-rad split dose (SHAH et al., 1981).

5 Technical Considerations

External irradiation in the present day is carried out with instruments capable of producing photons in excess of 1 MEV energies. This is on contrast to earlier days when energies of 250 KEV to 400 KEV were commonly used. Presently Co60 units operating at 80 cm SSD or 4 MEV Linacs operating at 80 or 100 SSD are most prevalent with higher energies of 8, 10, 12 and 25 MEV photons being available as well as electrons in energy ranges up to 40 MEV. The major advantages of the instruments with energies in excess of 1 MEV is the greater penetrability of the beam, predominant forward scatter of the secondary electrons and the point of electronic equilibrium deep to the skin surface that has eliminated the skin reaction as the dose limiting toxicity. It has decreased absorption of x-ray energies by bone because of the predominance of Comptom scattering, that is independent of the atomic number in this energy range.

5.1 Treatment Planning

5.1.1 Application of Computerized Tomography (CT)

A major acquisition of the modern age has been the computer. With this instrumentation dose, distribution simulation can be carved out by the physician, physicist and technologist readily without the laborious hand calculations that were necessary in the past. Plans can be done and discarded until an acceptable one is obtained based upon the data available. However, this planning system and the high energy treatment instruments rely on tumor localization techniques that are time honored, i.e. standard x-ray procedures, physical exam

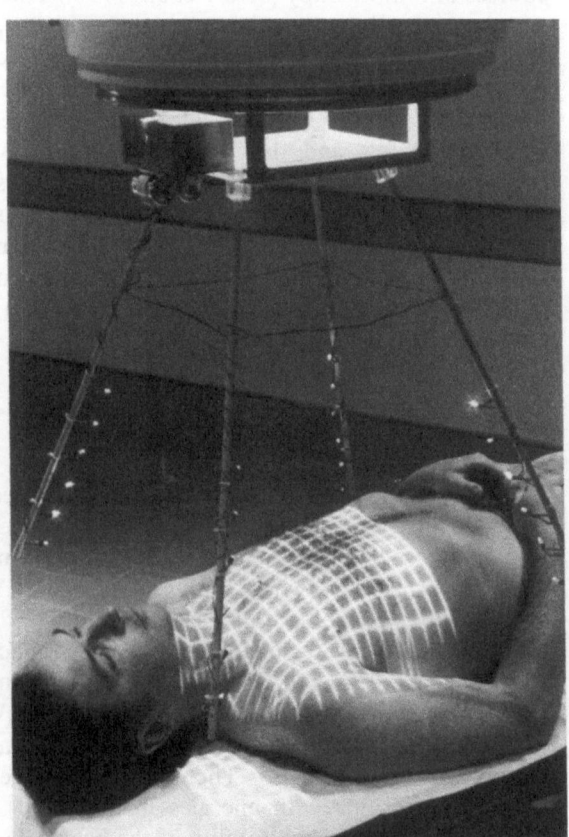

and surgical descriptions. Only with the addition of computerized tomography (CT) scanning did a new technology offer to the radiotherapist a new view of the patient that has the potential of seriously offering an improvement in outcome by better localization of the tumor, ensuring adequate radiation fields and by decreasing the risk of injury to consequential normal anatomy, e.g. the spinal cord, by more accurate planning.

One should never delude himself by asking a radiological tool to provide histological information. Therefore, to use a CT in place of tissue diagnosis is not appropriate. There is no doubt that due to physical limitation in the physical size of the pixel image, lesions less than a few millimeters in size cannot be detected. Lastly, there is no way to state that a normal image of a mediastinal node, for example, eliminates the possibility of metastases in that node. However, in the context of a known cancer of the lung, Occam's Razor is a valid thinking tool, i.e. that all abnormalities seen on the film are best related to the known diagnosis of cancer of the lung unless there are pathognomic findings indicating otherwise (Occam's razor). MUHM pointed this out in that 90% of additional nodules found on CT scan are metastases when found in the context of known malignancy (MUHM, 1980).

A useful and different view of the anatomy of the mediastinum is published by ZYLAK et al., in 1982. Rather that the usual divisions of the mediastinum that divides the area into the superior and inferior compartments with the latter being divided into anterior, posterior and middle, he divides it into three longitudinal spaces called the prevascular space, the vascular space and the post-vascular space. The prevascular space is anterior with the thymus, thyroid and parathyroids as its contents. The vascular space contains the pericardium and all its contents, the great veins, the anterior aorta and the major bronchus that continues into the neck. The post-vascular space contains the trachea, the esophagus, the descending aorta and the azygous vein. These divisions aid in the anatomical understanding of the mediastinum (ZYLAK et al., 1982).

Advantages to CT indicated by MIRA et al. are: 1) CT scan will show tumor 68% of the time when chest x-ray will not because of atelectasis. CT scan

Fig. 1. Light bulb frame and position of patient for stereo photogrammetric technique. Note how the top plate fits into the wedge slot of the radiotherapy unit. The bulbs are rigidly attached to the legs of the frame

showed unexpected extension in 78% of patients. 2) Mediastinal masses frequently extend anteriorly to the sternum and posteriorly toward the vertebrae and spinal cord. 3) Lung masses spread in one-third of the cases to the lateral costal pleura. Thus 1–2 cm margins are not necessarily sufficient. 4) Tumor size can be much larger than routine x-rays indicated. Hence, CT is useful for staging and treatment planning for cancer of the lung (MIRA et al., 1982).

The value of CT in evaluation and planning treatment for cancer of the lung was pointed out by EMAMI et al., when they were able to show a clearer demonstration of the tumor in 75%; a change in lesion size in 43%; a change in stage in 40%; inadequate treatment planning in 28% and changes of treatment to decrease irradiation of normal tissue in 40%. They estimated that the CT scan data was essentially for treatment planning in 53% of the patients (EMAMI et al., 1978). PRASAD et al. showed that 26% of their treatment plans were altered and optimization of plans in 64% with reduction of non-uniformity to less than 5% in 84% of their patients (PRASAD et al., 1981).

Every silver lining is associated with a cloud and that cloud is that tumor associated with atelectasis eliminates border definition. This was so in 50% of patients. Limited resolution of CT scanning prevents investigation of very small extensions of the tumor. In the post-treatment period CT is of limited usefulness in distinguishing between radiation fibrosis and tumor persistence or recurrent (SEYDEL et al., 1980; MIRO et al., 1982).

5.1.2 Compensators

Upon seeing a patient from a radiotherapy point, of view one realizes that the Creator was not one of us; otherwise, he would have made human beings cuboid and uniformly dense. Since we are neither, one cannot expect that the radiation distributions from a water phantom are not going to be true when treating a patient. Something needs to be done to allow for the curves and the indentation of the body surfaces as well as the inhomogeneities created by the lungs.

Clearly some method of tissue compensation is necessary so as to give some uniformity of dose within the patient. While there are alternative methods of varying degrees of labor, one of the simplest and most expedient is that described by RENNER et al. (1977). This method makes use of stereo photogrammetry to demonstrate the pa-

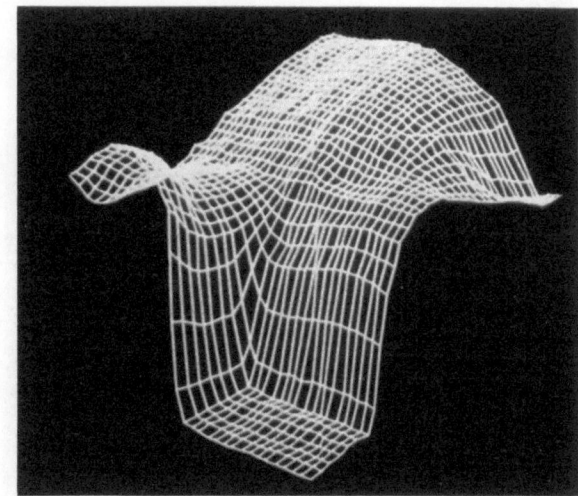

Fig. 2. Computer reconstruction of patient surface

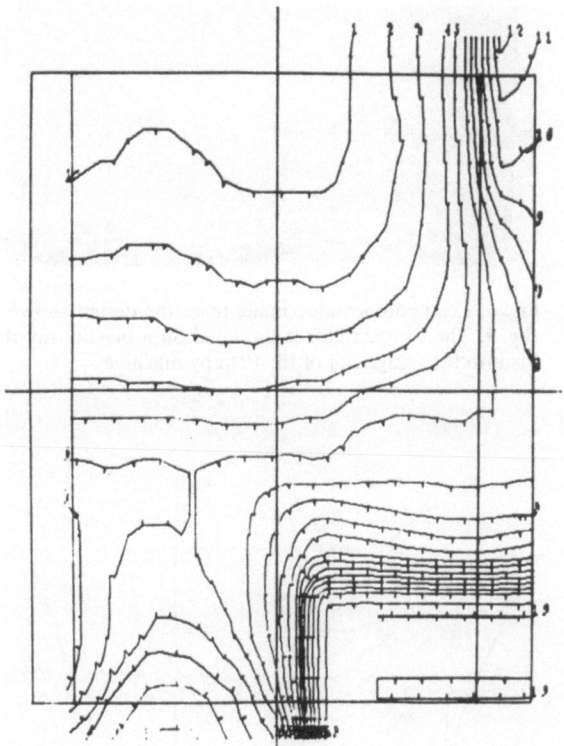

Fig. 3. Compensator designed by the computer from the photograph shown in Fig. 2. The design is basically a contour map of the patient's surface in the treatment field. The elevations between counter lines correspond to layers of sheet lead of 0.794 mm thick. The tick marks indicate increasing lead

tients' contour. This data is then digitized into a computer, e.g. Rad-8, and via appropriate software a template is printed out and then the lead sheet cut and fixed to the plastic plate for insertion

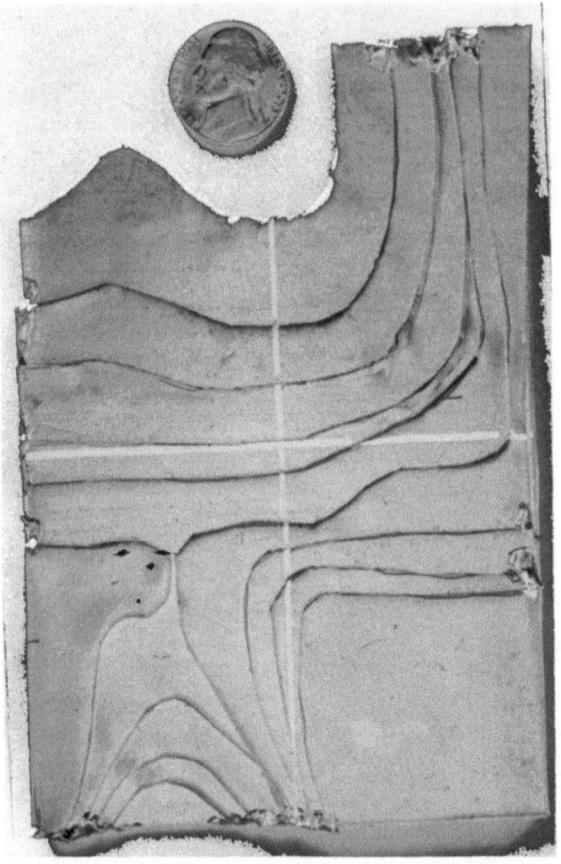

Fig. 4. Lead compensator made from the design shown in Fig. 3. The compensator is mounted on a plastic tray that fits into the wedge slot of the therapy machine

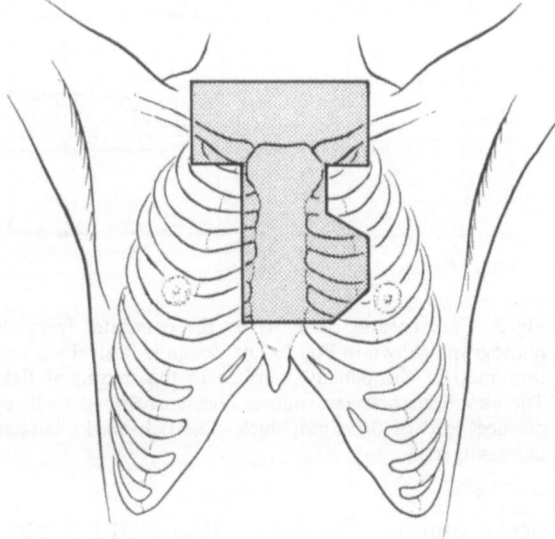

Fig. 5. Example of treatment field including primary (left lung), ipsilateral hilum, mediastinum and bilateral supraclavicular areas

into the treatment instrument head. This reduces the inhomogeneity due to the lung by less than 5% over the field (RENNER et al., 1982) (Fig. 1, 2, 3, 4).

5.1.3 Beam Orientation and Treatment Verification

Beam orientation that is simplest is anterior-posterior opposing fields. This has the advantage of minimizing all sorts of random errors and lends to the elimination of systematic error by simple repeated checking of verification films. It lends itself to field shaping with either standard blocks or with custom made blocks from low melting point material, e.g. cerro-bend. It allows for the incorporation of the entire mediastinum and the supraclavicular fields as well as the use of compensating filters. It also allows for the protection of the spinal cord with a thin posterior block to keep the dose to the cord at 4,500 rads or below (SHERMAN et al., 1981). Treating the entire tumor and the mediastinum with anterior-posterior fields with appropriate compensation filters to 4,500–5,000 rads allows maximum control of the radiation distribution and allows the boosting of the primary and mediastinum by oblique fields or rotational technique so as not to exceed the tolerance of large volumes of lung tissue and the spinal cord (Figs. 5, 6, 7, 8).

Lastly, all of the calculations made and the translation to actual treatment is subject to multiple possible errors. All of the planning is entirely speculation until the actual dose is confirmed by direct measurement. The entrance dose can easily be measured by a thermoluminescence dosimetry system or by a diode to confirm that the calculations and their translation into treatment are indeed correct. This plus weekly verification will produce good quality control over the patients treatment.

6 Brachytherapy

Brachytherapy for malignant tumors has been around for a very long time. In the 1930's when treatment for cancer of the lung by surgery was a tenuous undertaking, the use of interstitial implants was practiced. As previously mentioned in this chapter, the first successful pneumonectomy for cancer of the lung had a Radon implant of the bronchial stump done and that was 50 years ago in 1933 (GRAHAM and SINGER, 1983).

In 1937, R.C. OMEROD presented 100 patients treated by several methods. Sixty-seven patients underwent endobronchial implantation of Radon seeds through a bronchoscope. A total of 6–8 seeds of 2 millicuries each were put in place. Evaluation at that time showed 6 survivors free of disease in 1 year, with 4 more who died between 2 and 5 years from the implantation (OMEROD, 1937). A followup of these and additional cases in 1953 by OMEROD reported that in a group of patients not eligible for surgical resection, 8 survived 3 years or more, 4 survived 5 years or more and 3 remained free of tumor for more than 10 years. Thus, it was demonstrated that in unresectable patients there is a group who do not have distant metastases and are not doomed to death provided the primary tumor and local disease is controlled (OMEROD, 1953). HILARIS reported in 1979 patients with recurrence of their lung cancers treated with endobronchial implantation 2 out of 4 alive 2 and 6 years later (HILARIS et al., 1979).

A more usual approach to the use of interstitial implantation for cancer of the lung is at the time of surgery. In 1971, 53 patients reported by HILARIS with apical lung cancer were treated by partial resection and interstitial implants in 15 patients. The remainder were treated only with implantation with a variety of isotopes, I 125, Au 198, Rn 222, Ir 192. Nine patients survived for 5 years or more or 17% of the treated population (HILARIS et al., 1971).

In lesions other than apical lesions that have a superior prognosis to other lung cancer, results were reported using interstitial implantation with Rn 222 or I 125. Five patients survived for 5 years which is comparable with the outcome for external irradiation (HILARIS et al., 1975a). In a review of their 20-year experience with interstitial brachytherapy HILARIS reported 80% local control in

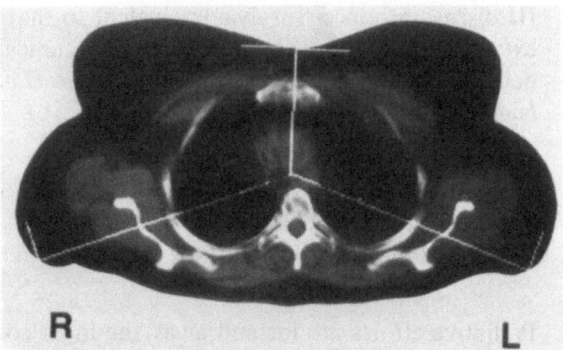

Fig. 6. Computerized tomography assisted treatment planning technique. Illustrates anterior and bilateral posterior oblique ports

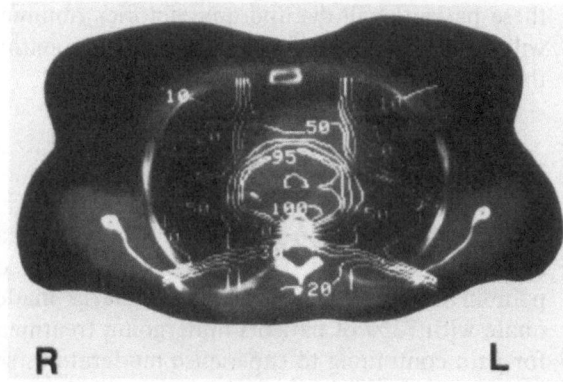

Fig. 7. Isoeffect lines plotted on computerized tomogram for entire treatment volume

Stage I and II and 60% local control in Stage III. The 5-year survival in Stage I was 46% and Stage III 7%. There were only 5 Stage II patients and one of these survived for 5 years (HILARIS et al., 1975a).

It seems clear that in Stage I, interstitial brachytherapy is equivalent of resection and in Stage

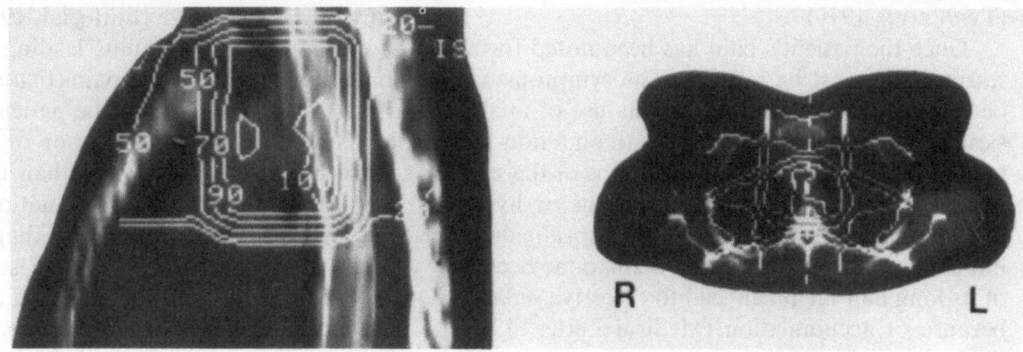

Fig. 8. Isoeffect lines plotted on computerized tomogram to the boost field of the primary tumor

III disease produces survival equivalent to that of external irradiation. The procedure is technically demanding with the details available in the *Handbook of Brachytherapy* (HILARIS et al., 1975b).

7 Evaluation and Radiotherapeutic Approach in the Palliation of Metastatic Disease

Palliative efforts are far and away the most common we will ever make in treating patients with cancer of the lung. It is here that our role as physician is broadest and most humane. Certainly, it is here that our skills are most taxed, our courage most tried and our judgment most needed for all these patients will die and any victories obtained will be in the relief of the symptoms tormenting the patients.

7.1 Pain Control

There is no obligation upon a physician so great as that of pain relief. However, the treatment of pain in hospitalized patients is regularly inadequate with 73% of patients undergoing treatment for pain continuing to experience moderate to severe discomfort (MARKS and SACHAR, 1973).

The explanation for this curious phenomenon in a survey of two teaching hospitals is a belief of great risk in the use of narcotics, that very low doses were effective against severe pain and higher doses would add nothing to the pain relief. The standard method of dosing was a prn (pro re nata) schedule so that the dose received by the patient was smaller than that ordered in spite of persistent pain (MARKS and SACHAR, 1973).

According to TWYCROSS the frequency of severe terminal pain is 50%. The general explanation is simply inadequate doses of narcotic analgesics (TWYCROSS, 1979).

Once the patient's pain has been noted for assessment, it must be relieved. The symptoms can be suppressed or eliminated by the use of analgesics. The use of morphine by mouth on a non-prn, round the clock basis, is the prototype of the satisfactory analgesic schedule. Methadone or hydromorphone can be substituted in appropriate doses, but caution must be used with methadone because of its long half life it can lead to excessive sedation because of accumulation (Medical Letter, 1982). Doses beginning at 10 mg of morphine elixir every 4 hours by mouth can be altered every 4 or 8 h

up or down to control the painful symptoms. With attention paid to bowel function with laxatives and metoclopramide significant constipation can be avoided. There are times when nausea is a problem from the morphine and prochlorperazine 5 mg every 4 h will satisfy controlling that problem.

For less pain the use of acetaminophen or salicylates every 4 h can be useful. The use of oxycodone or codeine plus acetaminophen or aspirin can produce a very adequate analgesic schedule in the situation of moderate pain. The judge of the adequacy of pain control is the patient, not the observer.

The goals to be attempted are pain relief at night which is very likely attainable, pain control at rest which can often be done and pain control in motion which is most difficult (TWYCROSS, 1979).

7.2 Bone Metastases

Bone metastases in lung cancer are a painful fact of life with the frequency of metastases being 29–42% depending on the cell type in BUDINGER's series of untreated patients. The most common sites of involvement were the vertebrae and skull, but no bones are spared including the phalanges of the hand (BUDINGER, 1958). The access of the lung cancer to the bones is through the hematogenous route and does not involve the lymphatics. In addition to their anatomical presence, bone metastases are quite able to elicit an osteolytic agent thought to be a prostaglandin that is a major factor in bone loss as well as the hypercalcemia seen in these individuals. This process offers an avenue of therapeutic approach in that non-steroidal anti-inflammatory drugs can be used to shut off prostaglandin manufacture via inhibition of prostaglandin synthetase. The most commonly used drugs are aspirin and indomethacin, although there are many others to choose (Editorial, 1976).

The iatrotropic stimulus leading to the suspicion of bone metastases is pain (FEINSTEIN, 1967a). In FOLEY's review 97% of the patients' pain complaints are related to the tumor or its treatment so one needs look no further than the presenting diagnosis of cancer for the explanation of the painful symptoms (FOLEY, 1979). The diagnostic procedures followed are the bone scan so as to define whether the metastases are present, and if present whether they are solitary or multiple. Radiographs of the symptomatic area will show the degree of bone destruction, and in the case of long bones the need for internal fixation prior to any other therapy.

If a pathologic fracture of a long bone is identified, then internal fixation needs to be undertaken immediately so as to give the patient a function limb, and irradiating a pathological fracture that is not fixed will result in a non-union (BONARIGO et al., 1967).

The presence of bone metastases in lung cancer is an ominous finding heralding the clinical onset of disseminated disease. The median survival from the time of diagnosis of a solitary metastases is 14 weeks and 12 weeks with evidence of multiple metastases (TONG et al., 1982).

The treatment for symptomatic osseous metastases from bronchogenic carcinoma is radiotherapy. Treatment schemes have been recently investigated by the Radiation Therapy Oncology Group. For solitary metastases 4,050 rads in 15 fractions and 2,000 rads in 5 fractions were equivalent with the exception that the 2,000 rads produced a more rapid pain relief and there was a high frequency of pathological fractures at the site when 4,050 rads were used. In patients with multiple metastases the schemes of 3,000 rads in 2 weeks and 1,500, 2,000 and 2,500 rads in 1 week were compared with similar outcomes in terms of pain relief (TONG et al., 1982).

Nearly 90% of patients had minimal relief of pain, 83% achieved partial relief of pain, but only 54% obtained complete relief of pain. Pain relief was least good in patients with lung cancer, lesions in the pelvis, patients with severe pain at the onset of treatment, and in those who were unable to complete their treatment. The frequency of failure to complete treatment was greatest in the longer schemes (TONG et al., 1982).

The relapse rate of pain was the same whether the patient had solitary or multiple metastases, although pain relief was more rapid in those with multiple metastases. Twenty-nine percent of patients, 41% of those with partial relief and 54% of those with complete relief, had recurrence of pain at the treatment site prior to death. The site of the primary did not affect the duration of minimal relief with lung cancer patients doing least well (TONG et al., 1982).

The treatment fields for patients should be arranged so as to be simple and avoid toxicity as much as possible. Single posterior fields will do well for the thoracic, lumbar and sacral spine with the dose calculated at 5–6 cm depth. The fields over the cervical spine ought to be right and left parallel and opposed to avoid irradiation the patients' mouth, larynx and salivary glands. Fields over the humerus can be single, and either anterior or posterior because of the usual lack of thickness of the arm. However, the fields for the femur ought to be parallel and opposed because of the thickness of the thigh and hip. Treatment fields for the pelvis need to be arranged and shielded so as to not irradiate the bowel or the bladder. The ribs and scapulae are best treated with electron beam since one can readily control the depth of penetration by energy selection. If electrons are not available, then tangential fields to avoid irradiating the lung are useful when using photon beams. For superficial flat bones the use of 250 KVP is very appropriate if it is available (Fig. 9).

With the single exception of the ribs, since that is not practical, the entire bone ought to be treated. This simply eliminates any uncertainty of the patient having undiagnosed disease within the marrow cavity that will rapidly be a source of local morbidity. When treating the vertebrae it is useful to take at least one vertebra above and below the site of the lesion.

Vigorous treatment of bone metastases and the associated pain with appropriate dosage and scheduling of analgesics plus prostaglandin inhibitors (NSAID) and radiotherapy will produce the most humane of all outcomes for these patients. For: "Pain is soul destroying ... the quality of mercy is essential to the practice of medicine; here, of all places it should not be strained" (ANGELL, 1982).

7.3 Neurological Manifestations

Neurological events and metastases in patients with bronchogenic carcinoma were noted in the 19th Century with patients showing paraplegia from spinal cord compression as a result of vertebral metastases and also brain metastases (ROSENBLATT, 1964). In a greatly detailed autopsy series OLSON demonstrated 20.8% of all patients with cancer of the lung to have vertebral metastases with squamous cell carcinoma being least frequent at 7% and adenocarcinoma and undifferentiated at 25–29% respectively. The incidence of metastases to the spinal meninges was 3% all in the patients with undifferentiated carcinoma (OLSON, 1935). Since the usual event of spinal cord compression is related to vertebral metastases the demonstration of these lesions is consequential. Of all the patients with spinal cord compression, patients with cancer of the lung are the most common (BRUCKMAN and BLOOMER, 1978).

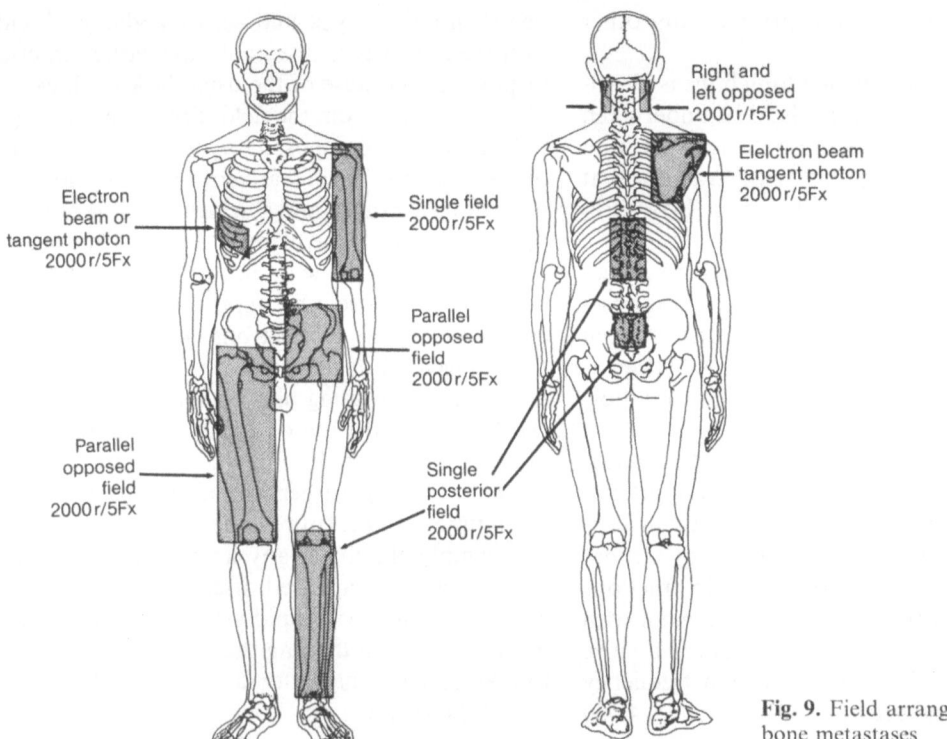

Electron beam or tangent photon 2000 r/5Fx

Single field 2000 r/5Fx

Parallel opposed field 2000 r/5Fx

Parallel opposed field 2000 r/5Fx

Single posterior field 2000 r/5Fx

Right and left opposed 2000 r/r5Fx

Elelctron beam tangent photon 2000 r/5Fx

Fig. 9. Field arrangements for treatment of bone metastases

At the time of first symptom 96% of the patients will have pain and only 2% will have weakness. At the time of diagnosis 96% will have pain, 76% weakness, 57% autonomic dysfunction (bladder and bowel), and 51% will have weakness (BRUCKMAN and BLOOMER, 1978).

The usual distribution of site for cord compression in lung cancer patients is the cervical spine 38%, dorsal spine 57% and lumbosacral spine 5% (GILBERT et al., 1978).

Once the diagnosis is suspected the sine qua non of diagnosis is a myelogram. While unusual, the lumbar puncture may precipitate paraplegia and arrangements for surgical decompression need to be at hand (TÖRMÄ, 1957).

The treatment undertaken is usually very high dose steroids based upon studies by USHIO et al., that experimentally showed a decrease in edema at the site of obstruction (USHIO et al., 1977). Since there have been no differences due to treatment, i.e. surgery and radiotherapy and radiotherapy alone, radiotherapy is undertaken (GILBERT et al., 1978). Radiotherapy was once feared to cause sufficient edema so as to compromise the spinal cord further. RUBIN showed that large fraction radiotherapy produced a response of tumor that was greater than the risk of any edema (RUBIN, 1969). The present treatment scheme is usually 400 rads

per day for 3 days with 200 rads per day to follow up to 4,000 rads. Other fractionation schemes produce the same result (GREENBERG et al., 1980). This plus doses of dexamethasone as high as 100 mg per day for 3 days with rapid tapering afterwards is well tolerated (GILBERT et al., 1978).

The prognosis for ambulation is dependent upon the state of the patient when he enters treatment (GILBERT et al., 1978). If one is ambulatory going in, then 79% will remain so; if parapetic then 34% will remain so; if paraplegic all will remain so except for occasional very radio-sensitive tumors. For lung cancer, specifically, 20% were improved by surgery and radiotherapy and 50% were improved by radiotherapy alone.

Brain metastases are common either as the presenting manifestation of lung cancer of as a later complication. In 1935 OLSON demonstrated a 36% prevalence of brain metastases in his autopsy series (OLSON, 1935). Thirty years later in patients surviving longer than one month after surgery 37% of patients in SPJUT's series demonstrated brain metastases at autopsy (SPJUT and MATEO, 1965). Of intracerebral metastases 604 of them are multiple (POSNER, 1977). The symptoms that the patient complains about when coming to a physician are headache, weakness, mental changes, seizures, ataxia and aphasia. The associated signs are hemiparesis, impaired thinking, sensory loss, papill-edema, ataxia and aphasia.

Once the diagnosis is suspected then the most useful of all radiological tools is the CT scan. It has made obsolete all other diagnostic tools in particular the invasive ones of angiography or pneumoencephalography. Skull films can be helpful, but only rarely, and are therefore not usually needed.

Prompt early relief as symptoms can be expected in 60–75% of patients with the use of large doses of steroids. Dexamethasone is a favored medication at a dose of 16 mg per day in divided doses. A steroid myopathy can intervene complicating the subsequent course of the patient's life. Cimetidine has frequently been used in an effort to prevent the peptic ulcer toxicity of steroids. One must remember that this drug rearranges the hepatic blood flow and thereby raises the effective blood levels of other drugs metabolized in the liver. Of particular interest in this regard is the fact that anti-convulsant blood levels can be raised by 60% and can thereby lead to an unexpected toxicity (MANGINI, 1982). Since seizures occur in 15% of patients the use of anti-convulsants is usually limited.

There are unusual cases of solitary lesions of the brain that lend themselves to surgery. This modality has been undertaken with a 29% survival and 15% survival at 1 and 2 years (WHITE et al., 1981). In general, patients will have other sites of metastases in 80% of the cases, and the interval for onset from the time of diagnosis was a median of 6 months (WEST and MAOR, 1980).

The usual treatment, however, is radiotherapy, most often in conjunction with steroids (BORGELT et al., 1980). The Radiation Therapy Oncology Group investigated multiple time dose relationships and determined that 2,000 rads in 1 week is the equivalent of 4,000 rads in 3 weeks when the whole brain is treated. Patients with lung cancer showed a 37% improvement in those who were less severely injured, and 72% in those more severely injured. Symptoms resolved in the majority of patients with headache being abolished in 82% of the patients. The median survival for ambulatory lung cancer patients was 16 weeks and 11 weeks for the non-ambulatory patient. The brain metastases was a cause of death in about 31% of the patients receiving 2,000 rads in 1 week 3,000 rads in 2 weeks, or 4,000 rads in 3 weeks. Individuals who have controlled primaries with the brain as the only site of metastases have a superior prognosis to their fellows (Fig. 10).

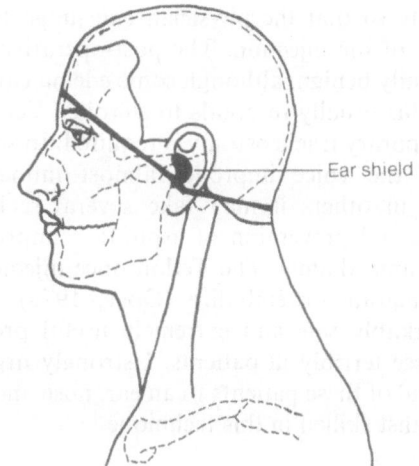

Fig. 10. Field arrangement for treatment of the whole brain

7.4 Vocal Cord Paralysis

The left vagus nerve passes into the thoracic cavity, passes in front of the aorta and then gives off the recurrent laryngeal nerve, that innervates the vocal cord on the left side. On the right, the vagus nerve does not go so deeply into the thoracic cavity, but gives off the recurrent branch that loops around the subclavian artery and then innervates the right vocal cord. The anatomical function of the vocal cords is to protect the trachea from foreign material. The evolved function is to allow us to speak. A physiological function is to allow pressure to generate in the chest for an effective cough. A cancer of the lung involving nodes at the aortic window can entrap the left recurrent laryngeal nerve and cause paralysis of the vocal cord leading to aspiration, hoarseness and an ineffective cough. The finding of a paralyzed cord in a patient with cancer of the lung eliminates him as a candidate for resection. External radiation will infrequently allow recovery of the function of the vagus nerve so the patient now cannot eat because he cannot swallow, particularly liquids, without coughing. He cannot effectively communicate, because of the loss of volume of his voice, and he cannot effectively cough. Aspiration, pneumonia, cachexia are the followers of this event.

This tragedy can be corrected by the injection of the affected vocal cord with Teflon (LEWY and MATTHEWS, 1965). The Teflon is injected by a special injector into the posterior two-thirds of the cord with the intent of causing approximation of the vocal cords. This procedure is done under local anesthesia with the patient awake and able to cooperate so that the physician can judge the adequacy of the injection. The post-operative course is usually benign, although some edema can develop. This usually responds to steroids. Very rarely a temporary tracheostomy is required. In some patients the voice improves almost immediately, while in others it may take several seeks. The cough and prevention of aspiration improves almost immediately. The Teflon once injected does not migrate or embolize (GOFF, 1973). It is a remarkably safe and extremely useful procedure in these terribly ill patients. I strongly urge early referral of these patients to an ear, nose and throat specialist skilled in this technique.

7.5   Superior Vena Caval Obstruction (SVCO)

The syndrome of superior vena caval obstruction was described as due to a bronchogenic carcinoma in 1844 (ROSENBLATT, 1964). In the present day, the most common cause of SVCO is malignancy with bronchogenic carcinoma the most frequent cause (PARISH et al., 1981). There are some benign iatrogenic causes related to thrombosis as a consequence of subclavian catheters, but in the face of a known cancer, the cancer is the cause, and most likely a demonstration of a cancer of the lung when it presents de novo. The patient will present with vein distention on the neck and the chest, edema of the face, tachypnea, plethora of the face, cyanosis and edema of the upper extremities depending upon the extent of the obstruction (PEREZ et al., 1978). There is almost always a right mediastinal mass on chest x-ray, or at least a demonstrable right hilar mass. Upon suspicion of the diagnosis the anatomical fact can be demonstrated by a radionuclide superior vena cavagram or by phlebography. If the histology is not yet known, the workup for histology is accomplished by the least invasive means so as not to risk the patient nor to interfere with his treatment.

The treatment for SVCO is considered to be an emergency procedure by the radiotherapist. The dose schedules that are selected are based upon experimental studies by GREEN et al. that demonstrated that radiation edema was non-consequential and that high doses of radiation delivered rapidly were maximally beneficial (GREEN et al., 1963). From their experiments they went to a clinical situation of delivering 400 rads for three days followed by a more conventional fractionation of 200 rads per day up to 400 rads or greater (RUBIN et al., 1963).

The present day treatment schemes are basically 400 rads per day for 3 or 4 days followed by 200 rads per day up to 4,000 rads to 6,000 rads. The portals encompass all known disease in the chest including the primary, the hilum, the mediastinum as well as the supraclavicular nodes.

The response rates vary in some measure with the author and the rate of presentation of the syndrome. Subacute presentation had a 79% response rate versus 47% with acute presentation (KANJI et al., 1980). SLAWSON et al. had a complete remission rate in 86–93% of their patients (SLAWSON et al., 1981), while PEREZ et al. had a complete response of 20% of patients with bronchogenic carcinoma, 50% partial response, 15% with minimal response and 15% with no response. Eleven of the 18 patients, 61% with bronchogenic carcinoma in this series had an excellent or good response with combination chemotherapy and radiation therapy. Persistent or recurrent SVCO occured in 10% of non-small cell cancer of the lung and 19% with small cell carcinoma. Thirty-three percent of those who did not have the supraclavicular area treated failed at that site while less than 10% of those who were treated failed there. The survival of the patients was 25% at 1 year and 10% at 30 months (PEREZ et al., 1978). While a rarity, long term survivors of patients with cancer of the lung have been reported at up to 13 years (NOGEIRE et al., 1979; PERCARPIO et al., 1979).

7.6   Pericardial and Pleural Effusion

Of tumors that metastasize to the pericardium and heart, cancer of the lung does so must frequently (BAKER, 1979). In fact, 20% of autopsied specimens had evidence for heart involvement in Kline's series. Hematogenous spread was very uncommon with the lymphatic route being the major route of involvement. There are two major syndromes related to heart and pericardial involvement by tumor. The least common is congestive heart failure due to involvement of the lymphatics of the heart, although this may be a consequence of lack of diagnosis since 20/61 patients with heart and pericardial involvement had signs of congestive heart failure that were probably the immediate cause of death. The second major syndrome is due to the constriction of the heart by either pericardial effusion or by a constrictive process from tumor or inflammation (KLINE, 1972).

The patients become symptomatic when the intrapericardial pressure exceeds the pressure of filling, i.e. the pressure in the inferior and superior vena cava (BAKER, 1979). This produces venous distention, a fall in cardiac output and hypotension. The findings of the now tamponaded heart are venous distention, distant heart sounds and a paradoxical pulse, i.e. one that diminishes in amplitude with inspiration. It is demonstrated by exceeding a 10–20 mm Hg fall in blood pressure at the end of inspiration. Evaluation of the heart is best done by chest x-ray and echocardiography. If a large effusion is present, then a pericardiocentesis can be done with rapid relief of symptoms. If a constrictive process has formed, then only a surgical pericardiectomy is possible and this must be considered in the face of the short term terminal prognosis. A pleuro-pericardial window may be tried for recurrent effusions. Instillation of 5 FU or tetracycline or external radiation to the heart and pericardial sac may be attempted. One needs to carefully define the short term goals that are being pursued so as not to subject a patient to a therapeutic misadventure.

Patients may develop effusion in the pleural space that arises from direct tumor extension, mediastinal involvement by tumor, atelectasis or congestive heart failure. When the process occurs late in the patient's course and respiration is hampered, the use of chest drainage by thoracostomy followed by tetracycline is appropriate. The tetracycline causes a pleuritis that causes the visceral and the parietal pleura to adhere together and thereby eliminates the space. The instillation of tetracycline can be very painful, and the use of liberal doses of meperidine 100 mg IM or morphine 15 mg IM is appropriate.

In the case of a serous effusion with mediastinal tumor involvement, the external irradiation of the mediastinum can alleviate this without further intervention.

8 Complications of Major Organs

When one irradiates a fellow human being afflicted with cancer of the lung, the intent is to do the individual some good. The ratio of the good done for the patient to the harm inflicted by the irradiation is the therapeutic ratio. So long as the good exceeds the harm, then we stand on good grounds. All of our efforts are directed by technique to enhance the good and minimize the harm.

The patient's cancer is him. It is not a foreign organism invading his body. It is him and differs from his normal tissue in minimal ways. It is our role to destroy the tumor as it sits within the host surrounded by normal tissue; that is, normal in the sense that is not overtly infiltrated by cancer, and not normal in the sense that all people, of all ages, in all states of physiological well being do not share the same identical response to irradiation.

When one undertakes to treat a patient, there are four and only four possible outcomes. They are:

1) Control of tumor without complications,
2) Control of tumor with complications,
3) Failure to control the tumor without complications,
4) Failure to control the tumor with complications.

This scenario for evaluation of outcome and complications is dependent upon the parameters of treatment, i.e. total dose, fractionation, volume treated, total time, other events, i.e. surgery, chemotherapy, concomitant illnesses and the length of time the patient lives, since one cannot demonstrate a complication that takes one year to develop if the patient dies in six months.

Absorption of x-rays by tissues causes the acceleration of secondary electrons by photoelectric effect, compton effect or pair formation and generates ions. These in turn generate free radicals that are highly reactive chemical moieties that produce chemical changes that in turn produce biological effects. Some of these changes are reversible; others are fixed into the molecules, e.g. DNA, to be demonstrated when that molecule is required to function as in mitosis (GROSS, 1977). Since radiation injury will, in general, demonstrate itself during mitosis, it follows that rapidly turning over tissue is the first to demonstrate injury. When treating the chest of a human being the most common early side effect is dysphagia secondary to esophagitis. Although reported to occur at varying frequencies from 30–90% (COX et al., 1978; SEALY et al., 1982; ABRAMSON et al., 1973), it undoubtedly is present in all patients once a dose of 3,000 rads is attained. It is more frequent in higher fraction, short course irradiation but occurs in both. However, there are few reports of chronic injury since the tolerance dose of the esophagus is about 6,000 rads at 1,000 rads per week (RUBIN et al., 1972).

When a patient with lung cancer is irradiated his pulmonary function, as measured by Forced

Vital Capacity (FVC) and Forced Expiratory Volume (FEV) at one second, improves during the course of therapy, perhaps as a consequence of the resolution of tumor and the opening of bronchi to ventilation, to be followed by a modest decrease of about 10% in six months (Meoz et al.; Shankar, 1980).

8.1   Lung – Pneumonitis

The effect of radiation on the lung appears to be dose-time related with the incidence of pneumonitis ranging from zero at 750 rets to 100% at doses greater than 1,200 rets (Wara et al., 1973). This led to an estimate of 2,500 rets in 20 fractions as a threshold for pneumonitis. The effect of volume in decreasing the tolerance to radiation is demonstrated clinically with upper half body irradiation. Fryer et al. demonstrated an acute radiation pneumonitis syndrome with cough and characteristic radiographic changes in 44/245 patients (17.5%). The median onset was 100 days and fatal in 84% of the 44. This effect was 83% for 1,000 rads uncorrected for transmission and 29% for 800 rads uncorrected for transmission (Fryer et al., 1978). Fowler observes that a threshold dose of 600–700 rads corrected for tissue inhomogeneity seems to be present and recommends doses be kept below that threshold (Fowler and Travis, 1978).

Radiation pneumonitis is reported at about 2–11% (Gross, 1977; Abramson et al., 1973; Choi et al., 1981). The acute syndrome may be associated with fever, dry cough, chest pain, friction rub, tachycardia, rales, cyanosis or clubbing in extreme situations, or it may be asymptomatic with the diagnosis being made on chest x-ray. The findings are those of increased interstitial markings related to the radiation fields. The histological changes of septal edema and hyaline membrane formation exist at this time. Complete resolution of this syndrome can occur aided by treatment with steroids or it may remit spontaneously.

The occurrence of radiological changes in patients with breast cancer treated with megavoltage radiation was 41%. The proportion of the total who had symptoms corresponding to radiation pneumonitis was 11%. Late radiological changes corresponding to fibrosis were 60% but rarely were accompanied by symptoms (Gross, 1977). The late changes of pulmonary fibrosis are asymptomatic depending upon the volume of lung treated and now fibrosed.

The paradox of cancer treatment by radiation is pointed out by Cohen (1982) in that normal tissue tolerance is dependent upon the total volume of tissue treated, i.e. large volumes will tolerate small doses and vice versa. Tumors on the other hand have larger cell population proportional to their volume and thereby require greater cell kill from a larger radiation dose for control (Choi et al., 1981).

8.2   Spinal Cord – Myelopathy

Radiation induced injury of the spinal cord, myelopathy, has a frequency in the literature of 1% to 13.3% with the highest frequency being present in patients with longer survival (Emami et al., 1979; Sealy et al., 1982; Abramson et al., 1973; Fitzgerald et al., 1981). The estimated tolerance dose of the spinal cord is 4,500 to 5,000 rads at 800 to 1,000 rads per week (Rubin et al., 1972) with the tolerance falling as greater lengths of the spinal cord are treated and as fraction size increases (Fitzgerald et al., 1981).

The myelopathy syndromes are recognized as four distinct types (Reagan et al., 1980): 1) Transient myelopathy with the Lhermitte's sign being a feature, i.e. shock like sensation in the extremities with flexion of the neck. It is thought to be due to demyelination from injury to oligodendrogliocytes. 2) Chronic progressive myelopathy involving the lateral columns and producing a Brown-Sequard syndrome. 3) Acute paraplegia or quadraplegia depending upon the level of injury. 4) A lower motor neuron lesion with flaccid paralysis after lumbar irradiation. Lhermitte's sign is an unusual event in the last three types of injury manifestation. Aside from the acute transient form of myelopathy, there is no recovery from the injury (Fajardo, 1982b; Reagan et al., 1968).

To entertain the diagnosis of a radiation induced myelopathy one must be able to show that the spinal cord has been irradiated, that the segment of the cord must have been in the irradiated area and that cord compression must be excluded as an alternative diagnosis (Pallis et al., 1961).

In order to avoid excess injury to the spinal cord, the dose of radiation to the spinal cord must be kept to tolerance levels. This is accomplished by shielding with anterior-posterior opposing fields and avoidance of the cord using oblique boosting fields if doses of 4,500 rads are to be exceeded. Meticulous planning in three dimensions to account for all of the dose distribution is necessary, since patients chests have varying diameters and the spinal cord moves anteriorly in the upper part of the chest. Compensation for increased lung transmission and for changing chest contours are necessary to insure uniformity of dose. Documentation of the dose by in vivo measurement when possible, transmission measurement or entrance measurement plus weekly anatomical verification films assure good quality control. All these things are necessary if the price of prolonged survival is not to be paralysis in a significant minority of our patients.

8.3 Heart and Pericardium

The clinical syndromes of RIHD (radiation induced heart disease) according to FAJARDO are: 1) Acute pericarditis during radiation. This is rare and usually associated with tumor involvement of the pericardium. 2) Delayed pericarditis presenting as an acute pericarditis syndrome or as a chronic pericardial effusion. 3) Pericarditis presenting with pericardial and myocardial fibrosis with or without endocardial fibroelastosis. 4) Coronary artery disease. 5) Functional valvular or conduction defects (FAJARDO, 1982a). It is of interest that cardiac or pericardial syndromes are not typically described on the lists of complications in treatment series of lung cancer patients. It is shown as isolated instances at autopsy, and it is commonly described in association with Hodgkin's disease patients, in particular, those who have been retreated (SCHNEIDER et al., 1979; STEWART et al., 1971).

The treatment for the RIHD is to avoid treating as much of the heart as possible and to recognize that the most common form of the disease is a pericardial syndrome with effusion that can be treated by evacuation of the fluid or pericardiectomy in the long term survivor with an otherwise good prognosis.

References

Abramson N, Cavanaugh PJ (1970) Short-course radiation therapy in carcinoma of the lung, Radiology 96:627–630.

Abramson N, Cavanaugh PJ (1973) Short-course radiation therapy in carcinoma of the lung: a second look, Radiology 108:685–687.

American Cancer Society (1980) Cancer of the lung, CA 39:199–207.

Angell M (1982) The quality of mercy, N Engl J Med 306:98–99.

Baker R (1979) Pleural and pericardial effusions. In: Abeloff Md (ed) Complications of cancer, The Johns Hopkins Univ Press, Baltimore London p 169–184.

Berry RJ, Laing AH, Newman CR, et al (1977) The role of radiotherapy in treatment of inoperable lung cancer, Int J Radiat Oncol Biol Phys 2:433–439.

Bloedorn FG, Cowley RA, Cuccia CA, et al (1961) Combined therapy: irradiation and surgery in the treatment of bronchogenic carcinoma, Am J Roentgenol Radium Ther Nucl Med 85:875–885.

Bloedorn FG, Bowley RA, Cuccia CA, et al (1964) Preoperative irradiation in bronchogenic carcinoma, Am J Roentgenol Radium Ther Nucl Med 92:77–87.

Boag JW, Haybittle JL, Fowler JF, et al (1971) The number of patients required in a clinical trial, Br J Radiol 44:122–125.

Bonarigo BC, Rubin P (1967) Nonunion of pathological fracture after radiation therapy, Radiology 88:889–898.

Borgelt B, Gelber R, Kramer S, et al (1980) The palliation of brain metastases: final results of the first two studies by the radiation therapy oncology group, Int J Radiat Oncol Biol Phys 6:(6):1–9.

Brashear RE (1978) Editorial: Should asymptomatic patients with inoperable bronchogenic carcinoma receive immediate radiotherapy? No. Am Rev Respir Dis 117:411–414.

Bruckman JE, Blomer WD (1978) Management of spinal cord compression, Semin Oncol 5:135–140.

Budinger JM (1958) Untreated bronchogenic carcinoma. A clinicopathological study of 250 autopsied cases, Cancer 11:106–116.

Butler AR, Leo JS, Lin JP, et al (1979) The value of routine cranial computed tomography in neurologically intact patients with primary carcinoma of the lung, Radiology 131:399–401.

Chapman GS, Kumar D, Redmond J III, et al (1982) Letter to the editor: Upper abdominal CT scanning in staging non-oat cell lung carcinoma, N Engl J Med 307:189.

Choi NC, Grillo HC, Gardiello M, et al (1980) Basis for new stategies in postoperative radiotherapy of bronchogenic carcinoma, Int J Radiat Oncol Biol Phys 6:31–35.

Choi NC, Doucette JA (1981) Improved survival of patients with unresectable non-small cell bronchogenic carcinoma by an innovated high-dose en-bloc radiotherapeutic approach, Cancer 48:101–109.

Choi NC (1982) Editorial: Reassessment of the role of postoperative radiation therapy in resected lung cancer, Int J Radiat Oncol Biol Phys 8:2015–2018.

Chung CK, Stryker JA, O'Neill M Jr, et al (1982) Evaluation of adjuvant postoperative radiotherapy for lung cancer, Int J Radiat Oncol Biol Phys 8:1877–1880.

Cohen L (1982) The tissue volume factor in radiation oncology, Int J Radiat Oncol Biol Phys 8:1771–1774.

Cox JD, Petrovich Z, Paig C, et al (1978) Prophylatic cranial irradiation in patients with inoperable carcinoma of the lung. Preliminary report of a cooperative trial, Cancer 42:1135–1140.

Cox JD, Yesner R, Mietlowoki W, et al (1979) Influence of cell type on failure pattern after irradiation for locally advanced carcinoma of the lung, Cancer 44:94–98.

Cox JD, Komaki R, Eierst LR (1980) Irradiation for inoperable carcinoma of the lung and high performance status. JAMA 244:1931–1933.

Coy P, Kennelly GM (1980) The role of curative radiotherapy in the treatment of lung cancer, Cancer 45:698–702.

Deeley TJ (1966) A clinical trial to compare two different tumour dose levels in the treatment of advanced carcinoma of the bronchus, Clin Radiol 17:299–301.

Deeley TJ (1967) The treatment of carcinoma of the bronchus, Br J Radiol 40:801–822.

Dunnick NR, Ihde DC, Johnston-Early A (1979) Abdominal CT in the evaluation of small cell carcinoma of the lung, AJR 133:1085–1088.

Durrant KR, Berry RJ, Ellis F, et al (1971) Comparison of treatment policies in inoperable bronchial carcinoma, Lancet 1:715–719.

Easson EC (1967) The management of Hodgkin's disease and allied disorders. In: Deeley TJ, Wood CAP (eds) Modern trends in radiotherapy, Butterworths London, p 579.

Editorial (1976) Osteolytic metastases, Lancet 2:1063–1064.

Einhorn L (1983) Reporting on chemotherapy of both small cell and non-small cell lung cancer, The Clin Cancer Let 6(2):4.

Eisert DR, Cox JD, Komaki R (1976) Irradiation for bronchial carcinoma. Reasons for failure. I. Analysis of local control as a function of dose, time, and fractionation, Cancer 37:2665–2670.

Emami B, Melo A, Carter B, et al (1978) Value of computed tomography in radiotherapy of lung cancer, AJR 131:63–67.

Emami B, Munzenrider JE, Lee DJ, et al (1979) Radical radiation therapy for advanced lung cancer, Cancer 44:446–456.

Fajardo LF (1982a) Cardiovascular system. In: Pathology of radiation injury, chap 3, Masson Publishing, USA, p 15–33.

Fajardo LF (1982b) In: Pathology of radiation injury, chap 16, Masson Publishing, USA, p 220–226.

Feinstein AR (1967a) In: Clinical judgement, Williams and Wilkins Co., Baltimore, p 317.

Feinstein AR (1967b) A new staging system for cancer and reappraisal of "early" treatment and cure by radical surgery, N Engl J Med 279(14):747–753.

Fidler IJ, Hart IR (1982) Biological diversity in metastatic neoplasms: origins and implications, Science 217:998–1003.

Fitzgerald RH, Marks RD, Wallace KM (1981) Chronic radiation myelitis, Radiology 144:609–612.

Foley KM (1979) Pain syndromes in patients with cancer. In: Advanced pain research and therapy, Raven Press, New York.

Fowler JR, Travis EL (1978) The radiation pneumonitis syndrome in half-body radiation therapy, Int J Radiat Oncol Biol Phys 4:1111–1113.

Fowler JR (1982) Fractionation of radiation dose in therapy, ASTR refresher course, Int J Radiat Oncol Biol Phys, Proc. Am Soc Ther Radiol, Orlando, Florida, 8 (Suppl 1):56, 1982.

Fryer CJH, Fitzpatrick PJ, Rider WD, et al (1978) Radiation pneumonitis: experience following a large single dose of radiation, Int J Radiat Oncol Biol Phys 4:931–936.

Gilbert RW, Kim JH, Posner JB (1978) Epidural spinal cord compression from metastatic tumor: diagnosis and treatment, Ann Neurol 3:40–51.

Goff WF (1973) Intracordal polytef (Teflon) injection. Histologic study of two cases, Arch Otolaryngol 97:371–372.

Graham EA, Singer JJ (1933) Successful removal of an entire lung for carcinoma of the bronchus, JAMA 101:1371–1374.

Green J, Rubin P, Holzwasser G (1963) The experimental production of superior vena caval obstruction, Radiology 81:406–415.

Green N, Kurohara SS, George FW, III (1971) Cancer of the lung: an in-depth analysis of prognostic factors, Cancer 28:1229–1233.

Greenberg HS, Kim JH, Posner JB (1980) Epidural spinal cord compression from metastatic tumor: results with a new treatment protocol, Ann Neurol 8:361–366.

Gross NJ (1977) Pulmonary effects of radiation therapy, Ann Intern Med 86:81–92.

Guttman RJ (1965) Results of radiation therapy in patients with inoperable carcinoma of the lung whose status was established at exploratory thoracotomy, AJR 93:99–103.

Hilaris BS, Luomanen RK, Manan GD, et al (1971) Interstitial irradiation of apical lung cancer, Radiology 99:655–660.

Hilaris BS, Martini N, Batata M, et al (1975a) Interstitial irradiation for unresectable carcinoma of the lung, Ann Thorac Surg 20:491–500.

Hilaris BS, Henschke UK (1975b) General principles and techniques of interstitial brachytherapy. In: Hilaris BS (ed) Handbook of interstitial brachytherapy, chap 5, Publishing Sciences Grp Inc., Acton, Massachusetts.

Hilaris BS, Martini N, Luomanen RK (1979) Endobronchial interstitial implantation, Clin Bull 9(1):17–20.

Jacobs L, Kinkel WR, Vincent RG (1977) 'Silent' brain metastasis from lung carcinoma determined by computerized tomography, Arch Neurol 34:690–693.

Jesse RH, Lindberg RD, Westbrook KC (1980) Neck nodes. In: Textbook of radiotherapy, 4th edn, Lea & Febiger, Philadelphia, p 339.

Johnson RJR, Walton RJ, Lim ML, et al (1973) A randomized study on survival of bronchogenic carcinoma treated with conventional or short fractionation radiation, Clin Radiol 24:494–497.

Kanji AM, Chao JH, Liebner EJ, et al (1980) Extrinsic compression of superior vena cava: an analysis of 41 patients, Int J Radiat Oncol Biol Phys 6:213–215.

Kirsh MM, Sloan H (1981) Treatment of bronchogenic carcinoma with mediastinal metastases: a 15-year experience. In: Controversies in Surgical Oncology, pp 69–74.

Kjaer M (1982) Radiotherapy of squamous, adeno- and large cell carcinoma of the lung, Cancer Treat Rev 9:1–20.

Kline IK (1972) Cardiac lymphatic involvement by metastatic tumor, Cancer 29:799–808.

Leddy ET, Moersch HJ (1940) Roentgen therapy for bronchogenic carcinoma, JAMA 115:2239–2242.

Lewy RB, Matthews R (1965) Immediate temporary restoration of glottic valve function, Laryngoscope 75:1348–1351.

Luomanen RKJ, Watson WL (1968) Autopsy findings. In: Watson, WL (ed) Lung Cancer: A study of five thousand Memorial Hospital cases. CV Mosby, Saint Louis, Mo., p 504.

Mangini RJ (1982) Clinically important cimetidine drug interactions, Clin Pharm 1:433–439.

Marks RM, Sachar EJ (1973) Undertreatment of medical inpatients with narcotic analgesics, Ann Intern Med 78:173–181.

Matthews MJ, Kanhowa S, Pickren J, et al (1973) Frequency of residual and metastatic tumor in patients undergoing curative surgical resection for lung cancer. Cancer Chemother Rep 4(2):63–67.

McBride CM, Brown BW, Thompson JR, et al (1983) Can patients with breast cancer be cured of their disease?, Cancer 51:938–945.

Medical letter (1982) Drug treatment of cancer pain, Med Lett Drugs Ther 24(621):95–96.

Meoz RT, Hudgins PT, Wright A (1978) Effect of pulmonary function of split course radiation therapy for carcinoma of the lung, Rev Interam Radiol 3:(1):15–19.

Meyer JA (1973) Growth rate versus prognosis in resected primary bronchogenic carcinomas, Cancer 31: 1468–1472.

Mira JG, Fullerton GD, Ezekiel J, et al (1982) Evaluation of computed tomography numbers for treatment planning of lung cancer, Int J Radiat Oncol Biol Phys 8:1625–1628.

Morrison R, Deeley TJ, Cleland WP (1963) The treatment of carcinoma of the bronchus. A clinical trial to compare surgery and radiotherapy, Lancet 1:683–684.

Mountain CF, Carr DT, Anderson WAD (1974) A system for the clinical staging of lung cancer, AJR 120:130–138.

Muhm JR (1980) Editorial: Role of computed tomography in evaluation of intrathoracic lesions, J Thorac Cardiovasc Surg 79:469–470.

Neilsen ME Jr, Heaston DK, Dunnick NR, et al (1982) Preoperative CT evaluation of adrenal glands in non-small cell bronchogenic carcinoma, AJR 139:317–320.

Nogeire C, Mincer F, Botstein C (1979) Long survival in patients with bronchogenic carcinoma complicated by superior vena caval obstruction, Chest 75:325–329.

Occam's razor, Webster's New Collegiate Dictionary, G & C Merriam Company, Springfield, Mass, USA.

Olson KB (1935) Primary carcinoma of the lung: a pathology study, Am J Pathol 11:449–468.

Ormerod FC (1937) The pathology and treatment of carcinoma of the bronchus, J Laryngol Otol 52:733–745.

Ormerod FC (1953) The late results of treatment, by interstitial radiation, of one hundred cases of carcinoma of the bronchus, J Laryngol Otol 67:406–416.

Pallis CA, Louis S, Morgan RL (1961) Radiation myelopathy, Brain 84:460–479.

Parish JM, Marschke RF, Dines DE, et al (1981) Etiologic considerations in superior vena cava syndrome. Mayo Clin Proc 56:407–413.

Pater JL, Loeb M (1982) Nonanatomic prognostic factors in carcinoma of the lung. A multivariate analysis, Cancer 50:326–331.

Percarpio B, Gray S (1979) Prolonged survival following the superior vena cava syndrome, Chest 75:639–640.

Perez CA, Presant CA, Van Amburg AL III (1978) Management of superior vena cava syndrome, Semin Oncol 5:123–134.

Perez CA, Stanley K, Rubin P, Kramer S, et al (1980) Patterns of tumor recurrence after definitive irradiation for inoperable non-oat cell carcinoma of the lung, Int J Radiat Oncol Biol Phys 6:987–994.

Perez CA (1982) Editorial: Is postoperative irradiation indicated in carcinoma of the lung? Int J Radiat Oncol Biol Phys 8:2019–2022.

Petrovich Z, Stanely K, Cox JD, Paig C (1981) Radiotherapy in the management of locally advanced lung cancer of all cell types: final report of randomized trial, Cancer 48:1335–1340.

Posner JB (1977) Management of central nervous system metastases, Semin Oncol 4(1):81–91.

Poste G, Doll J, Fidler IJ (1981) Interactions among clonal subpopulations affect stability of the metastatic phenotype in polyclonal population of big melanoma cells, Proc Natl Acad Sci USA 78(10):6626–6630.

Prasad SC, Pilepich MV, Perez CA (1981) Contribution of CT to quantative radiation therapy planning, AJR 136:123–128.

Reagan TJ, Thomas JE, Colby MY Jr, (1968) Chronic progressive radiation myelopathy. Its clinical aspects and differential diagnosis, JAMA 203:106–110.

Renner WD, O'Connor TP, Amtey SR et al (1977) The use of photogammetry in tissue compensator design, Part I: Photogrammetric determination of patient topography, Radiology 125:505–510, Part II: Experimental verification of compensator design, Radiology 125:511–516.

Renner WD, O'Connor TP, Bermudez NM (1982) An electronic device for digitizing radiotherapy films for the construction of tissue compensators, Med Phys 9:910–916.

Rosenblatt MB (1964) Lung cancer in the 19th century, Bull Hist of Med 38:395–425.

Rubin P, Green J, Holzwasser G, et al (1963) Superior vena cava syndrome. Slow low-dose versus rapid high-dose schedules, Radiology 81:388–401.

Rubin P (1969) Extradural spinal cord compression by tumor. Part I: Experimental production and treatment trials, Radiology 93:1243–1260.

Rubin P, Casarett GW (1972) A direction for clinical radiation pathology: the tolerance dose. In: Vaeth JM (ed) Frontiers of Radiation Therapy and Oncology, vol 6, University Park Press, Baltimore, London, pp 1–16.

Russell MH (1958) Contribution to symposium on presentation of results of cancer treatment, Seventh Intl Cancer Congress, London.

Salazar OM, Scarantino CW, Rubin P, et al (1980) Total (half-body) systemic irradiation for occult metastases in non-small cell lung cancer, Cancer 46:1932–1944.

Sandler MA, Pearlberg JL, Madrazo BL, et al (1982) Computed tomographic evaluation of the adrenal gland in the preoperative assessment of bronchogenic carcinoma, Radiology 145:733–736.

Schneider JS, Edwards JE (1979) Irradiation-induced pericarditis, Chest 75:560–564.

Sealy R, Lagakos S, Barkley T, et al (1982) Radiotherapy of regional epidermoid carcinoma of the lung: a study in fractionation, Cancer 49:1338–1345.

Selawry OS, Hansen H (1973) Lung cancer. In: Holland JF, Frei E (ed) Cancer Medicine, chap XXIII, Lea & Febiger, Philadelphia pp 1473–1518.

Seydel HG, Kutcher GJ, Steiner RM, et al (1980) Computed tomography in planning radiation therapy for bronchogenic carcinoma, Int J Radiat Oncol Biol Phys 6:601–606.

Shah K, Olson MH, Ray P, et al (1981) Comparison of dose-time-fractionation schemes in non-oat cell lung cancer, Cancer 48:1127–1132.

Shankar PS (1980) Split-course radiation therapy: effects on pulmonary function in patients with bronchogenic carcinoma, J Am Geriatr Soc 28:547–549.

Sherman DM, Weichselbaum R, Hellman S (1981) The characteristics of long-term survivors of lung cancer treated with radiation, Cancer 47:2575–2580.

Silverberg E (1983) Cancer statistics, CA 33(1):9–25.

Slawson RG, Prempree T, Viravathana T, et al (1981) Radiation therapy for superior vena cava syndrome due to lung cancer, Md State Med J 30(11):68–70.

Smart J (1966) Can lung cancer be cured by radiation alone?, JAMA 195:1034–1035.

Sontag S (1979) Illness as metaphor, Farrar, Straus and Giroux, New York.

Spjut HJ, Mateo LE (1965) Recurrent and metastatic carcinoma in surgically treated carcinoma of the lung, Cancer 18:1462–1466.

Stewart JR, Fajardo LF (1971) Radiation induced heart disease. Clinical and experimental aspects, Radiol Clin North Am 9:511–531.

Straus MJ (1974) The growth characteristics of lung cancer and its application to treatment design, Semin Oncol 1:167–173.

Tong D, Gillick L, Hendrickson FR (1982) The palliation of symptomatic osseous metastases. Final results of the study by the Radiation Therapy Oncology Group, Cancer 50:893–899.

Törmä T (1957) Malignant tumors of the spine and the spinal extradural space. A study of 250 histologically verified cases, Acta Chir Scand [Suppl] 225:1–138.

Twycross RG (1979) Advances in pain research and therapy. In: Bonica JJ, Ventafridda V (ed) Overview of analgesia, vol 2, Raven Press, New York, pp 617–633.

Ushio Y, Posner R, Posner JB, et al (1977) Experimental spinal cord compression by epidural neoplasms, Neurology 27:422–429.

Van Houtte P, Rocmans P, Smetz P, et al (1980) Postoperative radiation therapy in lung cancer: a controlled trial after resection of curative design, Int J Radiat Oncol Biol Phys 6:983–986.

Wara WU, Phillips TL, Margolis LW, et al (1973) Radiation pneumonitis: a new approach to the deviation of time dose factors, Cancer 32:547–552.

West J, Maor M (1980) Intracranial metastases: behavioral patterns related to primary site and results of treatment by whole brain irradiation, Int J Radiat Oncol Biol Phys 6:11–15.

White KT, Fleming TR, Laws ER Jr (1981) Single metastasis to the brain. Surgical treatment in 122 consecutive patients, Mayo Clin Proc 56:424–428.

Zylak CJ, Pallie W, Jackson R (1982) Correlative anatomy and computed tomography: a module on the medias terms, Radiographics 2(4):555–592.

Chapter VII Results of Clinical Trials and Basis for Future Therapeutics

FREDERICK RICHARDS and CHARLES W. SCARANTINO

CONTENTS

FREDERICK RICHARDS, II, M.D., Associate Professor of Medicine, Department of Medicine

CHARLES W. SCARANTINO, M.D., Ph.D., Associate Professor of Radiation Oncology, Department of Radiology

Bowman Gray School of Medicine of Wake Forest University, 300 South Hawthorne Road, Winston-Salem, NC 27103, USA

Cancer of the lung is the most common and most lethal form of human cancer in the United States. During 1983, there will be approximately 139,000 new cases and about 121,000 deaths from lung cancer in the United States (SILVERBERG, 1984). The overall five-year survival rate with this disease is less than five percent, a resultant from the fact that at diagnosis the disease is usually advanced.

Antineoplastic chemotherapy and irradiation therapy have been utilized to improve the control of bronchogenic carcinoma. Considerable progress has been made in the therapy of small cell carcinoma, and encouraging results are being seen with patients with the other tumor histologies. The natural history of the disease is still a powerful indicator of prognosis.

Lung cancer is currently divided into two major categories: those of the small cell anaplastic carcinoma variety and those of the non-small cell type (epidermoid, adenocarcinoma, and large cell anaplastic carcinoma). This broad categorization is based on the knowledge that the natural history and the clinical course of small cell lung cancer differs substantially from the non-small cell varieties (COHEN, 1982).

1 Main Problems Associated with the Treatment of Lung Cancer

1.1 Small Cell Lung Cancer

Small cell carcinoma of the lung comprises between 15 and 25% of all bronchogenic carcinoma. Therefore, it is estimated that there are approximately 20 to 35,000 new cases of small cell (oat cell) lung cancer annually. This disease is characterized by rapid tumor proliferation, high thymidine labeling index (range, 11%–30%), short doubling time, and a large proliferation or growth fraction (MUGGIA et al., 1974). Cell cycle time is similar to other human solid tumors but growth is much higher. It is more often associated with paraneoplastic syndromes than the other lung cancer types. This disease may originate from the Kulchitsky type cell (K-cell) of the amine precursor uptake and decarboxylation (APUD) system from the basal lining of the bronchial mucosa (TISCHLER, 1978; PETTENGILL et al., 1980; GAZDAR et al., 1980). Clinically, this disease is characterized by rapid growth, a short symptomatic period with abrupt presentation, early tumor dissemination, and a short median survival of 6 weeks (extensive disease) to 12 weeks (limited disease) in untreated patients. Small cell lung cancers are seldom resectable. These tumors are highly sensitive to chemotherapy and radiotherapy, and complete and partial responses are seen in a high percentage of cases. There is no relationships between TNM stage and survival because of its propensity for disseminated disease. However, the simple classification into limited disease (tumor confined to one hemithorax including ipsilateral supraclavicular fossa) and extensive disease (tumor outside this area) is of value in prognosis. About two-thirds of patients present with extensive and one-third with limited involvement.

Most physicians feel that chemotherapy is the most important modality in the therapy of small cell carcinoma of the lung because of its propensity for early dissemination. In limited disease, radiotherapy seems to be necessary for prolonged disease-free survival. The value of thoracic irradiation in extensive disease is less certain. Prophylactic cranial irradiation helps prevent cerebral disease but does not prolong survival. The role of surgery as a "debulking" modality in limited disease needs further investigation.

Recently, aggressive treatment using either combination chemotherapy alone or combination chemotherapy and chest irradiation, have resulted in a significant proportion of disease-free survivors and improvement in median survival (COMIS, 1982). The median survival of those with extensive disease is about 9 months and about 12–18 months for those with limited disease. More importantly, about 10–12% of small cell carcinoma patients (probably <3% with extensive disease and 10–25% with limited disease) may enjoy disease-free remissions of two years or longer; it is thought that many of these latter patients may be cured (GRECO and OLDHAM, 1979a). It has not yet been established whether these fortunate patients should be continuously maintained on some form of chemotherapy until relapse, or if therapy should be discontinued after patients have remained disease-free for a given period of time.

Complete response is essential to prolonged remission and survival. Bronchoscopy is helpful in substantiating complete response. Most patients who will achieve a complete response will usually do so within one to three treatment cycles. Important factors for complete response are good performance status, extent of disease, and number of metastatic sites of extensive disease (GRECO et al., 1979b; GINSBERG et al., 1979; MINNA et al., 1982). Further efforts, therefore, are necessary to achieve complete response and thereby improve the duration of longer term disease free survival. Furthermore, despite initial responses, a large percentage of patients continue to relapse and die of distant and local metastases. Relapses most commonly occur in the primary site and areas of previously documented metastases.

In addition to complete response to therapy, extent of disease, immune status, and performance status are important prognostic factors (BUNN et al., 1977; LIVINGSTON et al., 1978b). Some studies have reported females to live significantly longer than males (EDMONDSON et al., 1976). Prior therapy also influences response and survival. There is no significant alteration in prognosis associated with age, race, site of primary tumor (main bronchus, hilum, peripheral or apical), radiological appearance (solitary or multiple, circumscribed or noncircumscribed, presence or absence of pneumonitis, atelectasis), histological subtype, or mediastinal invasion (MOUNTAIN, 1978). Extent of disease is a very important factor both in regards to complete response and median survival (BUNN et al., 1977). In addition, performance status ("ambulatory" and "non-ambulatory" status) also significantly influences response to treatment and survival both independently and when used in conjunction with extent of disease (LIVINGSTON et al., 1978b). Although about 60–80% of patients with small cell lung cancer initially respond to therapy, probably less than five percent are potentially cured. In most studies both tumor response to therapy and survival are related to disease extent and performance status of the patient at diagnosis. Metastasis to the central nervous system or liver significantly shortens survival but involvement of bone, soft tissue, or bone marrow does not adversely affect survival (MINNA et al., 1982). A single metastatic site usually does not affect survival.

Small cell carcinoma comprises about 20% of lung cancers. Small cell carcinomas tend to be central lesions, but they may also occur peripherally.

Usually they grow submucosally and spread quickly to the regional (bronchial, hilar, and mediastinal) lymph nodes. Cavitation is rare. Cell growth studies using in vivo labelled tritiated thymidine have shown small cell carcinoma to have the most rapid doubling time of all tumors. These tumors have a propensity for rapid and early spread outside of the hemithorax with wide-spread metastases. There are two major histological types of small cell carcinoma of the lung: the classic lymphocyte like (oat cell) subtype and the intermediate cell subtypes (which include the fusiform, polygonal, and other varieties). There are no clinically significant differences in behavior of the various histological subtypes (COHEN and MATTHEWS, 1978). The lymphocyte-like and fusiform varities may have better survival (NIXON et al., 1979). Although cells are relatively small and have high nuclear-cytoplasmic ratios, the distinguishing features are the nuclear characteristics. Nuclear chromatin is dispensed in a uniform fine and coarse stippled pattern throughout the entire nucleus. Nucleoli are small and indistinct. Ultrastructurally, the characteristic feature is the presence of neurosecretory granules.

The cellular origin of small cell carcinoma of the lung is a matter of controversy. As already alluded to above, small cell lung cancer appears to be a distinct biological entity and the cells have APUD properties. In vivo and in vitro studies have shown that small cell lung carcinomas have many of the properties associated with APUD cells including neurosecretory granules, high specific activity of the APUD enzyme L-dopa decarboxylase, neuron-specific enolase, and the secretion of a variety of polypeptides and hormones (GAZDAR et al., 1980; BENSCH et al., 1968; BAYLIN et al., 1978; SORENSON et al., 1981; HANSEN et al., 1980b). Recent data as discussed below indicate a common origin for all bronchial carcinomas (Section 1.3).

A number of important biological studies of small cell carcinoma of the lung have identified markers that distinguish small cell lung cancer from the non-small cell varieties (MINNA et al., 1982). Of particular interest is the peptide hormone bombesin which stimulates small cell lung cancer lesions to grow. Bombesin is produced by tumor cells and is potentially a new blood marker for following small cell lung cancer (MOODY et al., 1983). In addition, it could be responsible for some of the paraneoplastic features of small cell lung cancer. Another new marker is the presence of a specific acquired chromosome defect, deletion 3 p (14–23) which appears to be specific for small cell lung cancer (WHANG-PENG 1982).

In addition, these cell clone cultures have been used for in vitro chemotherapy studies with encouraging correlations with clinical results. In vitro resistence was correlated with in vivo resistence in 100% of cases, while correlation of in vitro/in vivo sensitivity was 75% (MINNA et al., 1982).

In addition, several monoclonal antibodies using hybridoma technology have been prepared against small cell lung cancer. These monoclonal antibodies have been found to have potential applicability in treatment and diagnosis (MINNA et al., 1982).

1.2 Non-small Cell Lung Cancer

Non-small cell carcinoma of the lung constitutes approximately 75 to 85% of all lung cancers. In contrast to small cell lung cancer, non-small cell lung cancer (NSCLC) is a heterogeneous group, with distinct but overlapping histological features, clinical course, and biologic behavior. For NSCLC, careful staging is the most important factor in deciding treatment. Few, if any, biologic markers characterize non-small cell lung cancer. With the exception of surgical excision, response to treatment is limited and brief. They cannot be cured once they have spread beyond the thoracic cavity. At the present time, non-small cell lung cancers are usually combined into groups and treated as a single entity because our knowledge of the biology of non-small cell lung cancer is relatively limited. Eventually, the importance of delineating non-small cell lung cancer into histologic (or other) types will become apparent as we begin to understand the biology.

The great majority of lung cancer of all types (non-small cell lung cancer and small cell lung cancer) are aneuploid (RABER et al., 1980; BUNN et al., 1980; CARY et al., 1981) and have a relatively high proliferative activity as determined by the percentage of cells in S phase (mean 17.5%). Most have a single aneuploid peak suggesting monoclonal origin. Cytogenetic studies demonstrate that small cell lung cancer tumors and cell lines have a highly specific chromosomal abnormality (WHANG-PENG et al., 1982). In contrast, all non-small cell lung cancer cell lines are aneuploid with many numerical and structural chromosomal abnormalities, and that chromosomes 1, 2, 3, 9, 11, and 12 are frequently involved, and 8, 13, 20, and 21 less frequently (Gazdar et al., 1983).

1.2.1 Squamous Cell Carcinoma

Squamous cell carcinoma comprises 30 to 35% of lung cancers. Squamous cell carcinoma is the only bronchogenic carcinoma that has a recognized phase of dysplasia and carcinoma in situ distinct from invasive carcinoma. It is frequently multifocal. Over two-thirds arise centrally at the bifurcation of segmental on subsegmental bronchi. They tend to extend into the bronchus to form obstructing masses. Microscopic criteria for diagnosis requires epithelial stratification and obvious intercellular bridge formation. Better differentiated tumors elaborate keratin. These tumors tend to locally invade adjoining lung parenchyma and regional lymph nodes. They cavitate more frequently than other lung tumors. In about one-half of the case studies at autopsy, particularly the well differentiated types, no extrathoracic metastases can be identified (Matthews et al., 1983). Poorly differentiated tumors tend to metastasize outside the chest.

1.2.2 Adenocarcinoma

Adenocarcinomas of the lung are identified by the formation of glandular or papillary structures and/ or by mucin production. Desmoplasia may be seen. Adenocarcinomas appear to be increasing in frequency and now constitute 25 to 30% of lung cancer. Most adenocarcinomas present as circumscribed peripheral lung masses. There is a strong association between scarring of the lungs and adenocarcinomas, both diffuse and localized. It is thought that peripheral adenocarcinomas occur in association with scars and that they also produce typical central foci of scarring due to vascular involvement. Cellular distribution of glycoproteins after in vitro labelling suggests that adenocarcinomas arise from a cell type committed to differentiated into ciliated epithelium (Dermer, 1981). Bronchiolo-alveolar carcinoma, a relatively rare type of adenocarcinoma, arise from type II pneumonocytes or their precursors, the Clara cells. These peripheral masses are unrelated to bronchi except by local invasion, compression, or submucosal lymphatic spread (Matthews et al., 1983; Yesner and Carter, 1982). Adenocarcinomas spread early to the pleura and mediastinal lymph node and extrathoracic sites such as the adrenal,

liver, central nervous system, and bone (Matthews et al., 1983; Yesner and Carter, 1982). Its tendency to metastasize to the brain is particularly noteworthy, in that brain metastases may be the presenting symptoms and in about 10 to 15% of cases the brain may be the only site of metastases. Prophylactic brain irradiation may, therefore, be of value in adenocarcinoma (Yesner and Carter, 1982; Cox et al., 1978).

1.2.3 Large Cell Carcinoma

Large cell lung cancers are defined as non-small cell neoplasms without cellular maturation; they comprise about 15 to 20% of lung cancers and are usually peripheral in location (Mitchell et al., 1980). They lack the characteristic nuclear cytology of small cell lung cancer. Histological criteria of diagnosis include cells greater than 12 µm in diameter, no evidence of keratinization, and no evidence of tubule formation or mucin production. These tumors do not behave clinically like the small cell undifferentiated lung cancer. Giant cell carcinoma of the lung is a rare tumor that resembles the large cell undifferentiated tumor (Kallenberg and Jaqué, 1979). These tumors tend to grow quite large locally and metastasize late. They tend to have a high rate of cerebral metastases.

1.3 Interrelationships of Tumors

Despite fairly specific microscopic appearances and clinical behavior of the majority of lung cancers, there is evidence that all lung cancers including the small cell lung cancer may arise from a common stem cell or endoderm (Yesner and Carter, 1982; Berger et al., 1981; McDowell and Trump, 1981; Gazdar et al., 1981). All varieties of lung cancer may occur within a single tumor, and it is not usual for changes in cell type to occur following therapy with chemotherapy or radiation therapy or for in vitro transformation of lung cancer to occur with the passage of time. Electron microscopic features of small cell, squamous cell, and adenocarcinoma may be found within individual cells. Biochemical markers (histaminase, calcitonin, B-lipotropin, ACTH, l-dopa decarboxylase) may be found with both small and non-small cell lung tumors (Berger et al., 1981). These data suggest that there is a close ontogenic relationship among the various histological types and that they could well evolve from a common cell linkage.

2 Results of Clinical Trials

2.1 Small Cell Lung Carcinoma

2.1.1 Chemotherapy

Small cell lung carcinoma is a highly aggressive tumor, and most patients will die from the disease. Unlike the other histological subtypes of lung cancer, where surgical resection is the most effective therapy, small cell lung cancer is widely disseminated at diagnosis. Therefore, chemotherapy alone or in combination with radiation therapy is the only currently effective therapy available. Small cell lung cancer usually has an explosive course with most patients having systemic or extrathoracic symptoms such as weight loss, bone pain, or the consequences of ectopic hormone production. Dissemination occurs much earlier than in other types of lung cancer, and the great majority of patients have had their symptoms for less than two months. Distant metastases are found in about 65% of small cell lung cancer patients dying from non-tumor-related causes within 30 days of curative resection (MATTHEWS et al., 1973). At autopsy, tumor confinement to the chest is found in less than five percent of patients. Metastases are found with substantial frequency in almost every organ of the body with involvement of hilar and mediastinal lymph nodes, liver, adrenals, abdominal lymph nodes, bone marrow, pancreas, bone, contralateral lung, and central nervous system being especially common. The propensity to involve endocrine glands (including the adrenals, thyroid, pancreas, testis, and pituitary) is striking. An isolated peripheral nodule in small cell lung cancer amenable to surgical resection is rare.

The TNM staging classification is not applicable to small cell lung cancer because of its rapid dissemination and occult metastases are very common. Improved techniques such as the CT scan frequently identifies unsuspected tumor both in the abdomen and the chest (HARPER et al., 1981). The classification of small cell lung cancer into limited disease (tumor confined to one hemithorax including the ipsilateral supraclavicular region) and extensive disease (tumor outside this area) is of value in prognosis. About 25 to 30% of patients present with limited disease. The natural (untreated) history of limited disease is usually less than 35 weeks (median 12–14 weeks) and less than 20 weeks (median 5–7 weeks) in those with extensive disease. Patients with supraclavicular node involvement and/or superior vena cava syndrome have the same response rate and overall prognosis as limited disease while those with pleural effusions behave like extensive disease (LIVINGSTON, 1980a). Liver and CNS metastases are associated with a particularly poor prognosis. Overall, the median survival is about ten weeks with less than five percent alive at one year (GRECO, 1979a).

Combination chemotherapy has improved the natural history of small cell lung cancer (BUNN et al., 1977; GRECO et al., 1978; WEISS, 1978) (Table 1). Several chemotherapy agents have greater than 20% response rate in this disease including adriamycin, vincristine, cyclophosphamide, methotrexate, vindesine, and epipodophyllotoxin (VP-16-213). Duration of response with single agent is brief (median of 3 months), and less than 3% achieve a complete remission (BRODER et al., 1977). The median survival with single agent therapy is similar to that of local radiotherapy (5–6 months). Combining three or four drugs yields an objective response rate of 80 to 95% with an improvement of median survival in limited disease to about 12–16 months and extensive disease to 8–12 months. The attainment of a complete response or complete remission seems to be the most important factor in prognosis. The complete response rate for limited disease approaches 60% as compared to 20% for extensive disease (GRECO et al., 1978). About 20–25% of patients who achieve a complete response treated with chemotherapy alone or in combination with radiation therapy have a two year disease free survival. Overall, about 8 to 17% of patients with limited disease and 0–2% of patients with extensive disease are disease free at two years. Complete response is significantly more likely in fully ambulatory patients with limited disease (48 versus 21%, p<0.05), and complete or partial response is more likely in fully ambulatory patients with extensive disease (65 versus 46%, p<0.01) (LIVINGSTON et al., 1981).

Table 1. Results of chemotherapy in small cell lung cancer[a]

	Limited disease patients	Extensive disease patients
Complete response rate	50–60%	20–25%
Partial response rate	30–40%	40–50%
Median survival (Mo)	12–16	8–12
Two year survival	10–17%	0– 2%

[a] Adopted from COMIS, 1982; AISNER, 1982; MORSTYN, 1984

Complete responses are significantly longer than partial responses (median of 48 weeks versus 29 weeks for limited and 39 weeks versus 19 weeks for extensive disease, p=0.001). The duration of response for limited disease is greater than that for extensive disease. The relapse rate declines after 18 months, but failures continued to occur and continuous remission beyond four years is achieved in only 18% of limited disease and ten percent of extensive disease in patients who achieve an initial complete remission (Livingston et al., 1981).

Total intrathoracic tumor area correlates with response and survival (Harper et al., 1982). In one study, patients with T_1 or T_2 lesions (less than 30 cm^2) had a complete response rate of 62% and median survival of 58.8 weeks versus none for larger tumor and median survival of 34 weeks (p= 0.001).

Some studies suggest that all complete responses are evident by six weeks (two courses) whereas other studies indicate that it may take as many as six courses of chemotherapy (Cohen et al., 1977b; Aisner et al., 1982; Cohen et al., 1979). Some recent studies have suggested that intensive induction therapy for six courses without subsequent maintenance may provide for reasonable response and survival results (Feld et al., 1981; Natale et al., 1980). Thus, it appears that a minimum of six courses of chemotherapy may be necessary and maintenance may not be necessary to prolong response and survival.

The simultaneous administration of active drugs is more efficacious than their sequential administration. Intensive inductive chemotherapy in which drug doses are given irrespective of hematological toxicity results in a higher response rate and longer survival but is associated with increasing toxicity and mortality related to therapy (Bunn et al., 1977; Cohen et al., 1977b; Minna et al., 1980).

Other investigators have attempted to prevent drug resistance to increase the complete response rate and thereby improve survival by using alternating combinations of drugs that are not cross-resistant (Cohen et al., 1979; Aisner et al., 1980; Livingston and Mira, 1980b). There appears to be slight improvement in response duration and survival. Other investigators are attempting to increase the two-year survival percentage by intensive therapy after an initial response (Bunn et al., 1981).

The question of duration of therapy remains. Firm guidelines for continuation of therapy are not established and various studies have ended therapy at 6–30 months (Bunn et al., 1981). Results are similar suggesting that shorter periods of therapy may be as effective as longer periods. One study randomized complete responders at 6 months to continued versus no additional chemotherapy until relapse. Although survival was significantly improved in limited disease patients, response duration was not (Maurer et al., 1980). There are few relapses among patients with limited disease after 24 months. Patients with limited disease have similar patterns of failure whether they achieve complete or partial response. About two-thirds of relapses occur intially in the chest alone and at least one-third of these are in the irradiated field (Matthews et al., 1973). About 25% of the failures after response were *not* from clinical relapse: sudden death, radiation pneumonitis, a second squamous lung cancer, aspiration pneumonitis, other medical deaths, and one-third of relapses occurred outside of chest.

Patients with extensive disease also have similar recurrence patterns, regardless of type of response (CR/PR). Fifteen percent die without clinical evidence of recurrent disease. Among those who relapse, 24% fail intially in the chest alone. Failure at a single site (chest or prior metastatic involvement) occurs in 47%. Relapse in isolated non-brain CNS sites (meningeal, epidural) accounted for 5% of all and 11% of "new recurrences". About 32% had documented relapse in several sites (Feld et al., 1981; Maurer et al., 1980). In a recent study in which radiation therapy to the chest was not administered to patients with extensive disease, the incidence of "chest only" failure was greater than 50% with comparable response duration. This may indicate greater ability of the more recent, aggressive chemotherapy to cope with systemic micrometastases, coupled with poor local control because irradiation at the primary site was deleted (Livingston et al., 1981).

In a study of combined irradiation to the chest with radiotherapy McMahon et al. observed that 60% of limited disease and 20% of extensive disease patients had relapse in the chest alone, and the median time to relapse was twice as long (540 versus 270 days) in patients who received greater than 4,000 rads to the chest, compared to those who received only 3,000 rads (McMahon et al., 1979).

Preliminary studies utilizing intensive chemotherapy and TBI (total body irradiation) with autologons bone marrow transplantation in small cell lung cancer are encouraging (Stewart et al.,

Table 2. Toxic reactions of some of the more commonly used drugs in lung cancer

Agent	Trade name	Route of adminis- tration	Myelo- sup- pres- sion	Stoma- titis	Nausea and vomi- ting	Alo- pecia	Skin nec- rosis	Ana- phyla- xis	Other specific toxicities
Alkylating agents									
Mechlorethamine	Mustargen (HN$_2$)	IV	+	0	+	+	+	0	Hepatotoxic, ototoxic
Cyclophos- phamide	Cytoxan	IV, PO	+	±	+	+	0	0	Sterile hemor- rhagic cystitis
Chloroethyl- cyclohexyl- nitrosourea (CNNU)	Lomustine	PO	+	+	+	±	0	0	Hepatotoxic
Chlorethyl- methyl-cyclo- hexal-nitroso- urea (MeCCNU)	Semustine	PO	+	+	+	0	0	0	Hepatotoxic, renal toxicity
Antimetabolites									
Methotrexate (MTX)	Methotrexate	PO, IV, IM	+	+	±	±	0	0	Hepatotoxic, renal toxicity
5-fluorouracil (5-FU)	Fluorouracil	IV	+	+	±	0	0	0	Diarrhea, neurotoxic (rare)
Antibiotics									
Doxorubicin	Adriamycin	IV	+	+	+	+	+	0	Cardiotoxic, diarrhea
Bleomycin	Blenoxane	IM	±	±	0	+	0	+	Pulmonary fibrosis, skin rash
Mitomycin C	Mutamycin	IV	+	+	+	+	+	0	Renal toxicity
Natural Products									
Vincristine	Oncovin	IV	0	0	0	+	+	0	Neurotoxic
Vinblastine	Velban	IV	+	+	±	±	+	0	Neurotoxic
Vindesine		IV	+	+	+	+	+	0	Neurotoxic
VP-16		IV	+	0	+	+	0	+	Hypotension
Miscellaneous Drugs									
Procarbazine	Matulane	PO	±	+	+	0	0	0	Monoamine oxid- ase inhibitor, neurotoxic, skin reactions
Cis-platinum	Platinol	IV	+	0	+	0	0	+	Renal toxicity, peripheral neuropathy, ototoxicity
Hexamethyl- melamine		PO	+	0	+	±	0	0	Neurotoxic, skin reactions

1983). The addition of anticoagulation with warfarin to chemotherapy in small cell lung cancer has been reported to be of benefit in two separate trials (ZACHARSKI et al., 1981; CHAHINIAN et al., 1984). There has also been a lot of interest in immunotherapy (BCG, MER fraction of BCG, corynebacterium parvum, levamisole, thymosin, interferon) of lung cancer, but most of these agents have shown no efficacy (JACKSON et al., 1982; McCRACKEN et al., 1982; MORSTYN et al., 1984; JONES et al., 1983; COHEN et al., 1982).

2.1.1.1 Toxicity. Some of the common side effects or toxicities associated with cancer drugs that are employed for lung cancer are given in Table 2. Combinations of drugs are usually used in lung cancer, and there is often increased patient toxicity. The toxicities vary depending on the drugs used. The major toxic effect of the most commonly used chemotherapeutic programs is myelosuppression due in most part because virtually all drugs have hematological toxicity. Myelosuppression is the most common cause of morbidity and mortality. Prompt diagnosis, treatment, and patient awareness of treatment associated fever and infectious complications are necessary to reduce drug-related mortality. Severe thrombocytopenia or anemia is less common. Other common toxic effects include nausea and vomiting (generally tolerable), alopecia, diarrhea, and neuropathy. Nausea and vomiting can be severe, and patients may refuse further therapy because of gastrointestinal side effects.

Treatment toxicity is often one of the patient's main fears. The fear may be so profound that the patient may refuse initiation of therapy or withdraw from treatment at the first sign of toxicity. Patient and family education with explanation of the expected therapeutic effects and information about adverse reactions and side effects improve patient compliance.

2.1.2 Radiation Therapy

Radiation therapy is an effective modality for small cell lung cancer and has a major role in its management. Small cell lung cancer is one of the most sensitive tumors to irradiation. Local tumor regression almost always occurs with irradiation and often complete disappearance of local tumor is achieved (SALAZAR et al., 1976). In addition, radiation therapy in patients with limited disease increased median survival to about 9 to 11 months with a 30% one-year survival and may cure a small percentage of patients with disease confined to one hemithorax (FOX and SCADDING, 1973; SEYDEL et al., 1978; SALAZAR and CREECH, 1980; MATTHEWS et al., 1980; PETROVICH et al., 1978; LEE et al., 1976; GARRETT et al., 1979). Randomized trials indicate that radiation therapy alone is more effective than surgery in patients with localized disease (FOX and SCADDING, 1973). There is a dose-response relationship for local control by irradiation with about an 80 to 90% local control with doses of 4,800–6,000 rads (RISSANEN et al., 1968; CHOID and CAREY, 1976; BRODER et al., 1977). With combined-modality treatment (chemotherapy + radiation therapy), similar local control may be achieved with 3,000–4,000 rads (COX et al.,

1979). Despite local control of tumor with local irradiation in most patients, disease progression in extrathoracic areas remains a major cause of failure. With the high rate of response seen with combination chemotherapy for small cell lung cancer, some investigators have questioned the necessity of local chest irradiation (HANSEN et al., 1980a, COHEN, 1977a; COHEN, 1983; COHEN et al., 1979), but we feel as others that control of intrathoracic tumor is important for long-term survival, regardless of disease extent, provided there is a complete response to systemic chemotherapy (BYHARDT and COX, 1983; BLEEHEN et al., 1983).

Primary failure in the chest alone is quite common in patients treated with chemotherapy alone, although in most instances it is followed quickly with systemic relapse (COHEN et al., 1977a; COHEN et al., 1979). Although earlier trials using single drugs plus radiation therapy versus radiation therapy alone in limited disease patients produced no differences in median or in one or two year survival, more recent trials have used more effective drug combinations with radiation therapy (BUNN and IHDE, 1981; Med Res Council, 1979; MATTHIESSEN, 1978). These studies clearly show the superior results of combined radiation therapy – chemotherapy over radiation alone with one year survival of 18 to 28% and 2-year survival of 8 to 11%. Results of the third Medical Research Council small cell study suggested no significant survival advantage for either radiotherapy followed by chemotherapy or two pulses of chemotherapy and then radiotherapy followed by the rest of the chemotherapy in limited disease (Medical Research Council Lung Cancer Working Party, 1983). The Cancer and Leukemia Group B is presently prospectively investigating the value of simultaneous radiotherapy and chemotherapy.

In addition, when the results of all non-randomized trials using chemotherapy alone or both chemotherapy and radiation therapy are compiled, the potential benefit of combined modality treatment over chemotherapy alone is seen as an increase of long-term survival, although complete response rate and median survival are similar (BUNN et al., 1981).

Although the results of combination chemotherapy combined with radiation therapy are superior to those using radiation therapy plus single agent therapy or radiation therapy alone, the results are similar to those achieved in some recent trials with combination chemotherapy alone in those with limited disease (BUNN and IHDE, 1981). About 80 to 90% of patients respond with over

50% achieving a complete response; median survival in general range from 9–18 months and almost 20% have two year disease-free survival.

The results of combined modality therapy in patients with extensive disease is similar to combination chemotherapy alone (BUNN and IHDE, 1981; WILLIAMS et al., 1977) and clearly inferior to results in limited disease. Overall, only about 10 to 25% of patients with extensive disease have a complete response with a median survival of 6 to 11 months. Less than five percent of patients with extensive disease have a two year disease-free survival.

The appropriate dose, timing, and schedule of radiotherapy with chemotherapy is unknown (MORSTYN et al., 1984).

Salvage radiation therapy is helpful for patients with intrathoracic SCLC progressing on combination chemotherapy. Twenty-five patients with SCLC were given radiotherapy to progressive intrathoracic tumor after failing chemotherapy; five of 16 responders did not progress intrathoracially for the duration of their illness and there were two patients who had prolonged local control and survival beyond 18 months (OCHS et al., 1983).

Radiation therapy also has a very important role in the alleviation of symptoms of locally advanced or metastatic disease in small cell carcinoma of the lung. Radiotherapy is useful for the treatment of bone metastases, overt brain metastases, spinal cord compression, superior vena caval obstruction, and bronchial obstruction (SEYDEL et al., 1978; BUNN et al., 1978).

2.1.2.1 Toxicity

1. *Radiation therapy alone.* Radiation therapy for lung cancer may have toxicity and side effects. Pulmonary toxicity is seen in about 10% of patients and is related to the volume of lung irradiated and the dose rate of irradiation and can be divided into two phases (GROSS, 1977; LIPSHITZ and SOUTHARD, 1974). The acute phase of radiation pneumonitis is characterized by a hazy infiltration on chest x-ray, which usually develops within 6 to 12 weeks. Clinically, most patients have cough and dyspnea; fever and chest pain may also occur. Many patients have no or minimal symptoms. Usually the acute phase subsides gradually but in rare cases there may be gradual radiographic progression to fibrosis with respiratory failure, cor pulmonale, and death. Other pulmonary complications of radiation to the lung are spontaneous

pneumothorax, pleural effusion, and pneumonitis outside the irradiated field. It is important to differentiate radiation reactions from infection and recurrent or lymphangitic spread of malignancy. Mechanisms are not well understood but the current theory is that of depletion of the surfactant-containing lamellar bodies in the alveolar type II cell (RUBIN et al., 1981). Concommitant chemotherapy, repeat courses of radiation, and steroid withdrawal are exacerbating factors. Corticosteroids and antibiotics may help during the acute phase.

Radiation myelitis is a serious complication of radiation therapy for carcinoma of the lung and usually requires a year or more to become clinically apparent (LOCKSMITH and POWERS, 1968). Clinically, a Brown-Sequard syndrome is usually seen. Radiation-induced myocarditis and pericarditis are relatively rare and late sequelae (LAWSON et al., 1972). Drainage of the effusion by a pericardial window or pericardectomy may be necessary. Corticosteroids may benefit this complication (BRIAN, 1978).

In addition to these life-threatening complications, relatively minor complications may occur (GROSS, 1977; LIPSHITZ and SOUTHARD, 1974). Esophagitis with dysphagia is more frequent with increasing dose and occurs in about 40% of patients receiving greater than 50–55 Gy (HELLMAN et al., 1964). This dysphagia is usually transient and subsides spontaneously. Esophageal stricture is rare. Skin reactions are usually mild and include subcutaneous fibrosis. Radiotherapy rarely causes significant hematopoietic depression unless the marrow is already compromised because less than 25% of the active bone marrow is present in the hemithorax (RUBIN and SCARANTINO, 1978). General symptoms of anorexia, weakness, malaise, nausea, and vomiting may occur with irradiation for lung cancer.

Serious complications from radiation therapy are usually avoidable with special care to time-dose-volume relationships, excluding noncancerous tissue from radiation and avoiding overlapping fields.

2. *Combined radio-chemo therapy.* Toxicity is usually enhanced when radiation and chemotherapy are given in the combined modality approach to lung cancer. In some instances, the toxicities may be particularly enhanced by the concurrent administration of both modalities (AISNER and WIERNIK, 1981b; JOHNSON et al., 1976; CHABORA et al., 1977; LAMOUREUX, 1974; EINHORN et al., 1978).

In particular, there may be enhancement of dysphagia and esophagitis, desquamative skin reactions, pneumonitis, pulmonary fibrosis, cardiac toxicity, and hematopoietic toxicity. A transient "CNS" syndrome of recent memory loss, tremor, somnolence, and slurred speech have been reported with concurrent chemotherapy, chest irradiation, and cranial irradiation. These complications may result in fatalities usually in the range of 3–4% but may be higher (JOHNSON et al., 1976). These complications may be less frequent in trials employing radiotherapy prior to chemotherapy or in between chemotherapy cycles (MOORE et al., 1978). Leukemia and radiation myelitis also have been reported with combined modality treatment programs (SEYDEL et al., 1978; BRADLEY et al., 1982).

2.1.2.2 Prophylactic Cranial Irradiation.

Another area in which radiotherapy is being evaluated is prophylactic brain irradiation. Metastases to the central nervous system and leptomeninges in small cell lung cancer pose significant clinical problems. Cranial metastases are present at diagnosis in about 10% of patients and by two years about 60 to 70% will have metastases without cranial irradiation (NUGENT et al., 1979; KOMAKI et al., 1981). Pituitary metastases are frequent; they usually occur in the posterior pituitary, and may be the only site of CNS metastases. Intracranial and leptomeningeal metastases are significantly more likely to develop in patients with marrow or liver involvement at diagnosis. With longer survival of patients on chemotherapy there is an increasing incidence of brain metastases. Prophylactic cranial irradiation produces an appreciable decrease in the incidence of cerebral metastases (JACKSON et al., 1977; BUNN et al., 1978; BLEEHEN et al., 1983). Initially, drugs such as CCNU and procarbazine were included in chemotherapy regimens because they crossed the blood brain barrier, but with disappointing results in preventing CNS metastases. Although prophylactic cranial irradiation substantially reduces the incidence of brain metastases, it has not conferred a survival benefit since patients who develop CNS metastasis will usually develop progressive disease at other metastatic sites. Prophylactic cranial irradiation does not protect against leptomeningeal, spinal, or epidural metastases. Intrathecal methotrexate and/or cytosine arabinoside are being evaluated for treatment and prophylaxis of this condition. Radiation therapy is as effective as surgery in relieving symptoms of spinal cord compression (DRAKLEY et al., 1979).

There is little information regarding therapeutic irradiation in established cranial metastases in SCLC (NUGENT et al., 1979; BAGLAN and MARKS, 1981; CRANE et al., 1983). BAGLAN and MARKS (1981) concluded that symptomatic cranial irradiation controls CNS disease as well as prophylactic therapy. Approximately 47 to 92% of patients who receive a full course of therapeutic irradiation will be benefited. Another study evaluated all patients who developed brain metastases (40–45%) while undergoing treatment without cranial irradiation (COX et al., 1980). Despite very early recognition of brain metastases, the disease can be so rapidly progressive that prompt irradiation can be too late. They concluded that therapeutic brain irradiation was not sufficiently effective to preclude prophylactic irradiation.

Acute and chronic effects of cranial irradiation have been reported (SHELINE et al., 1980; CATANE et al., 1981). Alopecia occurs in all patients. Adverse effects of irradiation of the human brain have been considered according to the time of appearance. Acute reactions are those that occur during the course of irradiation and are thought to be a result of cerebral edema. Recent memory loss, myoclonus, tremor, and slurred speech have been reported. This transient syndrome may be more frequent with concommitant chemotherapy (JOHNSON et al., 1976; BAGLAN and MARKS, 1981). These effects are usually of little clinical importance and usually improve with corticosteroid therapy. An early delayed reaction is probably a result of demyelinization; it is usually transient and disappears within several weeks, although fatalities may occur. Leukoencephalopathy is probably a variant of the early delayed reaction. The late delayed reaction is the major CNS hazard. The injury tends to be more severe in the white matter. The onset may be from several months to years after exposure. It is generally irreversible and frequently leads to deaths from brain necrosis. CATANE et al. (1981) reported only minimal CCT abnormalities (mild atrophy or encephalomalacia) in patients receiving CNS prophylaxis without significant clinical abnormalities or EEG changes. CRAIG et al. (1984) reported that almost all patients develop CCT abnormalities after chemotherapy and cranial irradiation including atrophy, ventricular dilatation and decreased coefficient of absorption.

We reserve prophylactic cranial irradiation for those patients who achieve a response with chemotherapy and radiation therapy as they have the best chance for prolonged survival. The reason for this is that the brain can only tolerate a defined maximal dose of radiation, and the possibility of having to retreat the brain if systemic disease has not been controlled because the systemic disease may reseed the brain. It should begin before the 12 weeks of therapy because brain metastases become more frequent after that date (LIVINGSTON et al., 1980a; NUGENT et al., 1979). The use of prophylactic cranial irradiation in patients with SCLC who achieved a complete response reduced the incidence of CNS metastases from 52% to 25% at two-years and improved the two-year survival rate from 16% to 38% compared to a comparable group who did not receive prophylactic cranial irradiation (ROSEN, 1983). In another randomized study of prophylactic cranial irradiation which was restricted to patients in complete response, the frequeny of brain relapse was significantly reduced by prophylactic cranial irradiation and one patient in the control arm died with brain metastases as the sole site of tumor (AISNER, 1982).

Disturbances of mentation have also been described with chemotherapy alone (SILVERFARB, 1983).

2.1.3 Surgery

Small cell lung cancer is generally regarded as a surgically incurable disease. The five-year survival rate is less than one percent for patients undergoing surgical resection. Even in patients with apparent solitary peripheral lesions, most patients are found to be inoperable at the time of thoracotomy. Most studies show that surgical resection has little or no effect on survival, however, in small, highly selective series in which "curative resection" was possible, the five-year survival has ranged from 10% to 36% (DRAKLEY, 1979; HIGGINS et al., 1975; SHORE and PANETH, 1980). Almost all patients had small peripheral lesions, stage I or II disease with no hilar involvement. These results are better than those patients with limited disease and good performance status treated with chemotherapy with or without radiation therapy. Most investigators feel that a complete response is a prerequisite for long-term survival. When radiation therapy is given along with chemotherapy, there is a reduction in the relapse rate at the primary site from 70% to 30 to 40% but without definite evidence of prolongation in survival in patients with limited disease. The role of surgery as a cytoreductive technique in combination with chemotherapy and/or radiotherapy in palliative resected

or curatively resected patients with limited small cell lung cancer needs to be evaluated in a comparative randomized trial. SHORE and PANETH (1980) reported a five year survival of 25% (10 patients) in 40 patients who were resected for cure. Neither chemotherapy or radiotherapy were used; most investigators now would advise adjunctive chemotherapy (see below). The Veteran Administration study concluded that definitively resected small cell lung cancer patients treated with adjuvant cytoxan had a better survival than the untreated group (SHIELDS, 1973; HIGGINS, 1972). KARRER (1982) reported a 13% increase in the five year survival rate in 53 surgically resected patients with small cell lung cancer with adjuvant chemotherapy over the control arm. Others have reported no benefit from this approach (Reported by Med Res Council, 1971). TAKITA et al., (1973) reported a 55.6% one-year survival when incomplete (palliative) resection was combined with radiation therapy/chemotherapy.

An improved ability to stage disease by chest CT scanning and the failure of radiotherapy at tolerable doses to control local disease in 30 to 40% of cases has led to renewed interest in surgery for the control of the primary lesion (HARPER et al., 1981). Recent pilot studies which employ surgery as an adjuvant or as the primary local modality with chemotherapy and/or irradiation for selected limited disease patients have practically eliminated local relapse as a major site of failure (COMIS et al., 1981; HOFFMAN et al., 1982; MANDELBAUM et al., 1978; MEYER et al., 1979; VALDIVIESO et al., 1982b). In 1982, SHIELDS et al., (1982), reviewed the results of the Veteran Administration Groups experience in 148 patients with SCLC who had resection for cure. The five year survival in these patients was 23%, all in early stage patients. MEYER et al. (1982) reported on ten stage I and II SCLC patients (four T_2-N_1, four T_2-N_0, two T_1-N_0) who were resected for cure, eight received postoperative multiple drug chemotherapy, one died in the postoperative period, and the remaining nine were in complete remission from 7 to 69 months postoperatively. MARCHELLO reported on 4 resected patients (one T_2-N_1, two T_2-N_0, and one T_1-N_0) with SCLC, all of whom are alive and free of disease from 10 to 55 months (MARCHELLO et al., 1984). MEYER, also reported on 6 stage II (N_2, M_0) patients who had good initial response to chemotherapy followed by subsequent surgical resection (MEYER et al., 1982). The results were that five of six patients remained free of disease 5 to 25 months after the start of treatment, and one relapsed at 26 months with hepatic metastases. FOSTER et al. (1983) have found that only about 28% of limited disease patients (11 of 40 patients) were able to undergo thoracotomy after chemotherapy; and only 8 could actually be resected. Further studies are required to determine the value, if any, of cytoreductive surgery in limited small cell lung cancer.

2.2   Non-small Cell Lung Cancer

2.2.1   Surgery

Surgical resection of patients with non-small cell lung cancer is the most effective method of therapy and offers the only chance for long-term survival. Unfortunately, surgical resection is only possible in about 20 to 25% of patients at the time of diagnosis. Of these patients, about 20 to 30% or 6 to 8% overall will have a five-year survival because of the presence of occult disease. The ten-year survival is about 16–18% (PAULSON and REISCH, 1976; SMITH, 1970). In patients with stage I disease, the five-year survival is much greater, 55–70%, particularly with squamous cell carcinoma (MARTINI and BEATTIE, 1977; MOUNTAIN 1977a; WILLIAMS et al., 1981). The surgical mortality rate is about 4 to 8%. Overall, about 30 to 35% of stage II and 20 to 25% of stage III survive five years. The cell type, the extent of the disease process (the stage), and the cardiopulmonary status determine resectability and are important factors in survival (MOUNTAIN, 1983a). The size of the tumor and extent of regional lymph node involvement are important in prognosis.

Definitive surgical resection is the treatment of choice presently for all stage I and II patients and selected stage III patients who have adequate cardiopulmonary physiologic status. Stage I disease comprises about 15 to 20% and Stage II about 5 to 10% of carcinomas. The optimal operation for stage I and II disease is lobectomy with careful and complete interlobular, hilar, and mediastinal lymph node dissection. Wedge and/or segmental resections can be curative procedures in stage I patients and may be the procedure of choice in those patients with compromised pulmonary function (WILLIAMS et al., 1981; HOFFMAN and RANSDELL, 1980; LE ROUX, 1972). Five-year survival rates of 30 to 50% have been reported with low morbidity and mortality with wedge/segmental procedures. Assessment of regional lymphatics is vital for determining the adequacy of

the procedure (HOFFMAN and RANSDELL, 1980; JENSIK et al., 1979; BENNETT and SMITH, 1979). Pneumonectomy may be required to remove all disease in patients with stage II disease and for centrally located stage I disease. Postoperative morbidity and mortality are greater with pneumonectomy. The one-year survival is about 80% and five-year survival about 55% in patients with stage I disease (MARTINI and BEATTIE, 1977a; MOUNTAIN, 1977a). Cell type does not appear to influence survival for stage I disease. Within stage I disease, patients with $T_1 N_0$ have a significantly improved survival than those with $T_2 N_0$ tumors or those with $T_1 N_1$ disease (MARTINI and BEATTIE, 1977; WILLIAMS et al., 1981; MOUNTAIN, 1983b; SHIELDS et al., 1980).

In stage II (T_2 lesion, positive hilar nodes, negative mediastinum) disease, surgery is much less effective with a median survival of resected patients of 18 months. The five year survival varies from about 20% for adenocarcinoma and large cell undifferentiated carcinoma to about 35% for squamous carcinoma (MOUNTAIN, 1977a).

About one-third of patients with apparent curative resection for stage I, II, III disease have a recurrence due to the presence of occult disease. Seventy-two percent of those who failed did so in sites outside the ipsilateral hemithorax with an additional seven percent having both distant and regional failure and 21% with only regional failure (MOUNTAIN, 1983b).

In patients with stage I and II disease whose physiological status precludes surgical therapy or who refuse this therapy definitive radiotherapy results in a five year survival or about 16 to 25% (MOUNTAIN, 1983b; BARKLEY and MAOR, 1980).

The median survival for resectable stage III disease is about one year with 19% of those who had squamous lesions alive at five years (MOUNTAIN, 1977a). Twenty-seven percent of stage III patients with T_3 lesion only (N_0, N_1) survived five years compared with only eight percent with positive mediastinal nodes (N_2). Death from recurrent disease occurred in 60% with epidermoid histology and 71% with other histology which implies that two out of three patients with stage III disease may benefit from adjuvant therapy.

At the present time, there does not seem to be a role for adjuvant chemotherapy or adjuvant immunotherapy for patients with resectable disease (MOUNTAIN, 1982; LIVINGSTON, 1982). Several uncontrolled studies have suggested a role for post-operative radiation therapy for patients with positive hilar and mediastinal nodes especially for squamous cell carcinoma (GREEN et al., 1975; KIRSCH et al., 1976), and preoperative radiation therapy may be of benefit in selected patients with marginally resectable non-small cell lung cancer (SHERMAN et al., 1978). Two studies with preoperative radiation therapy in patients with all stages of disease with variation in radiation technique failed to show an advantage for preoperative radiation therapy (A Collaborative Study, 1975; SHIELDS et al., 1970).

Involvement of the chest wall may occur by direct extension of the lung cancer. The five-year survival rate is approximately 20 to 25% with adequate surgical resection (MARTINI and BEATTIE, 1982). Preoperative irradiation therapy does not appear to affect survival. For superior sulcus tumors, preoperative irradiation therapy favorably increased resectability and resulted in a 30 to 35% five-year survival (PAULSON, 1975; MILLER et al., 1979; HILLARIS et al., 1974). On the negative side KIRSCH et al. (1973) and MORRIS (1979) felt that chest wall resection was not worthwhile. We feel that superior pulmonary sulcus tumors without evidence of hilar or mediastinal nodes should be operated on after irradiation on the basis of clinical diagnosis. Patients with hilar or mediastinal nodes should receive irradiation for symptomatic relief. Incomplete resectable tumors can be treated with interstitial implantation of radioactive material.

In very rare instances, a combined approach to a resectable primary and a solitary cerebral metastases may be justified (MAGILLIGAN et al., 1976). The overall one-year survival rate was 45% with an improved quality of survival.

2.2.2 Radiation Therapy

Radiation therapy is important in the management of patients with non-small cell lung cancer. Radiotherapy has been utilized in several ways in the treatment of non-small cell lung cancer (i.e. by itself, preoperative, post-operatively, in combination with chemotherapy, and palliatively). Radiotherapy can improve the survival rate and the quality of life for patients with non-small cell lung cancer. Irradiation effectively relieves symptoms caused by the primary tumor or by mediastinal metastases or distant metastases in the majority of instances. A substantial proportion of patients (60–80%) who have intrathoracic symptoms from inoperable lung cancer (i.e. thoracic pain, hemoptysis, superior vena cava obstruction, cough dyspnea, dysphagia) will have improvement with irradiation therapy (COX et al., 1983; KJAER 1982; SLAWSON and SCOTT, 1979). Radiation therapy is less effective with vocal cord paralysis (6%) and atelectasis (23%). Radiotherapy has also been shown to be effective in improving ventilation and perfusion abnormalities in greater than 80% of instances with amelioration of breathlessness (FAZIO et al., 1979). This improvement was subsequently followed by a very slow progressive deterioration in regional pulmonary function due in part to radiation fibrosis.

In addition, distressing symptoms in patients with disseminated cancer can often be alleviated with local irradiation. Bone pain from metastases is effectively relieved with irradiation; and irradiation may also help to prevent pathological fractures. Although brain metastases are less frequent in non-small cell lung carcinoma than small cell lung carcinoma, it is not uncommon for the brain to be the only metastatic site (NEWMAN et al., 1974; DEELEY and EDWARDS 1968; LIVINGSTON and HEILBRUN 1978). Patients usually present with headache, confusion, lethargy, and impairment of motor function. Sensory loss, seizures, and cerebellar dysfunction are also common. The computed cranial tomography (CCT) scan is currently the best way to diagnose brain metastases. Nuclear scans, angiography, and pneumoencephalography may be used if a CCT scan is not available. There is a higher incidence of brain metastases with adenocarcinoma and large cell undifferentiated carcinoma than with squamous cell carcinoma. The incidence of brain metastases at autopsy by cell type was as follows: adenocarcinoma 59% (69/129); small cell carcinoma 45% (37/82); large cell carcinoma 52% (28/54); mixed cell carcinoma 25% (3/12); and squamous cell carcinoma 13% (16/123). In addition, brain metastases were the only metastatic site in 4% of squamous cell carcinomas, 6% of small cell carcinomas, and 12% of adenocarcinomas. The value of radiation therapy for brain metastases was established in the 1950's (CHAO et al., 1954). The palliative effects of a short intensive course of brain irradiation (3,000 rads in two weeks) was as effective as a high-dose course (5,000 rads in 4 weeks) in a randomized RTOG clinical trial for palliating symptoms, controlling metastatic foci, effect on median survival (17 weeks), and less expensive and more convenient (KURTZ et al., 1981). Steroids (Dexamethasone, i.e. 4 mg–16 mg/day) may be a useful adjunct to treatment (POSNER, 1977). The combination of surgery with radiation therapy might be the best approach for the patient with the solitary brain metastases (ZIMM, 1981). The results of treatment of clinically apparent brain metastases are often poor (NEWMAN and HANSEN 1974; BORGELT et al., 1980); and prophylactic cranial irradiation is effective in reducing the incidence of clinical metastases (COX et al., 1978). Extradural metastases, cardiac metastases, liver metastases, or an impending or actual ulceration of a subcutaneous mass may be treated with irradiation.

Most patients present with advanced disease because of difficulties in making an early diagnosis and the propensity for lymphatic and hematogenous metastases. Complete resection is only possible in about one-third of cases of operable bronchogenic carcinoma. In these patients about 30–40% will be alive at five years. The surgical mortality rate is approximately 5 to 10% (MOUNTAIN, 1977b). Radiotherapy offers a chance for cure in stage I and stage II patients who cannot be treated with surgery. The five year survival for these patients varies from 7 to 23% and these series may have included patients whose lesions thought to be operable would have proven unresectable at thoracotomy (a common occurrence) (SMART, 1966; MORRISON et al., 1963). These are substantial survival rates but are lower than surgical survival rates.

Preoperative radiotherapy has not been shown to benefit non-small cell lung cancer, and, in fact, may be accompanied by significant morbidity (BLOEDORN et al., 1964; RUBIN et al., 1970; SHIELDS 1972). Others have reported favorable results with preoperative radiation therapy (SHERMAN et al., 1978). Post-operative irradiation does not confer survival benefit when regional (hilum/mediastinal) lymph nodes are not involved; however, post-operative irradiation does improve disease-free survival when there is involvement of the regional lymph nodes especially with adenocarcinoma of the lung (GREEN et al., 1975; KIRSCH et al., 1976; VAN HOUTTE et al., 1980; CHOI et al., 1980). Survival is worse for patients with mediastinal nodal metastases than when only hilar and/or lobar nodes are involved (KIRSCH et al., 1976; SHIELDS et al., 1975).

Radical radiotherapy or irradiation for cure in patients with unresectable non-small cell lung cancer may be attempted under certain circumstances in patients with limited stage III disease. The median survival after radical radiotherapy is 5 to 6 months. The one year survival is 29 to 57% and the five year survival is only 3 to 10% (KJAER, 1982; LEE, 1983; WHITE and BOLES, 1981). Patients

with good performance status, small lesions, weight loss < 10 pounds, and squamous histology have a much better prognosis (COY and KENNELLY, 1980). Most patients who expire have local persistence or recurrence of tumor in the chest (especially epidermoid) and in others, distant metastases with or without local recurrence (adenocarcinoma/large cell) is more important (STANLEY et al., 1981). Several studies have shown that even in cases without cure "tumor sterilization" (area encompassed by treatment) frequently occurs. The sterilization rate has been reported to range between 30 to 50% (BLOEDORN et al., 1974; BLOEDORN, 1966; RISSANEN et al., 1968; ABADIR and MUGGIA, 1975; SHIELDS, 1972). Several studies have shown that there is a direct relationship between control of the local-regional tumor, survival, and the dose of irradiation. The safest and most effective approach to definitive irradiation is a continuous regimen with at least five fractions per week to a total dose of at least 6,000 rads (COX et al., 1983; PEREZ et al., 1982; PETROVICH et al., 1977; EISERT et al., 1976).

In 1968, ROSWIT and associates randomized radiotherapy (308 patients) versus placebo (246 patients) versus a variety of chemotherapeutic agents (246 patients) and demonstrated a statistically significant improved survival at the end of one year (18.2% vs. 13.9%, p = 0.05) for patients receiving radiation therapy (ROSWIT et al., 1968; WOLF et al., 1966). This study is often quoted as showing no difference in survival groups. Ninety percent of the irradiated group were treated with orthovoltage radiation (conventional x-irradiation or x-rays) with 1/3 of patients receiving doses less than 40 Gy.

A number of factors have emerged as being of prognostic importance for survival in patients with loco-regional inoperable lung cancer. Histology, mediastinal node involvement, weight loss, supraclavicular metastases, age, vocal cord involvement, pain, and malignant pleural involvement all affect response and survival in patients with region non-small (oat)-cell carcinoma (LANZOTTI et al., 1977; STANLEY, 1980; CALDWELL et al., 1968; PEREZ et al., 1980). Other factors of major importance in tumor control and survival in patients with unresectable non-oat cell carcinoma of the lung include irradiation techniques (i.e. variation in ipsilateral and contralateral nodal irradiation), dose of irradiation (6,000 rads > 5,000 rads > 4,000 rads), continuous vs. split course techniques, and size of the lesion (PEREZ et al., 1982; PEREZ et al., 1980). Of major importance in survival is the achievement of local control of the tumor (PEREZ et al., 1982; EISERT et al., 1976; PEREZ et al., 1980). The median survival of patients with complete or partial responses is about 50 weeks compared with 31 weeks for patients who fail to response (PETROVICH et al., 1981). Therefore, treatments directed at improving local control would have significant impact on survival (COX et al., 1983b).

A number of efforts to improve local control of lung cancer by irradiation are under investigation (FOWLER, 1979; KAPLAN, 1979; GEORGE, 1977): 1) biologic response modifier (levamisol); 2) electron-affinic hypoxic cell sensitizers-metronidazole (Flagyl), Misonidazole (R0-07-0582); 3) high-LET (linear energy-transfer particles) radiation; 4) hyperfractionated radiotherapy; 5) hemibody and whole body radiotherapy (SALAZAR et al., 1981); 6) hyperthermia. Results are preliminary and further investigation is needed to determine their ultimate role. Of interest is a recent report of a randomized double-blind study in 62 patients with non-oat cell lung carcinoma, predominantly squamous cell, utilizing the radiosensitizing drugs, misonidazone, and 3,500 cGy, there was no difference in response (SAUNDERS, 1984a, b). Survival was similar to other studies, with 78% survival at 12 months for complete responders versus 39% for the remaining patients. In addition to total regression of tumor, time to regrowth showed a highly significant correlation with survival ($p < 0.0005$). Tumor persisted or recurred at the primary site in 95% (58/61) of patients while 39% (24/61) showed no evidence for distant metastases. For these patients, improvement in control of the primary tumor would be important in improving survival.

Another approach to improve local control of regional unresectable lung cancer is the implantation of various types of radioactive sources directly into the tumor itself. Currently, the most commonly used radioactive source is iodine-125 (HILARIS et al., 1975; GIBBONS, 1976; MARTINI and MCCORMACK, 1983), but Iridium-192, Gold-198, and Radon-222 have been used. This procedure has the advantage of delivering very high doses of radiation to the tumor while limiting damage to the normal surrounding tissue.

Chemotherapy has also been added to irradiation in localized disease in an attempt to improve long-term survival by improving local control rate and by controlling subclinical distant metastases in patients with non-small cell lung cancer. Studies of combined radiotherapy and single agent chemo-

therapy (i.e. 5-FU, nitrogen mustard, cytoxan, vinblastine, methotrexate, hydroxyrea) has not resulted in improved results in relation to those treated with irradiation alone (BERGSAGEL et al., 1972; PALMER and KROENING, 1978; FINGERHUT and BARNETT, 1966). Initial reports of programs using combination chemotherapy with irradiation have suggested improved results in non-small cell lung cancer. However, the long-term survival effects of these studies are not yet fully determined and relatively high incidence of local and systemic relapse emphasize the need to improve the efficacy of both the irradiation and the chemotherapy (EAGEN et al., 1981; ISRAEL et al., 1982; VALDIVIESO et al., 1982a; ISRAEL et al., 1979).

KATZ (1983) has recently presented data to support a reappraisal of the role of combined resection and irradiation in non-small cell lung cancer in an attempt to reduce the high rate of local failure in potentially curable patients treated by irradiation alone. Over a 10 year period (1/69 to 12/79), he compared 176 patients who received high dose definitive radiotherapy alone to 53 patients who completed a course of definitive postoperative radiotherapy after undergoing resection of the primary tumor. A comparison of the incidence of local failure as the first site of failure for T_1, T_2 tumor demonstrated a statistically significant decrease in local failure in patients whose primary tumor was resected; local failure was decreased in patients with clinical T_3 tumor who underwent resection, but the difference was not significant.

Recurrent endobronchial lesions after standard therapy can be a life-threatening situation. The YAG and the carbon dioxide laser have been used successfully for opening obstruction of major airways by tumor (MCDOUGALL, 1983; DUMAN, 1982). Photoradiation utilizing the photodynamic action of hematoporphyrin derivative has also been successful (VINCENT, 1984). These methods are also being used for carcinoma in situ.

2.2.3 Chemotherapy

Greater than 50% of patients with non-small cell lung cancer present with evidence of metastatic disease and metastases or local progression will occur in most of the others following failure of initial treatment to control the disease with radiation therapy and/or surgical resection. Non-small cell lung cancer is relatively refractory to chemotherapy and evidence for worthwhile prolongation on survival is scant (RICHARDS et al., 1980; VO-SIKA, 1979). The achievement of complete response is necessary for significant influence on survival.

Performance status, degree of weight loss, and extent of disease are important prognostic indicators for survival in non-small cell lung cancer (STANLEY, 1980; AISNER and HANSEN, 1981 a). The median survival will vary from 6 to 72 weeks when these three prognostic factors are considered. In one study which considered seventy-seven prognostic factors, fifty prognostic factors were identified and the relative contribution to survival identified. The patient's initial performance status is at least as important as the disease extent, and seems to be more important than the histological subtype (FEINSTEIN et al., 1974). A Veteran Administration Lung Study Group (VALSG) study with supportive care alone in patients with extensive squamous cell lung cancer revealed a median survival of 20, 10, and 2.5 weeks, respectively, depending on whether they were fully ambulatory, partially ambulatory, or essentially non-ambulatory (ZELEN, 1973). Extent of disease is also an important factor both for response and survival (RICHARDS et al., 1984). Such factors must be recognized when evaluating chemotherapy trials.

With single agent chemotherapy, complete remissions are rare in non-small cell lung cancer. Objective responses with the most active agents have been reported to occur in 20 to 35% of patients but the range may vary considerably. For example, one study reported a 20 to 45% response rate to doxorubicin alone depending on dosage, whereas a larger study reported response rates less than 10% (CONTES et al., 1974; KNIGHT et al., 1976). These variations may be the result of different patient selection (performance status, extent of disease, previous chemotherapy, etc), drug dose, or response criteria. Palliation with single agent chemotherapy is short lived and survival impact is minimal. The median duration of response is about to two to four months (SELAWRY, 1974). No single agent has yet been demonstrated to influence survival. In a study of single agents versus placebo, patients receiving either had a similar duration of median survival (GREEN et al., 1969; DURRANT et al., 1971). Survival for responders is improved over that of non-responders. Some agents may have more meaningful activity than others in a specific histologic subtype. Most responses are seen in those patients with good performance status and limited tumor load. It is conceivable that further improvement can be made by means of dose scheduling or by developing rescue techniques that allow escalation of doses.

A recent prospective study has demonstrated that combination chemotherapy was significantly superior to placebo (CORMIER et al., 1982). Another prospective study failed to demonstrate survival prolongation with combination chemotherapy (LAING et al., 1975). In particular, over the past five to ten years, many combination chemotherapy regimens have been tried in non-small cell lung cancer with varying therapeutic results even when various investigators or groups used the same combination. There are a number of different combinations of drugs that have reportedly caused remission in up to 40 to 45% of patients with prolongation of median survival to 6 to 7 months as opposed to an expected 3 to 4 months in pilot studies (HOFFMAN et al., 1983). Unfortunately, there appears to be a lack of reproducibility of results for some of these combinations. Furthermore, toxicity from these combinations are frequently considerable or excessive in view of minimal response. Major toxic effects include bone marrow suppression, mucositis, fever, and/or sepsis, renal toxicity, cardiac toxicity, and skin rash. Table 1 lists the toxicities associated with some of the more commonly used drugs in the treatment of non-small cell lung cancer. Some of this lack of corroboration is due to the heterogenous nature of patient groups with respect to previous radition or chemotherapy, performance status, stage of disease, and histology.

The results of repeated trials of variation combination chemotherapy regimens in non-small cell lung cancer vary a great deal. For example, MACC (methotrexate, doxorubicin, cyclophosphamide, and lomustine) has been reported to give a response rate of 44% with an 8.3 months median survival versus a 12% response rate and 3.5 month survival (CHAHINIAN et al., 1979; VOGL et al., 1979). With CAP (cyclophosphamide, adriamycin, and cisplatinum) the response rate has varied from 4% to 44% with a median survival of 3.5 months to 5.8 months (EAGEN et al., 1980; DAVIS et al., 1981).

The wide variation in response rates and survival seen with the same combination of chemotherapy seem to be due to differences in response criteria and patient selection. In addition, such results need to be compared with the natural history of the disease. The natural history of inoperable lung cancer without treatment is 5 to 6 months for ambulatory patients and 2 to 3 months for non-ambulatory patients (GREEN et al., 1969; HYDE et al., 1973; HIGGINS and BEEBE, 1969). Many studies have shown that pretreatment performance status affects response rate and survival.

Also, patients with limited disease survive longer than patients with extensive disease and may have a higher response rate (RICHARDS et al., 1982; RICHARDS et al., 1979; VINCENT et al., 1980). In addition, some histological subtypes may be more responsive than others, but results are not consistent (VALDIVIESO et al., 1982a; RICHARDS et al., 1982; RICHARDS et al., 1984). Patients are more likely to respond if they have limited disease, good performance status, loss <6% body weight, have received no prior chemotherapy, and are immunocompetent.

In summary, response to chemotherapy is more likely in the fully ambulatory patients and usually occurs within one to two cycles of chemotherapy (RICHARDS et al., 1979; LIVINGSTON and HEILBRUN, 1978a). Relapse usually occurs in sites of previously evident disease (LIVINGSTON and HEILBRUN, 1978a). In addition, those patients who respond to treatment have a longer survival (RICHARDS et al., 1982).

At present, no presently available combination chemotherapy regimens can be recommended as standard therapy for inoperable non-small cell lung cancer. Patients responding to therapy clearly appear to benefit from treatment. However, as previously mentioned, patients who are ambulatory with little or no symptoms (i.e. better initial performance status) are more likely to respond and this is also the group with the longest survival when untreated. Thus, at present, there is little evidence that chemotherapy is superior to no treatment or produces such an effect independent of prognostic factors (AISNER and HAUSER, 1981a).

2.3 Summary

Prognostic factors which relate both to response to treatment and survival in small cell lung cancer include extent of disease and performance status. Currently therapy in patients with limited disease produce complete response rates of 50 to 60% with median survival of 12 to 16 months; about 10 to 17% of limited disease patients now have a two year survival. Complete response rates of 20 to 25% and median survivals of 8 to 12 months are being achieved in patients with extensive disease. Combined modality therapy with radiation therapy, and chemotherapy have increased the two-year disease free survival. The optimal duration of chemotherapy and the role of maintenance chemotherapy has not been defined. Prophylactic cranial irradiation can decrease the frequency of development of clinically detectable brain metastases, but has no effect on survival, except perhaps in patients who achieve a complete response to treatment. Surgical resection of tumor in selected patients with stage I, II, and III M_0 disease may be a useful adjuvant to chemotherapy, but its role has not been established. Recently, advances in understanding the biology of SCLC including the identification, characterization of growth factors, development of monoclonal antibodies to tumor associated antigens and the tumor stem cell assay may well lead to new approaches in diagnosis, staging, and therapy of small cell lung cancer.

Careful staging is the most important factor in deciding therapy of non-small cell lung cancer. Important prognostic factors such as performance status, extent of disease, weight loss and possibly histology have become much better defined. We should continue to carefully select patients who can obtain surgical cure as well as inoperable patients who will benefit from radiotherapy and chemotherapy. Radiation therapy continues to have a major and expanding role in the management of patients with non-small cell lung cancer. Radiation therapy effectively palliates cancer related symptoms and contributes to improved survival in unresectable and resectable patients who have regional lymph nodes. Prophylactic cranial irradiation in non-small cell lung cancer and systemic irradiation may have an increasing role in the future. Combination chemotherapy achieves a survival benefit in responding patients but the majority of patients do not respond. Hopefully, a better understanding of the biology of non-small cell lung cancer will lead to more effective therapy.

3 Rational Basis for New Approaches in Combined Modality Therapy

3.1 Statement of the Problem

The rational approach to any significant problem must take into account all the known factors regarding the origin and perpetuation of the problem. Lung cancer, its natural history, patterns of failure, and results of treatment, is considered a significant challange because of its prevalence in man today, for the significant effects it has on the patient and because of the lack of improvement in results over the past several decades. As with other disease sites, the treatment approach has been confined mostly to empirical considerations. It is often difficult to consider a more rational based approach to therapy because of ethical and technical limitations. However, even with these limitations, advances in the treatment of patients with small cell carcinoma of the lung have extended their median survival. Other examples can be found in the scope of oncologic malignancies and do attest to the importance of the empirical approach. It does appear, however, that more inclusions and reflections upon experimental therapeutics can improve results if carefully analyzed and properly transferred to the clinical situation.

PLUME (Chapter 3) has presented a detailed view of the basic anatomical construct of the lung and has reminded us of the many pathways available to the malignant cell(s) located in the thorax. The metastatic potential of lung cancer has been well established by several authors (MATTHEWS, 1973) and represents an important facet in the natural history of lung cancer. This fact alone is responsible for eliminating a number of patients for surgical excision and is reason for some to question the need for systemic therapy. However, local failure continues to be a problem not only in resected lesions but also after radical irradiation (PEREZ, 1982). Most recently SAUNDERS (1984) reported persistant or recurrent tumor at the primary site in 95% of patients (58 of 61, 42 with autopsy) with lung cancer receiving 3,500 rad alone or in combination with misanidazole. Thus we are faced with the dual task of controlling local and distant disease, a fact that has not eluded investigators and has been the driving force for continued clinical trials and new innovative approaches.

The results of clinical trials have failed to influence the overall survival in spite of reported excellent response rates. Whether this is due to the fact that we do not understand completely the biology of lung cancer or that we have not identified certain characteristics of the "responding" tumors is not known. It is possible that what is known is not being utilized in the most efficient manner. It is the purpose of this section to explore some of that which is known regarding tumor cell kinetics and propose an alternative approach to the treatment of lung cancer. The approach will attempt to incorporate results from a) experimental studies on tumor cell kinetics and b) clinical studies utilizing similar methods. More specifically it is the concept of pertubation kinetics following single high-dose irradiation and the subsequent administration of a second systemic cytotoxic agent during the post-irradiation proliferative phase. The incorporation of single high dose irra-

diation (SHDI) and a drug is not new to the experimentalist, however, in light of recent reports utilizing SHDI clinically, the experimental information must be re-examined and evaluated to determine its feasibility and application to the clinical arena.

3.2 Tumor Cell Growth and Kinetics

Alterations in tumor cell kinetics with growth have been observed by a number of investigators who have reported a decrease in the S-phase and growth fraction. Some have attributed this to a decrease in cell production and an increase in cell loss coincident with increasing tumor size (SCHABEL 1969). The work of EVANS et al. (1981) suggests a decrease in proliferative activity to be a function of tumor burden since changes in kinetics were noted on tumors of various sizes and independent of vascular considerations. LALA (1972) using Ehrlich ascites tumor felt that invironmental factors were important in the regulation of cell proliferation. The important observation is that of a decrease in cell proliferation coincident with increased cell burden. Assuming this to be true and realizing that increased cell kill occurs most efficiently during active proliferation, then if one can alter the kinetics and increase the proliferative fraction, an increased cell kill could be accomplished through the administration of further cytotoxic agents. The denoument to this approach and one that is fundamental in producing the desired cytotoxic effect rests on discerning the cytokinetic changes following pertubation in order to administer the various cytotoxic agents at the most opportune time which will result in decreased normal tissue toxicity while achieving greater tumor cell kill. Although both aspects are important it is the alteration of cell kinetics will be discussed in detail since the approach to the latter (determination of proper time based on cell cycle age distribution) has been more difficult to determine clinically. However, some insight to future possibilities will be discussed.

In this section, the application of single high-dose irradiation (SHDI) will be explored as a modality which can produce the necessary kinetic changes discussed above. The rationale and utilization of SHDI is based on experimental evidence and clinical experience and is presented solely as a model for a more rational approach in the treatment of solid tumors in general and for lung cancer in the current context.

3.3 Experimental Results of Single High Dose Irradiation (SHDI)

The two most significant findings observed after SHDI are a) an immediate high cell kill and b) a period of rapid or active cell proliferation. HERMENS and BARENDSEN (1969) studied the effects of a single dose of 2,000 rad on a rat rhabdomyosarcoma and observed a reduction in the clonogenic fraction to 0.8% of normal immediately following irradiation to day four post irradiation. From day four through day nine they observed an increase in the clonogenic fraction which returned to normal levels by day ten. Similarly, VAN PEPERZEEL (1972) observed a reduction in the "effective" volume of tumors followed by a period of accelerated growth three to six days following a single dose of irradiation for lung metastases in mice, dogs, and humans. More recently, ROFSTAD et al. (1980) reported on the results of 500 and 1,000 rad on the proliferation kinetics of a human malignant melanoma xenograph in athymic nude mice. A slight delay in tumor regrowth was noted after 500 rad whereas after 1,000 rad the delay lasted for eight days and slowly returned to normal. During this time the clonogenic fraction was reduced to 5% of normal immediately following 1,000 rad, reaching a nadir at three to four days followed by a gradual return to normal at twenty-two days. The increase in volume noted after day eight correlated with the increase in clonogenic fraction.

The results of these studies show that although SHDI results in a significant immediate reduction in the clonogenic fraction, it does not eliminate or sterilize this fraction. Rather, there is a delay followed by a period of renewed proliferative activity with an increase in the clonogenic fraction. Thus, the goal of increased cell kill can be achieved by the administration of a cytotoxic agent after SHDI, which is in keeping with the premise of the current suggested approach.

VAN PEPERZEEL (1972) following his initial observations on the effect of SHDI, tested the validity of the hypothesis that the sensitivity of a tumor was related to its growth rate by observing a greater volume reduction in a tumor which initially received a moderately high dose of irradiation and a subsequent dose of irradiation when in an accelerated period of growth compared to the volume reduction achieved with one single dose of irradiation. BRAUNSCHWEIGER et al. (1979) studied the effects of acute high doses of irradiation on the T1699 mouse mammary tumor cell kinetics with tritiated thymidine (^{3}H-TdR) labeling index, DNA synthesis time and primary dependent DNA polymerase labeling index and described four phases of the response (eluded to above):

a) initial phase characterized by a decrease in the labeling index and an increase in the DNA polymerase labeling index.
b) a second phase characterized by the variable dose dependent interval of decreased cell proliferation.
c) a recovery phase characterized by increased cell proliferation.
d) a final phase characterized by re-establishment of normal proliferative patterns.

Following these initial observation on the kinetics of SHDI they found the most effective schedule for local tumor control was one in which a second dose of irradiation was delivered three days following a single dose of 600 rad. Day three corresponded to the time just prior to the initiation of recovery. If the second dose is given on day four (time of maximum recovery of the labeling index), local tumor control was significantly worse.

Similar results of local tumor control and cure have been reported by LOONEY in a series of studies (LOONEY et al., 1983, 1979). Using the same reasoning and logic described above, he has given cytotoxic drugs at various times following initial high dose of irradiation and achieved similar results of increased local tumor control and cures. Thus it appears that increased cell kill, manifested by improved local tumor control and cure, can be accomplished experimentally following SHDI through delivery of a second cytotoxic agent at the time of increased cellular proliferation.

These patterns of responses following SHDI have also been observed to occur in normal tissue, particularly the bone marrow and gut, two of the most important dose limiting organs in cytotoxic therapy. SCARANTINO et al. (1984) and JOHNKE et al. (1984) observed an immediate and high ($>80\%$) cell kill of the committed granulocyte-macrophage bone marrow stem cell compartment (CFU_c-GM) after 500, 600 and 1,000 rad half-body irradiation of normal animals. The response after pertubation was similar to that described for neoplastic systems except there was return to pretreatment values by seven days compared to a delay of 10–12 days in the neoplastic systems studied (VAN PEPERZEEL, 1972; ROTSTAD 1981; BRAUNSCHWEIGER et al. 1979). Thus, there appears to be a 3–5 day period (7–10 day post irradiation) after the return to normal of bone marrow stem cells

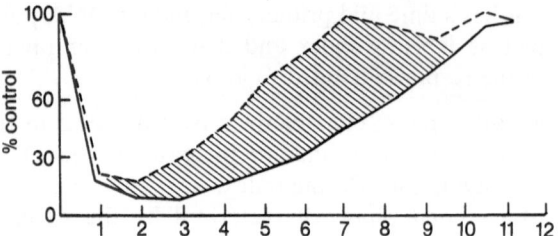

Fig. 1. Effects of single high dose irradiation on: a) hemato-poietic system as determined by CFU_c-GM (----); pretreatment values achieved at seven days, and b) solid tumors (——) which represents results from a variety of studies and suggests active proliferation from 7–10 days

during which time there is active tumor proliferation (Fig. 1). It is during this time when the administration of a second cytotoxic agent should result in increased tumor cell kill and decrease normal tissue toxicity due to the difference in proliferative activity of both compartments.

3.3.1 Pertinent Aspects of Kinetic-directed Therapy

The problem clinically is the lack of techniques to determine the time of most active cell proliferation for both the normal and tumor tissue. In most instances this would require repeated biopsies for in-vitro analysis of the tissue(s) under study, however, the practical and ethical considerations limit this approach in most patients. In those instances where it has been possible to obtain repeated tumor samples from patients and direct therapy based on kinetic changes the results of such an approach have been effective. The recent report by Barranco et al. (1983) suggests that kinetic-directed therapy can be a viable clinical approach. After exposing Chinese hampster overy cells to 1,2:5,6-dianhydrogalactitol (DAG) they observed an increase in the S-phase cell compartment followed by a similar increase in G_2M after release of DAG. Administration of bleomycin (effective against cells in G_2M) at that time demonstrated greater cell kill. These kinetic studies were followed by flowmicro-fluorometry. Using a similar technique to study cell kinetic changes they reported similar but not consistant increases in the S-phase fraction on 14 of 17 human tumors. The response of each tumor to DAG was different, stressing the importance of obtaining cell kinetic data during cytotoxic therapy in each individual patient. In addition, the data illustrates the influ-

ence that kinetic alterations have on selecting the most opportune time to administrate specific cytotoxic agents. Such tumor cell kinetic directed therapy should lead to more individualized therapy and improved therapeutic response and survival. Therefore at the present time while an empirical approach is necessary and important it does eliminate the prospect of an individualized therapeutic approach. To improve the emperical approach the incorporation of sufficient experimental evidence would make a stronger case when approaching the clinical application of combined modality therapy.

The discussion thus far has a) identified an important problem in the treatment of solid tumors related to cell kinetic factors b) presented evidence that single high dose irradiation can be an effective modality in altering tumor cell kinetics by producing an immediate high cell kill with a subsequent increase in proliferative activity and c) suggest that following pertubation and with proper timing the administration of cytotoxic agents can achieve increase cell kill and tumor cure.

These points provide the experimental basis upon which a more rational approach to the treatment of lung cancer has been formulated. The pertinent clinical experience and corollaries with SHDI will be presented in the following discussion.

3.4 Clinical Experience with Single High Dose-Half Body Irradiation

3.4.1 Palliation

The clinical application of single high dose irradiation (half-body irradiation-HBI) for palliation of multiple areas of cancer related pain was first reported by Fitzpatrick and Rider in 1976. Excellent pain relief occured in most patients within 24 h with a variety of tumor types. A number of other reports followed which substantiated the subjective findings of Fitzpatrick and Rider (Salazar et al., 1978; Epstein et al., 1979; Keen et al., 1980; Jaffee et al., 1979; Quasim 1981; Pene et al., 1981; Rowland et al., 1981, 1983). In addition several investigators reported findings of objective responses after a single high dose of radiation (Quasim 1981; Salazar et al., 1978; Jaffee et al., 1979; Rowland et al., 1983; Lombardi et al., 1982).

The major toxicity of these early reports was pneumonitis. The incidence in most reports varied between 10–20% since most investigators utilized doses of 800 rad. Prato et al. (1976) found an increased incidence from 0% at 600 rad at 40% at 1,000 rad. FRYER et al. (1978) subsequently updated these results and found a 12% incidence at 600 rad, 19% at 800 rad and 52% at 1,000 rad. It must be pointed out that most patients treated with SHDI to the upper half body received previous cytotoxic therapy (irradiation and or chemotherapy) and were treated without consideration for increased lung transmission. Two important considerations which could account for the pulmonary toxicity and which have definitely influenced subsequent investigators to reduce the dose to the upper half body to 600 rad. This has resulted in a decrease in the incidence of pneumonitis to less than 10%.

The second major and not unexpected toxicity was hematological, particularly the white blood cells and platelets. The nadir response usually occured within 2–3 weeks following HBI but returned to pre-treatment values within 4–6 weeks depending on amount of previous cytotoxic therapy.

3.4.2 Adjuvant

The clinical results (immediate pain relief) reported after half body irradiation (HBI) can be explained by the experimental findings of an immediate high cell kill noted experimentally. If this explanation is correct then the patterns of recovery noted experimentally, should also occur clinically. Thus, one would expect a high but not complete cell kill following HBI and symptoms and signs of tumor regrowth should return if only high dose irradiation were used. When single high dose irradiation was used alone clinically to determine its effectiveness as a "systemic" agent in eliminating occult disease ($<10^9$ cells) a delay of 3–5 months was noted in the onset of clinically apparent metastatic disease (SALAZAR 1980). This data suggested that HBI alone produced a 1–2 log cell kill (findings noted experimentally by SUTHERLAND who observed the 90% or 1–2 logs cell kill with single high dose irradiation in his spheroid model (SUTHERLAND 1976) and tumor regrowth occured. Both findings, especially the latter are similar to and support those results observed experimentally. If these observations and assumptions are correct, the next logical step in the treatment program employing high dose irradiation would be the administration of a cytotoxic agent following SHDI to obtain a further increase in cell kill. Since it is difficult to determine the precise optimal time to administer a 2nd cytotoxic agent which would re-

sult in tumor cell kill, the approach must employ results of experimental studies. From the bone marrow and tumor data presented above and summarized in Fig. 1, the "ideal" time for administration of the second agent appears to be between 7 and 10 days following HBI in the previously untreated patient which should not result in greater toxicity to normal tissue, since the CFU_c-GM stem cell content will have returned to pretreatment levels. In addition, experimental results indicate most tumor systems to be in a proliferative state 7–10 days following SHDI.

3.5 Incorporation of Half Body Irradiation and Chemotherapy in Bronchogenic Carcinoma

Currently, our approach to the treatment of nonsmall cell bronchogenic carcinoma takes into account all above considerations. Treatment is initiated with 600 cGy to the upper half body with opposite uninvolved lung shielded as well as the eyes and oral cavity (Fig. 2). One week following HBI, cyclophosphamide (350 mg/M²) for three days and concurrent local-regional irradiation (200 cGy per day × 5 days) are administered. Fol-

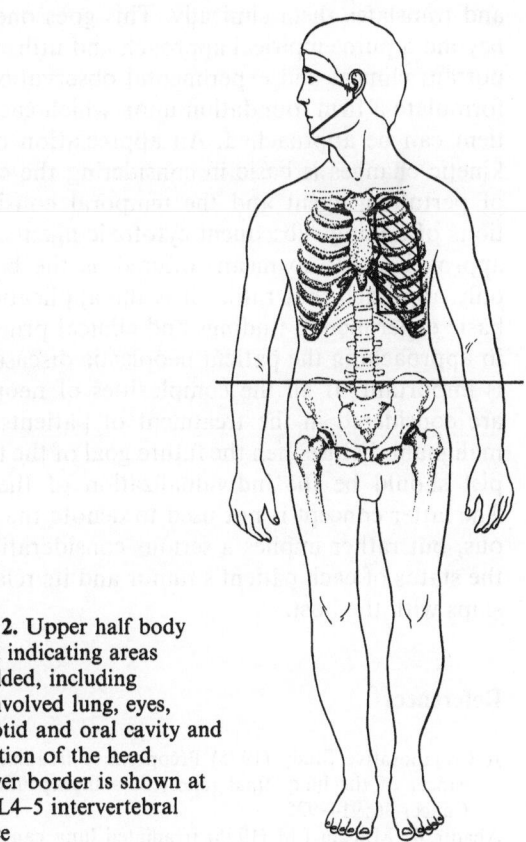

Fig. 2. Upper half body field indicating areas shielded, including uninvolved lung, eyes, parotid and oral cavity and position of the head. Lower border is shown at the L4–5 intervertebral space

lowing two weeks rest, cyclophosphamide and local regional irradiation (200 cGy × 10 fractions) are resumed. Cyclophosphamide is then repeated every 3 weeks for two additional cycles. Total dose of irradiation to the tumor is 3,600 rad. Preliminary results (Scarantino 1983) show this regament well tolerated clinically and hematologically. No instance of hematological toxicity has been noted in 20 patients completing protocol, suggesting the experimental findings are operative and relevant at least in previously untreated patients. In addition, a response rate of 70% has been noted in 20 patients. This is approximately twice that observed by Perez et al. (1980) in patients receiving 4,000 rad split course therapy suggesting a higher cell kill with smaller doses of irradiation in "proper" combination and more rational timing with chemotherapy. It cannot be determined if a delay in time of onset of metastatic disease or survival has been increased at the present time. Analysis of patterns of failure will obviously be important in determining more precisely the ability of high dose irradiation and cyclophosphamide to control occult overt disease.

In summary, an approach to the treatment in bronchogenic carcinoma has been suggested which integrates a number of experimental observations and translates them clinically. This goes one step beyond a pure empirical approach and utilizes important clinical and experimental observations to formulate a firm foundation upon which each patient can be approached. An appreciation of the kinetic changes is basic in considering the choice of pertubing agent and the temporal considerations of adding subsequent cytotoxic agents. This approach is by no means offered as the best or only approach, but rather it is the application of basic experimental findings and clinical principles in approaching the patient neoplastic disease that is important. If all the complexities of neoplasia are considered in the treatment of patients with malignant disease then the future goal of the therapist should be the individualization of therapy. The latter concept is not used to denote the obvious, but rather implies a serious consideration of the status of each patient's tumor and its relationships with the host.

References

A Collaborative Study (1975) Preoperative irradiation of cancer of the lung: final report of a therapeutic trial. Cancer 36:914–925.

Abadir R, Muggia FM (1975) Irradiated lung cancer. An autopsy analysis of spread pattern, Radiology 114:427–430.

Aisner J, Whitacre M, Van Echo DA, et al (1982) Combination of chemotherapy for small cell carcinoma of the lung: continuous versus alternating non-cross-resistant combinations, Cancer Treat Rep:221–230.

Aisner J, Whitacre M, Van Echo DA, et al (1980) Alternating non-cross resistant combination chemotherapy for small cell carcinoma of the lung (SSCL), Proc AACR-ASCO 21:453. (abstract C-528)

Aisner J, Hansen HH (1981a) Commentary: current status of chemotherapy for non-small cell lung cancer, Cancer Treat Rep 65:979–986.

Aisner J, Wiernick PH (1981b) Complications of treatment and of improved survival in patients with small cell carcinoma of the lung. In: Greco FA, Oldham RK, Bunn PA (eds) Small cell lung cancer. Grune and Straton, New York, pp. 381–398.

Baglan RJ, Marks JE (1981) Comparison of symptomatic and prophylactic irradiation of brain metastases from oat cell carcinoma of the lung, Cancer 47:41–45.

Barkley HT, Maor MH (1980) Radiotherapy in the treatment of bronchogenic carcinoma, Cancer Bull 32:113–116.

Barranco SC, May JT, Boerwinklew, et al (1982) Enhanced cell killing through use of cell kinetics-directed treatment schedules for two drug combinations in-vitro, Cancer Res 42:2894–2898.

Barranco SC, Townsend CM, Constanzi JJ, et al (1982) Use of 1,2:5,6-dianhydrogalactitol in studies on cell kinetics-directed chemotherapy schedules in human tumors in-vivo, Cancer Res 42:2899–2905.

Baylin SB, Weisburger WR, Eggleston JC, et al (1978) Variable content of histaminase, l-dopa decarboxylase and calcitonin in small-cell carcinoma of the lung. Biologic and clinical implications, N Engl J Med 299:105–110.

Bennett WF, Smith RA (1979) Segmental resection for bronchogenic carcinoma: a surgical alternative for the compromised patient, Ann Thorac Surg 27:169–172.

Bensch KG, Corrin B, Pariente R, et al (1968) Oat-cell carcinoma of the lung. Its origin and relationship to bronchial carcinoid, Cancer 22:1163–1172.

Berger CL, Goodwin, G, Mendelsohn G, et al (1981) Endocrine-related biochemistry in the spectrum of human lung carcinoma, J Clin Endocrinol Metab 53:422–429.

Bergsagel DE, Jenkin RDT, Pringle JF, et al (1972) Lung cancer: clinical trial of radiotherapy alone vs. radiotherapy plus cyclophosphamide, Cancer 30:621–627.

Biran S (1978) Corticosteroids in radiation-induced pericarditis, Chest 74:96–98.

Bleehen NM, Bunn PA, Cox JD (1983) Role of radiation therapy in small cell anaplastic carcinoma of the lung, Cancer Treat Rep 67:11–19.

Bloedorn FG (1966) Rationale and benefit of preoperative irradiation in lung cancer, JAMA 196:340–341.

Bloedorn FG, Cowley RA, Cuccia CA, et al (1964) Preoperative irradiation in bronchogenic carcinoma, AJR 92:77–87.

Borgelt B, Gelber R, Kramer S, et al (1980) The palliation of brain metastases: final results of the first two studies by the radiation therapy oncology group, Int J Radiat Oncol Biol Phys 6:1–9.

Bradley EC, Schechter GP, Matthews MJ, et al (1982) Erythroleukemia and other hematologic complications of intensive therapy in long-term survivors of small cell lung cancer, Cancer 49:221–223.

Braunschweiger PG, Schenken LL, Schiffer LM (1979) The cytokinetic basis for the design of efficacious radiotherapy protocols, Int J Radiat Oncol Biol Phys 5:37–47.

Broder LE, Cohen MH, Selawry OS (1977) Treatment of bronchogenic carcinoma. II. Small cell cancer, Cancer Treat Rev 4:219–260.

Bunn PA Jr, Ihde DC (1981a) Small cell bronchogenic carcinoma: a review of therapeutic results. In: RB Livingston (ed) Cancer Treatment and Research, volume 1, Lung Cancer, Martinus Nijhoff Publishers, Haque, Boston, London, pp. 169–208.

Bunn PA Jr, Lichter AS, Glatstein E, et al (1981) Results of recent studies in small cell bronchogenic carcinoma and prospects for future studies. In: FA Greco, RK Oldham, PA Bunn (eds) Small cell lung cancer. Grunn & Straton Inc., New York, pp. 413–446.

Bunn P, Schlam M, Gazdar A (1980) Comparison of cytology and DNA content analysis by flow cytometry (FCM) in specimens from lung cancer patients, Proc AACR/ASCO 21:40. (abstract #160)

Bunn PA Jr, Nugent JL, Matthews MJ (1978) Central nervous system metastases in small cell bronchogenic carcinoma, Semin Oncol 5:314–322.

Bunn PA Jr, Cohen MH, Ihde DC, et al (1977) Advances in small cell bronchogenic carcinoma, Cancer Treat Rep 61:333–342.

Byhardt RW, Cox JD (1983) Is chest radiotherapy necessary in any or all patients with small cell carcinoma of the lung? Yes, Cancer Treat Rep 67:209–215.

Caldwell WL, Bagshaw MA (1968) Indications for and results of irradiation of carcinoma of the lung, Cancer 22:999–1004.

Carey DN, Gazdar AF, Bunn PA Jr, et al (1981) Demonstration of the stem cell nature of clonogenic tumor cells from lung cancer patients, Stem Cells 1:149–164.

Catane R, Schwade JG, Yarr I, et al (1981) Follow-up neurological evaluation in patients with small cell lung carcinoma treated with prophylactic cranial irradiation and chemotherapy. Int J Radiat Oncol Biol Phys 7:105–109.

Chabora BMcC, Hopfan S, Wittes R (1977) Esophageal complications in the treatment of oat cell carcinoma with combined irradiation and chemotherapy, Radiology 123:185–187.

Chahinian AP, Ware JH, Zimmer B, et al (1980) Evaluation of anticoagulation with warfarin and of alternating chemotherapy in extensive small cell carcinoma of the lung (SCCL), Proc Am Soc of Clin Oncol 3:225. (abstract C879)

Chahinian AP, Mandel EM, Holland JF, et al (1979) MACC (methotrexate, adriamycin, cyclophosphamide and CCNU) in advanced lung cancer, Cancer 43:1590–1597.

Chao JH, Phillips R, Nickson JJ (1954) Roentgen-ray therapy of cerebral metastases, Cancer 7:682–689.

Choi NCH, Grillo HC, Gardiello M, et al (1980) Basis for new strategies in postoperative radiotherapy of bronchogenic carcinoma, Int J Radiat Oncol Biol Phys 6:31–35.

Choi CH, Carey RW (1976) Small cell anaplastic carcinoma of the lung. Reappraisal of current management, Cancer 37:2651–2657.

Cohen MH (1983) Is thoracic radiation therapy necessary for patients with limited-stage small cell lung cancer, No, Cancer Treat Rep 67:217–221.

Cohen MH, Chretien PB, Jonston-Early A, et al (1982) Thymosin fraction V prolongs survival of intensively treated small cell lung cancer patients. In: Immunotherapy of Human Cancer. Terry WC, Rosenberg SA (eds.) New York, Excerpta Medica, pp 141–145.

Cohen MH, Ihde DC, Bunn PA Jr, et al (1979) Cyclic alternating combination chemotherapy for small cell bronchogenic carcinoma, Cancer Treat Rep 63:163–170.

Cohen MH, Matthews MJ (1978) Small cell bronchogenic carcinoma: a distinct clinicopathologic entity, Semin Oncol 5:234–243.

Cohen MH (1977a) Small cell bronchogenic carcinoma, a prolonged remission following chemotherapy, JAMA 237:2528.

Cohen MH, Creaven PJ, Fossieck BE, et al (1977b) Intensive chemotherapy of small cell bronchogenic carcinoma, Cancer Treat Rep 61:349–354.

Comis RL (1982) Small cell carcinoma of the lung, Cancer Treat Rev 9:237–258.

Comis R, Meyer J, Ginsberg S, et al (1981) Effectiveness of combination chemotherapy (CTH) plus adjuvant surgery in small cell anaplastic lung cancer (SCALC), Proc AACR-ASCO 22:509. (abstract C-692)

Cormier Y, Bergerson D, La Forge J, et al (1982) Benefits of polychemotherapy in advanced non-small-cell bronchogenic carcinoma, Cancer 50:845–849.

Cortes EP, Takita H, Holland JF (1974) Adriamycin in advanced bronchogenic carcinoma, Cancer 34:518–525.

Cox JD, Byhardt RW, Komaki R (1983a) The role of radiotherapy in squamous, large cell, and adenocarcinoma of the lung, Semin Oncol 10:81–94.

Cox JD, Komaki R, Byhardt RW (1983b) Is immediate chest radiotherapy obligatory for any or all patients with limited stage non-small cell carcinoma of the lung? Yes, Cancer Treat Rep 67:327–331.

Cox JD, Komaki R, Byhardt RW, et al (1980) Results of whole-brain irradiation for metastases from small cell carcinoma of the lung, Cancer Treat Rep 64:957–961.

Cox JD, Byhardt R, Komaki R, et al (1979) Interaction of thoracic irradiation and chemotherapy on local control and survival in small cell carcinoma of the lung, Cancer Treat Rep 63:1251–1255.

Cox JD, Petrovich Z, Paig C, et al (1978) Prophylactic cranial irradiation in patients with inoperable carcinoma of the lung, Cancer 42:1135–1140.

Coy P, Kennelly GM (1980) The role of curative radiotherapy in the treatment of lung cancer, Cancer 45:698–702.

Craig J, Jackson D, Moody, et al (1984) Prognostic evaluation of changes in computerized cranial tomography (CCT) in patients with small cell carcinoma (SCLC) treated with chemotherapy and cranial irradiation, Proc Am Assoc Clin Oncol 3:224(C-875).

Crane J, Lichter A, Ihde D, et al (1983) Therapeutic cranial radiation (RT) for brain metastases in small cell lung cancer (SCLC), Proc Am Assoc Cancer Res 24:145(C-574).

Davis S, Rambotti P, Park YK (1981) Combination cyclophosphamide, doxorubicin, and cisplatin (CAP) chemotherapy for extensive non-small cell carcinomas of the lung, Cancer Treat Rep 65:955–958.

Deeley TJ, Edwards JMR (1968) Radiotherapy in the management of cerebral secondaries from bronchial carcinoma, Lancet 1:1209–1213.

Dermer GB (1981) Autoradiography of cellular glycoproteins reveals histogenesis of bronchogenic adenocarcinomas, Cancer 47:2000–2006.

Drakley MJ, Matthews HR, Watson D (1979) Oat cell carcinoma of bronchus-is there a place for surgery?, Thorax 34:427. (abstract)

Dumon JF, Reboud E, Garbe L, et al (1982) Treatment of tracheobronchial lesions by laser photoresection, Chest 81:278–283.

Durrant KR, Ellis F, Berry RJ, et al (1971) Comparison of treatment policies in inoperable bronchial carcinoma, Lancet 1:715–719.

Eagen RT, Lee RE, Fryta S, et al (1981) Thoracic irradiation therapy and adriamycin/cisplatin containing chemotherapy for locally advanced non-small-cell lung cancer, Cancer Clin Trials 4:381–388.

Eagen RT, Frytak S, Ingle JN, et al (1980) Phase II evaluation of the combination of triazinate, cyclophosphamide, doxorubicin, and cis-diamminedichloroplatinum (11) in patients with advanced adenocarcinoma of the lung, Cancer Treat Rep 64:925–928.

Edmonson JH, Lagakos SW, Selawry OS, et al (1976) Cyclophosphamide and CCNU in the treatment of inoperable small cell carcinoma and adenocarcinoma of the lung, Cancer Treat Rep 60:925–932.

Einhorn LH, Bond WH, Hornbach N, et al (1978) Long-term results in combined-modality treatment of small cell carcinoma of the lung, Semin Oncol 5:309–313.

Eisert DR, Cox JD, Komaki R (1976) Irradiation for bronchial carcinoma: reasons for failure. I. Analysis of local control as a function of dose, time, fractionation, Cancer 37:2665–2670.

Epstein LM, Stewart BH, Antunez AR, et al (1979) Half and total body radiation for carcinoma of the prostate, J Urol 122:330–332.

Evans MJ, Kovacs CJ, Schenken LL, et al (1981) Modification of the intestinal postirradiation proliferative response by intra-abdominal H-4-II-E$_2$ tumors, Radiat Res 88:552–564.

Fazio F, Pratt TA, McKenzie CG, et al (1979) Improvement in regional ventilation and perfusion after radiotherapy for unresectable carcinoma of the bronchus. AJR 133:191–200.

Feinstein AR, Gelfman NA, Yesner R (1974) The diverse effects of histopathology on manifestations and outcome of lung cancer, Chest 66:225–229.

Feld R, Evans WK, Yeoh JL, et al (1981) Combined modality induction therapy without maintenance chemotherapy for small cell carcinoma of lung (SCCL), Proc AACR-ASCO 22:494. (abstract-C631)

Fingerhut AG, Barnett MB (1966) X-ray therapy and combined therapy (x-ray and 5-fluorouracil) in the treatment of cancer of the lung, Dis Chest 49:393–395.

Fitzpatrick PJ, Rider WD (1976a) Half-body radiotherapy of advanced cancer, J Canad Assoc Radiol 27:75–79.

Fitzpatrick PJ, Rider WD (1976b) Half body radiotherapy, Int J Radiat Oncol Biol Phys 1:197–207.

Foster JM, Prager RL, Hainsworth JD, et al (1982) Limited-stage small cell carcinoma (SCC): prospective evaluation regarding the feasibility of adjuvant surgery. Proc Amer Soc Clin Oncol 2:196(C-766).

Fowler JF (1979) New horizons in radiation oncology, Br J Radiol 52:523–535.

Fox W, Scadding JG (1973) Medical research council comparative trial of surgery and radiotherapy for primary treatment of small-celled or oat-celled carcinoma of bronchus. Ten-year followup, Lancet 2:63–65.

Fryer CJH, Fitzpatrick PJ, Rider WD, et al (1978) Radiation pneumonitis: experience following a large single dose of radiation, Int J Radiat Oncol Biol Phys 4:931–936.

Garrett GG, Bradfield JS, Bagwell JC, et al (1979) Small

cell carcinoma of the lung: results of combination chemotherapy and radiation therapy, South Med J 72:1548–1553.

Gazdar AF, Carney DN, Minna JD (1983) The biology of non-small cell lung cancer, Semin Oncol 10(1):3–19.

Gazdar AF, Carney DN, Guccion JG, et al (1981) Small cell carcinoma of the lung: cellular origin and relationship to other pulmonary tumors. In: Greco FA, Oldham RK, Dunn PA (eds) Small cell lung cancer. Grune and Stratton, Inc, New York, pp. 145–175.

Gazdar AF, Carney DN, Russell EK, et al (1980) Establishment of continuous, clonable cultures of small-cell carcinoma of the lung which have amine precursor uptake and decarboxylation cell properties, Cancer Res 40:3502–3507.

George FW III (1988) Current status and recent advances in the radiotherapy of lung cancer, Chest 71:635–637.

Gibbons JRP (1976) Interstitial irradiation in carcinoma of the lung, Panminerva Med 18:62–63.

Ginsberg SJ, Comis RL Gottlieb AJ, et al (1979) Long-term survivorship in small-cell anaplastic lung carcinoma, Cancer Treat Rep 63:1347–1349.

Greco FA, Oldham RK (1979a) Current concepts in cancer: small-cell lung cancer, N Engl J Med 301:355–358.

Greco FA, Richardson RL, Snell JD, et al (1979b) Small cell lung cancer. Complete remission and improved survival, Am J Med 66:625–630.

Greco FA, Einhorn LH, Richardson RL, et al (1978) Small cell lung cancer: progress and perspectives, Semin Oncol 5:323–335.

Green N, Kurohara SS, George FW, et al (1975) Postresection irradiation for primary lung cancer, Radiology 116:405–407.

Green RA, Humphrey E, Close H, et al (1969) Alkylating agents in bronchogenic carcinoma, Am J Med 46:516–525.

Gross NJ (1977) Pulmonary effects of radiation therapy, Ann Intern Med 86(1):81–92.

Hansen M, Hansen HH, Dombernowsky P (1980a) Long term survival in small cell carcinoma of the lung, JAMA 244:247–250.

Hansen M, Hansen HH, Hirsch FR, et al (1980b) Hormonal polypeptides and amine metabolites in small cell carcinoma of the lung with special reference to stage and subtypes, Cancer 45:1432–1437.

Harper PG, Souhami RL, Spiro SG, et al (1982) Tumor size, response rate, and prognosis in small cell carcinoma of the bronchus treated by combination chemotherapy, Cancer Treat Rep 66:463–470.

Harper PG, Houang M, Spiro SG, et al (1981) Computerized axial tomography in the pretreatment assessment of small-cell carcinoma of the bronchus, Cancer 47:1775–1780.

Hellman S, Klingerman MM, von Essen CF, et al (1964) Sequellae of radical radiotherapy of carcinoma of the lung, Radiology 82:1055–1061.

Hermens AF, Barendsen GW (1969) Changes of cell proliferation characteristics in a rat rhabdomyosarcoma before and after x-irradiation. Eur J Cancer 5:173–189.

Higgins GA, Shields TW, Keehn RJ (1975) The solitary pulmonary nodule. Ten-year follow-up of veterans administration-armed forces cooperative study, Arch Surg 11:570–575.

Higgins GA Jr (1972) Use of chemotherapy as an adjuvant to surgery for bronchogenic carcinoma, Cancer 30:1383–1387.

Higgins GA, Beebe GW (1969) Bronchogenic carcinoma. Factors in survival, Arch Surg 94:539–549.

Hilaris BS, Martini N, Batata M, et al (1975) Interstitial irradiation for unresectable carcinoma of the lung, Ann Thorac Surg 20:491–500.

Hilaris BS, Martini N, Luomanen RKJ, et al (1974) The value of preoperative radiation therapy in apical cancer of the lung. Surg Clin North Am 54:831–840.

Hoffman PC, Bitran JO, Golomb HM (1983) Chemotherapy of metastatic non-small cell bronchogenic carcinoma, Semin Oncol 10:111–122.

Hoffman PC, Weiman OS, Bitran JO, et al (1982) Surgical resection in patients with stage II Mo small cell carcinoma of the lung, Proc AACR-ASCO 1:152. (abstract C593)

Hoffman TH, Ransdell HT (1980) Comparison of lobectomy and wedge resection for carcinoma of the lung, J Thorac Cardiovasc Surg 79:211–217.

Hyde L, Wolf J, McCracken S, et al (1973) Natural course of inoperable lung cancer, Chest 64:309–312.

Israel L, Depiere A, Dalesio O (1982) Interim results of EORTC protocol 08742: comparison, after irradiation of locally advanced squamous cell bronchial carcinoma, of abstention, immunotherapy, combination chemotherapy, or chemoimmunotherapy, Recent Results Cancer Res 80:214–218.

Israel L, Bonadonna G, Sylvester R (1979) Controlled study with adjuvant radiotherapy, chemotherapy, immunotherapy, and chemoimmunotherapy in operable squamous carcinoma of the lung. In: Muggia F, Rozenzweig M (eds) Lung Cancer (Progress in Therapeutic Research, vol 11). Raren, New York, New York, pp. 443–452.

Jackson DV Jr, Paschal BR, Ferree C (1982) Chemotherapy – radiotherapy with and without the methanol-extraction residue of bacillus calmette-guerin (MER) in small cell carcinoma of the lung, Cancer 50:48–52.

Jackson DV Jr, Richards F II, Cooper MR, et al (1977) Prophylactic cranial irradiation in small cell carcinoma of the lung. A randomized study, JAMA 237:2730–2733.

Jaffe JP, Bosch A, Raich PC (1979) Sequential hemi-body radiotherapy in advanced multiple myeloma, Cancer 43:124–128.

Jensik RJ, Faber LP, Kittle CF (1979) Segmental resection for bronchogenic carcinoma, Ann Thorac Surg 28:475–483.

Johnke RM, Scarantino CW, Kovacs CJ, Emma DA (1984) The effects of high dose half-body irradiation or cytoxan treatment on rabbit bone marrow hematopoiesis, (unpublished data).

Johnson RE, Brereton HD, Kent CH (1976) Small-cell carcinoma of the lung: attempt to remedy causes of past therapeutic failure, Lancet 2:289–291.

Jones DH, Bleehan NM, Slatr AJ, et al (1983) Human lymphoblastoid interferon in the treatment of small cell lung cancer, Br J Cancer 47:361–366.

Kallenberg F, Jaqué J (1979) Giant-cell carcinoma of the lung. Clinical and pathological assessment. Comparison with other large-cell anaplastic bronchogenic carcinomas, Scand J Thorac Cardiovasc Surg 13:343–346.

Kaplan HS (1979) Historic milestones in radiobiology and radiation therapy, Semin Oncol 6:479–489.

Karrer K, Denck H, Obermair H, et al (1982) Combination of surgery and polychemotherapy for cure in early small-cell bronchial carcinoma, Bull Cancer 69(1): 94–97.

Katz HR (1983) The effect of resection on local failure in irradiated non-oat cell carcinoma of the lung, Int J Radiat Oncol Biol Phys 9:1793–1805.

Keen CE (1980) Half body radiotherapy in the management of metastatic carcinoma of the prostate, J Urol 123:713–715.

Kirsch MM, Rotman H, Argenta L, et al (1976) Carcinoma of the lung: results of treatment over ten years, Ann Thorac Surg 21:371–377.

Kirsch MM, Dickerman R, Fayos J, et al (1973) The value of chest wall resection in the treatment of superior sulcus tumors of the lung, Ann Thorac Surg 15:339–346.

Kjaer M (1982) Radiotherapy of squamous, adeno- and large cell carcinoma of the lung, Cancer Treat Rev 9:1–20.

Knight EW, Lagakos S, Stolbach L, et al (1976) Adriamycin in the treatment of far-advanced lung cancer, Cancer Treat Rep 60:939–941.

Komaki R, Cox JD, Whitson W (1981) Risk of brain metastases from small cell carcinoma of the lung related to length of survival and prophylactic irradiation, Cancer Treat Rep 65:811–814.

Kurtz JM, Gelber R, Brady LW, et al (1981) The palliation of brain metastases in a favorable patient population: a randomized clinical trial by the radiation therapy oncology group, Int J Radiat Oncol Biol Phys 7:891–895.

Laing AH, Berry RJ, Newman CR (1975) Treatment of inoperable carcinoma of bronchus, Lancet 2:1161–1164.

Lala PK (1972) Age-specific changes in the proliferation of Ehrlich ascites tumor cells grown as solid tumors, Cancer Res 32:628–636.

Lamourex KB (1974) Increased clinically symptomatic pulmonary radiation reactions with adjuvant chemotherapy, Cancer Chemother Rep 58:705–708.

Lanzotti VJ, Thomas DR, Boyle LE, et al (1977) Survival with inoperable lung cancer. An integration of prognostic variables based on simple clinical criteria, Cancer 39:303–313.

Lawson RAM, Ross WM, Gold RG, et al (1972) Postradiation pericarditis: report on four more cases with special reference to bronchogenic carcinoma, J Thorac Cardiovasc Surg 63:841–847.

Lee RE (1983) Radiotherapy for lung cancer. In: Straus MJ (ed) Lung Cancer Clinical Diagnosis and Treatment. Grune and Stratton, New York, pp. 213–243.

Lee RE, Carr DT, Childs DS Jr (1976) Comparison of split-course radiation therapy and continuous radiation therapy for unresectable bronchogenic carcinoma: 5 year results, AJR 126:116–122.

Le Roux BT (1972) Management of bronchial carcinoma by segmental resection, Thorax 27:70–74.

Libshitz HI, Southard ME (1974) Complications of radiation therapy: the thorax, Semin Roentgenol 9:41–49.

Livingston RB (1982) Combined-modality therapy for non-small-cell carcinoma of the lung: an experimental approach. In: SK Carter, E Glatstein, RB Livingston (eds) Principles of Cancer Treatment. McGraw Hill-Book Company, New York, pp. 367–372.

Livingston RB, Trauth CJ, Greenstreet RL (1981) Small cell carcinoma: clinical manifestations and behavior with treatment. In: FA Greco, RK Oldham, PA Bunn (eds) Small cell lung cancer. Grune and Stratton Inc, New York, pp. 285–300.

Livingston RB (1980a) Small cell carcinoma of the lung, Blood 56:575–584.

Livingston R, Mira J (1980b) Non-cross-resistant combinations in patients (pts) with extensive small-cell lung cancer, Proc AACR-ASCO 21:449. (abstract C-512)

Livingston RB, Heilbrun LH (1978a) Patterns of response and relapse in chemotherapy of extensive squamous carcinoma of the lung, Cancer Chemother Pharmacol 1:225–227.

Livingston RB, Moore TN, Heilbrun L, et al (1978b) Small cell carcinoma of the lung: combined chemotherapy and radiation. A southwest oncology group study, Ann Intern Med 88:194–199.

Locksmith JP, Powers WE (1968) Permanent radiation myelopathy, Am J Roentgenol, Radium Ther Nucl Med 102:916–926.

Lombardi F, Lattuada A, Gasparini M, et al (1982) Sequential half-body irradiation as systemic treatment of progressive Ewing sarcoma, Int J Radiat Oncol Biol Phys 8:1679–1682.

Looney WB, Hopkins HA, Longerbeam MB, et al (1983) Comparison of effects of daily versus hyperfractionated split-course radiation schedules with and without cyclophosphamide on median survival, metastatic dissemination, tumor cure and growth rates, Cancer Res 43:60–67.

Looney WB, Hopkins HA, MacLeod MS et al (1979) Solid tumor models for the assessment of different treatment modalities – XIV: the evaluation of host and tumor response to cyclophosphamide and radiation, Int J Radiat Oncol Biol Phys 5:1461–1465.

Lowenbraun S, Bartolucci A, Smalley RV, Lynn M, Krauss S, Durant JR, and The Southeastern Cancer Study Group (1979) The superiority of combination chemotherapy over single agent chemotherapy in small cell lung carcinoma, Cancer 44:406–413.

Magilligan DJ Jr, Rogers JS, Knighton RS, et al (1976) Pulmonary neoplasm with solitary cerebral metastasis. Results of combined excision, J Thorac Cardiovasc Surg 72:690–698.

Mandelbaum I, Williams SD, Hornback NB, et al (1978) Combined therapy for small cell undifferentiated carcinoma of the lung, J Thorac Cardiovasc Surg 76:292–296.

Marchello B, Hammond N, Teel P, et al (1984) Resectability of small cell lung cancer (SCLC), timing, and incidence in a community setting, Proc Am Soc Clin Onc 3:233. (abstract C-911)

Martini N, McCormack P (1983) Therapy of stage III (Non-metastatic disease), Semin Oncol 10:95–110.

Martini N, Beattie EJ (1982) The surgical treatment of lung cancer, Semin Resp Med 4:1–8.

Martini N, Beattie EJ Jr (1977) Results of surgical treatment in stage I lung cancer, J Thorac Cardiovasc Surg 74:499–505.

Matthews MJ, Mackay B, Lukeman J (1983) The pathology of non-small cell carcinoma of the lung, Semin Oncol 10(1):34–35.

Matthews MJ, Rozencweig M, Staquet MJ, et al (1980) Long-term survivors with small cell carcinoma of the lung, Eur J Cancer 16:527–531.

Matthews MJ, Kanhouwa S, Pickren J, et al (1973) Frequency of residual and metastatic tumor in patients undergoing curative surgical resection for lung cancer, Cancer Chemother Rep, part 3, 4(2):63–67.

Mattiessen W (1978) Controlled clinical trial of radiotherapy alone, against radiotherapy plus chemotherapy in small-cell carcinoma of the lung. Comparison of radiation damage. Preliminary results, Scand J Respir Dis [Suppl] 102:209–211.

Maurer LH, Tulloh M, Weiss RB, et al (1980) A randomized combined modality trial in small cell carcinoma of the lung. Comparison of combination chemotherapy-radition therapy versus cyclophosphamide-radiation therapy effects of maintenance chemotherapy and prophylactic whole brain irradiation, Cancer 45:30–39.

McCracken JD, Chen T, White J, et al (1982) Combination chemotherapy, radiotherapy, and BCG immunotherapy in limited small cell carcinoma of the lung, a southwest oncology group study, Cancer 49:2252–2258.

McDougall JC, Cortese DA (1983) Neodymium-YAG laser therapy of malignant airway obstruction, May Clin Proc 58:35–39.

McDowell EM, Trump BF (1981) Pulmonary small cell carcinoma showing tripartite differentiation in individual cells, Hum Pathol 12:286–294.

McMahon LJ, Herman TS, Manning Mr, et al (1979) Patterns of relapse in patients with small cell carcinoma of the lung treated with adriamycin-cyclophosphamide chemotherapy and radiation therapy, Cancer Treat Rep 63:359–362.

Medical Research Council Lung Cancer Working Party of the Third Small-Cell Study (1983) Cytotoxic chemotherapy before and after radiotherapy compared with radiotherapy followed by chemotherapy in the treatment of small cell carcinoma of the bronchus: the results up to 36 months. Br J Cancer 48:755–761.

Medical Research Council Lung Cancer Working Party (1979) Radiotherapy alone or with chemotherapy in the treatment of small-cell carcinoma of the lung, Br J Cancer 40:1–10.

Meyer JA, Comis RL, Ginsberg SJ, et al (1982) Phase II trial of extended indications for resection in small cell carcinoma of the lung, J Thorac Cardiovasc Surg 83:12–19.

Meyer JA, Comis RL, Ginsberg SJ, et al (1979) Selective surgical resection in small cell carcinoma of the lung, J Thorac Cardiovasc Surg 77:243–248.

Miller JI, Mansour KA, Hatcher CR Jr (1979) Carcinoma of the superior pulmonary sulcus, Ann Thorac Surg 28:44–47.

Minna JD, Bunn PA Jr, Carney DN, et al (1982) Experience of the national cancer institute (USA) in the treatment and biology of small cell lung cancer, Bull Cancer 69:83–93.

Minna J, Ihde D, Bunn P, et al (1980) Extensive stage small cell carcinoma of the lung (SCCL): effect of increasing intensity of induction chemotherapy, Proc AACR-ASCO 21:448. (abstract C-510)

Mitchell DM, Morgan PGM, Ball JB (1980) Prognostic features of large cell anaplastic carcinoma of the bronchus, Thorax 35:118–122.

Moody TW, Russell EK, O'Donohue TL, et al (1983) Bombesin-like peptides in small cell lung cancer: biochemical characterization and secretion from a cell line, Life Sci 32:487–493.

Moore TN, Livingston R, Heilbrun L, et al (1978) An acceptable rate of complications in combined doxorubicin-irradiation for small cell carcinoma of the lung: a southwest oncology group study, Int J Radiat Oncol Phys 4:675–680.

Morris RW, Abadir R (1979) Pancoast tumor: the value of high dose radiation therapy, Radiology 132:717–719.

Morrison R, Deeley TJ, Cleland WP (1963) The treatment of carcinoma of the bronchus. A clinical trial to compare surgery and supervoltage radiotherapy, Lancet 1:683–684.

Morstyn G, Ihde DC, Lichter AS, et al (1984) Small cell lung cancer 1973–1983: early progress and recent obstacles, Int J Radiat Oncol Biol Phys 10:515–539.

Mountain CF (1983a) Biologic, physiologic, and technical determinants in surgical therapy in lung cancer. In: MJ Straus (ed) Lung Cancer. Clinical Diagnosis and Treatment. Grune and Straton, New York, pp. 245–260.

Mountain CF, (1983b) Therapy of stage I and stage II non-small cell lung cancer, Semin Oncol 10:71–80.

Mountain CF (19827) The role of adjuvant therapy in the surgical treatment of lung cancer, Semin Resp Med 4:9–16.

Mountain CF (1978) Clinical biology of small cell carcinoma: relationship to surgical therapy, Semin Oncol 5:272–279.

Mountain CF, (1977a) Assessment of the role of surgery for the control of lung cancer, Ann Thorac Surg 24:365–373.

Mountain CF (1977b) Biologic, physiologic, and technical determinants in surgical therapy for lung cancer. In: Straus MJ (ed) Lung Cancer: Clinical Diagnosis and Treatment. Grune and Stratton, New York, pp. 185–198.

Muggia FM, Krezoski SK, Hansen HH (1974) Cell kinetic studies in patients with small cell carcinoma of the lung, Cancer 34:1683–1690.

Natale R, Hilaris B, Wittes R (1980) Prolonged remission of small cell lung carcinoma (SCLC) with intensive chemotherapy induction and high dose radiation therapy without maintenance, Proc AACR-ASCO 21:452. (abstract C-525).

Newman SJ, Hansen HH (1974) Frequency, diagnosis, and treatment of brain metastases in 247 consecutive patients with bronchogenic carcinoma, Cancer 33:492–496.

Nixon DW, Murphy GF, Sewell CW, et al (1979) Relationship between survival and histologic type in small cell anaplastic carcinoma of the lung, Cancer 44:1045–1049.

Nugent JL, Bunn PA Jr, Matthews MJ, Ihde DC (1979) CNS metastases in small cell bronchogenic carcinoma. Increasing frequency and changing pattern with lengthening survival, Cancer 44:1885–1893.

Ochs JJ, Tester WJ, Cohen MH, et al (1983) "Salvage" radiation therapy for intrathoracic small cell carcinoma of the lung progressing on combination chemotherapy. Cancer Treat Rep 67:1123–1126.

Palmer RL, Kroening PM (1978) Comparison of low dose radiation therapy alone or combined with procarbazine (NSC-77213) for unresectable epidermoid carcinoma of the lung, state T3, N1, N2 or M1, Cancer 42:424–428.

Paulson DL, Reisch JS (1976) Long-term survival after resection for bronchogenic carcinoma, Ann Surg 184:324–332.

Paulson DL (1975) Carcinomas in the superior pulmonary sulcus. J Thorac Cardiovasc Surg 70:1095–1104.

Pene F, Schlienger M, Schmitt T, et al (1981) Half-body irradiation for pain relief, Eur J Cancer Clin Oncol 17:753–758.

Perez CA, Stanley K, Grundy G, et al (1982) Impact of irradiation technique and tumor extent in tumor control and survival of patients with unresectable non-oat cell carcinoma of the lung. Report by the radiation therapy oncology group, Cancer 50:1091–1099.

Perez CA, Stanley K, Rubin P, et al (1980) A prospective randomized study of various irradiation doses and fractionation schedules in the treatment of inoperable non-oat cell carcinoma of the lung, Cancer 45:2744–2753.

Petrovich Z, Stanley K, Cox JD, et al (1981) Radiotherapy in the management of locally advanced lung cancer of all cell types. Final report of a randomized trial, Cancer 48:1335–1340.

Petrovich Z, Ohanian M, Cox J (1978) Clinical research on the treatment of locally advanced lung cancer. Final report of VALG protocol 13 limited, Cancer 42:1129–1134.

Petrovich Z, Mietlowski W, Ohanian M, et al (1977) Clinical report on the treatment of locally advanced lung cancer, Cancer 40:72–77.

Pettengill OS, Sorenson GD, Wurster-Hill DH, et al (1980) Isolation and growth characteristics of continuous cell lines from small-cell carcinoma of the lung, Cancer 45:906–918.

Posner JB (1977) Management of central nervous system metastases, Semin Oncol 4:81–91.

Prato FS, Kurdyak R, Saibh EA, et al (1976) The incidence of radiation pneumonitis as a result of single fraction upper half body irradiation, Cancer 39:71–78.

Quasim MM (1981) Half body irradiation (HBI) in metastatic carcinomas, Clin Radiol 32:215–219.

Raber M, Barlogie B, Farquhar D (1980) Determination of pooidy abnormality and cell cycle distribution in human lung cancer using DNA flow cytometry, Proc AACR/ASCO 21:40. (abstract #159)

Report By A Medical Research Council Working Party (1971) Study of cytotoxic chemotherapy as an adjuvant to surgery in carcinoma of the bronchus, Br Med J 2:421–428.

Richards F II, Case LD, Jackson D, et al (1984) Prognostic factors as determinants of response and survival in advanced non-small cell carcinoma of the lung (NSCLC) treated with CMAP (CCNJ, methotrexate, adriamycin, cis-platinum), Proc Am Soc Clin Oncol 3:230. (abstract C-899).

Richards F, Case LD, Jackson D, et al (1982) CMAP (CCNU, methotrexate, adriamycin, platinum) in non-small cell lung cancer, Proc AACR-ASCO 1:144. (abstract C-604)

Richards F II, Cooper MR, White D, et al (1980) Advanced epidermoid lung cancer: prolonged survival after chemotherapy, Cancer 46:34–37.

Richards F II, White DR, Muss HB, et al (1979) Combination chemotherapy of advanced non-oat cell lung carcinoma of the lung, Cancer 44:1476–1581.

Rissanen PM, Tikka U, Holsti LR (1968) Autopsy findings in lung cancer treated with megavoltage radiotherapy, Acta Radiol Ther Phys Biol 7:433–442.

Rofstad EK, Lindmo T, Brunstad T, (1981) Effect of single dose irradiation on the proliferation kinetics in a human malignant melanoma in athymic nude mice, Acta Radiol (Oncol) 19:261–269.

Rosen ST, Makuch RW, Lichter AS, et al (1983) Role of prophylactic cranial irradiation in prevention of central nervous system metastases in small cell lung cancer, Am J Med 74:615–624.

Roswit B, Patno ME, Rapp R, et al (1968) The survival of patients with inoperable lung cancer: a large-scale randomized study of radiation therapy versus placebo, Radiology 90:688–697.

Rowland CG, Bullimore JA, Smith PJB, et al (1981) Half-body irradiation in the treatment of metastatic prostatic carcinoma, Br J Urol 53:628–629.

Rowland CG, Garrett MJ, Crowley FA (1983) Half body radiation in plasma cell myeloma, Clin Radiol 34:507–510.

Rubin P, Shapiro DL, Finkelstein JN, et al (1980) The early release of surfactant following lung irradiation of alveolar type II cells, Int J Radiat Oncol Biol Phys 6:75–77.

Rubin P, Scarantino CW (1978) The bone marrow organ: the critical structue in radiation drug ineraction, Int J Radiat Oncol Biol Phys 4:3–23.

Rubin P, Ciccio S, Setisarn B (1970) The controversial status of radiation therapy in lung cancer, Proc Natl Cancer Conf 6:855–865.

Salazar OM, Creech RH (1980) "The state of the art" toward defining the role of radiation therapy in the management of small cell bronchogenic carcinoma, Int J Radiat Oncol Biol Phys 6:1103–1117.

Salazar OM, Rubin P, Keller B, Scarantino CW (1978) Systemic (half-body) radiation therapy: response and toxicity, Int J Radiat Oncol Biol Phys 4:937–950.

Salazar OM, Scarantino CW, Rubin P, et al (1980) Total (half-body) systemic irradiation for occult metastases in non-small cell lung cancer: an eastern cooperative oncology group pilot report, Cancer 46:1932–1944.

Salazar OM, Rubin P, Brown, JC, et al (1976) Predictors of radiation response in lung cancer. A clinico-pathobiological analysis, Cancer 37:2636–2650.

Saunders MI, Bennett MH, Dische S, et al (1984) Primary tumor control after radiotherapy for carcinoma of the bronchus, Int J Radiat Oncol Biol Phys 10:499–501.

Saunders MI, Barltrop MA, Obst D, et al (1984) The relationship between tumor response and survival following radiotherapy for carcinoma of the bronchus, Int J Radiat Oncol Biol Phys 10:503–508.

Scarantino CW, Richards F II, Raben M, et al (1983) Non-small cell bronchogenic carcinoma (NSCBC); response and tolerance to sequential upper half body (HBI) cyclophosphamide (CP) and local radiation therapy (LRT), Int J Radiat Oncol Biol Phys 9(1):176.

Scarantino CW, Rubin P, Constine LS (1984) The paradoxes in patterns and mechanisms of bone marrow regeneration after irradiation. Part I: different volumes and doses, Radiotherapy and Oncology (in press).

Schabel FM Jr (1969) The use of tumor growth kinetics in planning "curative" chemotherapy of advanced solid tumors, Cancer Res 29:2384–2389.

Selawry OS (1974) The role of chemotherapy in the treatment of lung cancer, Semin Oncol 1:259–272.

Seydel HG, Cruch RH, Mietlowski W, et al (1978) Radiation therapy in small cell lung cancer, Semin Oncol 5:288–298.

Sheline GE, Wara WM, Smith V (1980) Therapeutic irradiation and brain injury, Int J Radiat Oncol Biol Phys 6:1215–1228.

Sherman DM, Neptune W, Weichselbaum R, et al (1978) An aggressive approach to marginally resectable lung cancer, Cancer 41:2040–2045.

Shields TW, Higgins GA Jr, Matthews MJ, Keehn RJ (1982) Surgical resection in the management of small cell carcinoma of the lung, J Thorac Cardiovasc Surg 84:481–488.

Shields TW, Humphrey EW, Matthews M, et al (1980) Pathological stage grouping of patients with resected carcinoma of the lung, J Thorac Cardiovasc Surg 80:400–405.

Shields TW, Yee J, Conn JH, et al (1975) Relationship of cell type and lymph node metastasis to survival after resection of bronchial carcinoma, Ann Thorac Surg 20:501–510.

Shields TW (1973) Status report of adjuvant cancer chemotherapy trials in the treatment of bronchial carcinoma, Cancer Chemother Rep, part 3, 4:119–124.

Shields TW (1972) Preoperative radiation therapy in the treatment of bronchial carcinoma, Cancer 30:1388–1394.

Shields TW, Higgins GA, Lawton R, et al (1970) Preoperative x-ray therapy as an adjuvant in the treatment of bronchogenic carcinoma, J Thorac Cardiovasc Surg 59:49–61.

Shore DF, Paneth M (1980) Surival after resection of small cell carcinoma of the bronchus, Thorax 35:819–822.

Silberfarb PM (1983) Chemotherapy and cognitive defects in cancer patients, Annu Rev Med 34:35–46.

Silverberg E (1984) Cancer statistics, CA-A Cancer Journal for Clinicians, 1:7–23.

Slawson RG, Scott RM (1979) Radiation therapy in bronchogenic carcinoma, Radiology 132:175–176.

Smart J (1966) Can lung cancer be cured by irradiation alone?, JAMA 195:1034–1035.

Smith RA (1970) Long-term clinical follow-up after operation for lung carcinoma, Thorax 25:62–76.

Sorenson GD, Pettengill OS, Brinck-Johnsen T, et al (1981) Hormone production by cultures of small-cell carcinoma of the lung, Cancer 47:1289–1296.

Stanley K, Cox JD, Petrovich Z, et al (1981) Patterns of failure in patients with inoperable carcinoma of the lung, Cancer 47:2725–2729.

Stanley KE (1980) Prognostic factors for survival in patients with inoperable lung cancer, JNCI 65:25–32.

Stewart P, Buckner DC, Thomas ED, et al (1983) Intensive chemoradiotherapy with autologous marrow transplantation for small cell carcinoma of the lung, Cancer Treat Rep 67:1055–1059.

Sutherland RM, Durand RE (1976) Radiation response of multicell spheroids: an in vitro tumour model, Curr Top Radiat Res Q 11:87–139.

Takita H, Brugarolas A, Marabella P, et al (1973) Small cell carcinoma of the lung. Clinicopathological studies, J Thorac Cardiovasc Surg 66:472–477.

Tischler AS (1978) Small cell carcinoma of the lung: cellular origin and relationship to other neoplasms, Semin Oncol 5:244–252.

Valdivieso M, Farha P, Umsawasdi T, et al (1982a) Antineoplastic chemotherapy of advanced lung cancer, Semin Respir Med 4:28–41.

Valdivieso M, McMurtrey MJ, Farha P, et al (1982b) Increasing importance of adjuvant surgery in the therapy of patients with small cell lung cancer, Proc AACR-ASCO 1:148. (abstract C-576)

Van Houtte P, Rocmans P, Smets P, et al (1980) Postoperative radiation therapy in lung cancer: a controlled trial after resection of curative design, Int J Radiat Oncol Biol Phys 6:983–986.

van Peperzeel HA (1972) Effects of single doses of radiation on lung metastasis in man and experimental animals, Eur J Cancer 8:665–675.

Vincent RG, Dougherty TJ, Rao U, et al (1984) Photoradiation therapy in advanced carcinoma of the trachea and bronchus, Chest 85:29–33.

Vincent RG, Mehta CR, Tucker RD, et al (1980) Chemotherapy of extensive large cell and adenocarcinoma of the lung. A randomized trial in 210 patients, Cancer 46:256–260.

Vogl SE, Mehta CR, Cohen MH (1979) MACC chemotherapy of adenocarcinoma and epidermoid carcinoma of the lung. Low response rate in a cooperative group study, Cancer 44:864–868.

Vosika GJ (1979) Large cell bronchogenic carcinoma. Prolonged disease-free survival following chemotherapy, JAMA 241:594–595.

Weiss RB (1978) Small-cell carcinoma of the lung: therapeutic management, Ann Intern Med 88:522–531.

Whang-Peng J, Kao-Shan CS, Lee EC (1982) Specific chromosomal defect associated with human small-cell lung cancer: deletion 3 p (14–23), Science 215:181–182.

White JE, Boles M (1981) The role of radiation therapy in the treatment of regional non-small (oat)-cell carcinoma of the lung. In: Livingston RB (ed) Cancer Treatment and Research. Vol 1: Lung Cancer I Martinus Nijhoff Publishers, Hague Boston London, pp. 113–156.

Williams DE, Pairolero PC, Davis CS, et al (1981) Survival of patients surgically treated for stage I lung cancer, J Thorac Cardiovasc Surg 82:70–76.

Williams C, Alexander M, Glatstein EJ, et al (1977) Role of radiation therapy in combination with chemotherapy in extensive oat cell cancer of the lung: a randomized study, Cancer Treat Rep 61:1427–1431.

Wolf J, Patno ME, Roswit B, et al (1966) Controlled study of survival of patients with clinically inoperable lung cancer treated with radiation therapy, Am J Med 40:360–367.

Yesner R, Carter D (1982) Pathology of carcinoma of the lung. Changing patterns. Symposium on recent advances in lung cancer, Clin Chest Med 3(2):257–289.

Zacharski LR, Henderson WG, et al (1981) Effect warfarin on survival in small cell carcinoma of the lung, JAMA 245:831–935.

Zelen M (1973) Keynote address on biostatistics and data retrieval, Cancer Chemother Rep, part 3, 4(2):31–42.

Zimm S, Wampler GL, Stablein D (1981) Intracerebral metastases in solid-tumor patients: natural history and results of treatment, Cancer 48:384–394.

Chapter VIII Redefining Clinical Research

CHARLES J. KOVACS

CONTENTS

1 Introduction

Unlike many other pathological states, the treatment of neoplasia has not been blessed with major "breakthroughs". Cancer treatment today is the result of a slowly evolving, quasi-empirical, methodological search for specific agents that (1) kill tumor cells, (2) have unique mechanisms of action, and (3) are assessed to be disease-effective and tolerated. Therefore, achievements in cancer treatment have required, and continue to require sound financial support, long hours in the laboratory and clinic, and cooperation and communication between an "army" of preclinical, clinical and basic scientists with a common goal. Despite this absence of major breakthroughs, however, the clinical management of cancer has evolved such that today, it represents a sophisticated, knowledgeable approach to health care.

The "cure rates" and "five-year survival" for a majority of cancer patients remains severely limited, and therefore the battle for the complete management of cancer through new, innovative treatment approaches continues. It is the goal of this section of the text to provide the framework necessary for future directions in the area of clinical cancer research by considering pertinent achievements of experimental treatment that have "immediate potential" for the oncologist. While recognizing that research areas even remotely related to the treatment of neoplasia may eventually make a contribution, an attempt to assess all the specific areas encompassed under the heading of "cancer research" would be, nonetheless, a monumental task. Therefore, the subject matter has been selected, albeit subjectively, to cover only those areas that are, or potentially have, some basis for clinical cancer research. Every attempt has been made to document the immediacy of the material and to avoid unnecessary subjective reinterpretation.

CHARLES J. KOVACS, Ph. D., Associate Professor and Director, Radiation Oncology Laboratories, Department of Radiology, Section of Radiotherapy

Bowman Gray School of Medicine of Wake Forest University, 300 South Hawthorne Road, Winston-Salem, NC 27103, USA

Present Address: C.J. KOVACS, Dr., Professor and Director, Division of Radiation Biology and Oncology East Carolina University, School of Medicine, Greenville, NC 27894, USA

2 Historical Considerations of Experimental Therapy

A brief summary of the development of radiotherapy at this time is intended to facilitate discussions of the overall direction of this treatment modality. These discussions are by no means comprehensive, and many of the topics are superficially presented.

Where appropriate, the reader will be referred to review articles on the topic. For the most part, those areas considered to have sufficient substance for future development are considered in depth.

2.1 Radiobiological Translation: Successes, Failures, and the Future

Radiotherapy has evolved from a clinical art to a highly technical therapeutic modality with a sound basis in radiobiology. At its inception, radiotherapy was essentially descriptive. An absence of appreciation for the quantitative aspects of radiotolerance led to many failures in the clinic. Although it had a scientific basis in physics, physics only taught how a radiation dose was distributed. The biological effects were only recognized through experience. Anyone who has had even a brief exposure to the "science of radiobiology" will recognize the postulates of BERGONIE and TRIBONDEAU (1906) as the first biological interpretations of radiation. However, they again were descriptive and provided little basis for the quantitative assessment of radiation effects observed in the clinic, let alone for predictive radiotherapeutic planning. Nonetheless, the advent of quantitative radiobiology has substantiated, with little modification, these descriptive postulates.

While the first report of quantitative experimental radiobiology was the clinical work of STRANDQUIST (1944), true interpretative radiobiology had its basis in the pioneering work of PUCK and MARCUS (1956). Their work, using experimental in vitro methods to assess cell survival and subsequent refinement notably by ELKIND and his colleagues (ELKIND and WHITMORE, 1967), led to an exponential increase in the quantitation and therefore, definition of both molecular and cellular radiation effects during the golden "60's and 70's".

The backbone of these studies, along with the development of tritiated thymidine (^{3}H-TdR), was the radiation survival curve and survival curve theory. The survival curve has served as the framework for describing most, if not all, of the recent advances in radiation therapy and radiobiology (e.g. hypoxic cell resistance, radiosensitization and more recently protection). Furthermore, the radiation survival curve, along with the classical tools of cell proliferation kinetics, were collectively believed to hold the key to successful radiotherapy.

Volumes of experimental data have accumulated over the last 15 years for optimizing the radiotherapy of animal tumors and normal tissues.

In general, this experimental data has substantiated the fundamental laws of radiobiology. Unfortunately, ethical considerations have prevented similar data from being obtained from patients in most cases. Quantitation of human tumor response, therefore, has been limited. In addition, many of the problems of cellular radiobiology have not been resolved. These complicating problems, along with the concept of radiation toxicity which will be addressed in a later section, are just some of the major limitations that are confronted in quantitative human radiation biology and therapy.

Overall, radiotherapy has been less than convincing as an effective method of treatment for most cancers. This has increasingly led clinicians to administer more aggressive therapeutic regimens using a combination of treatment modalities. The objective of these aggressive regimens has been to achieve enhanced tumoricidal activity at the primary disease site and better control of disseminated occult disease. Another promising trend in cancer therapy has been the administration of single, high-dose, half-body irradiation (SALAZAR et al., 1978, 1980) and more recently, intra-operative high-dose thoracic or abdominal irradiation (GOLDSON, 1978; ABE et al., 1980). These new approaches to radiotherapy are also being considered as one component of combined mode therapeutic scheduling, an approach already demonstrating the complexities of its multiplicity.

Obviously, these new approaches to treatment are based on established scientific principles or, at the least, available experience or knowledge which brings up the question "What has radiobiology contributed to the radiotherapy of human tumors?" Whereas the radiosensitivity of cells and tissues depends on their proliferative activity, cell proliferation in the form of reproductive integrity does not represent the only factor determining whether a tumor can be cured with ionizing radiation. In the discussions to follow, such concepts as delayed toxic effects, reoxygenation, host defense mechanisms and the hypoxic cell fraction, in addition to cellular damage, will be recognized as an undercurrent included in the components of neoplastic control. Clinical radiotherapy can no longer be considered an empiric science where neoplastic tissue must be irradiated to the limits of tolerance. Radiobiology has, over the years, defined the limits of radiotherapeutic dosage based on each of these components including a consideration of the type, location and biology of each tumor. The radiotherapist can, therefore, approach each patient with, at the very least, a better appreciation of his limitations.

The most underdeveloped area of tumor management for all oncologic specialists lies in the initial diagnosis of the presenting patient. Major decisions at this time depend on an appreciation of the histopathologic grading of the tumor as well as the primary anatomic site. These two guidelines have emerged as widely applicable tools for planning therapy and for assessing prognosis. Unfortunately, relatively few tumors can be categorically described, suggesting that the early concept of the "wild cell" would more aptly be applied at the tissue level. For this reason, predicting optimal radiotherapeutic responsiveness (and approach) for individual patients is often difficult, if not impossible.

Within the broad field of diagnostic oncology, a cognizance of a rapidly developing area occupied by a heterogeneous group of tumors that are collectively referred to as "poorly differentiated tumors" (PDT) is developing. PDT include not only those neoplasms lacking a differentiated histology, but also include those neoplasms that are recognizable as to a particular category (e.g. breast) while lacking differentiated characteristics. Frequently recognized PDT of this type include both tumors of the lung as well as the breast, but certainly do not exclude other tumor types. The problems associated with PDT are further complicated by the rapidly evolving concept of tumor heterogeneity which will be discussed in depth in a later section.

Several earlier studies by radiobiologists have attempted to establish characteristics of tumors that are accurately related to "tumor responsiveness". DENEKAMP and THOMLINSON (1971) and DENEKAMP (1972) have attempted to define the immediate response of a solid tumor to radiation by postulating a relationship between "response" and "cell loss factor". Clinically, however, the immediate response may not occur rapidly, due to the "slow growth rate" of many tumors, or be apparent at all if clonogenic repopulation occurs rapidly, obscuring extended regression. KOVACS et al. (1977), from studies of rapidly, moderately, and slowly growing tumors, have concluded that prediction of tumor response to radiation requires an understanding of both cell production and cell loss as well as histopathology and relative tissue composition of each tumor. Thus, important distinctions must be made between radiosensitivity (and perhaps chemosensitivity) of a tumor cell population and the clinical radioresponsiveness of a neoplasm. The question of solid tumor radio-

sensitivity or radioresistance is therefore more than just an academic exercises. There is a pressing need to establish generalities concerning solid tumors and the predictability of response to both single and multiple modality therapy.

As far back as 1966, BREUR, in a review of tumor radiosensitivity, stressed the need for laboratory experiments where radioresponsiveness could be assessed as a function of multiparimetrical end points. The clinical implications of a less than specific pathological diagnosis can result in inaccurate, and expensive treatment planning. The surgical pathologist, as charged by BREUR, is responsible for accurate and rapid identification of tumors. Until recently, histological grading resulted from light microscopic analyses of paraffin sections with some special staining techniques. Today, the pathologist has, in addition to the light microscope, a battery of advanced laboratory technology including the electron microscope, various fluorescent markers establishing differentiation and in vitro clonogenic methods for the growth of tumor cells, with which to make exact tumor identification a possibility. Collaborative studies between the pathologist, tumor biologist, radiation biologist and therapist, using these new technologies, should aid in establishing predictive markers of tumor radioresponsiveness as well as facilitating an understanding of various subsets within histologically and anatomically well-defined cancers.

2.2 Combined Drug Radiation Studies: Mechanisms and Sequencing

For many years, cancer treatment was the sequential usage of single modalities such as surgery, irradiation and chemotherapy. In more recent years, however, there has been an increasing use of approaches in which two (2) or more of the modalities are used in combination to achieve superior results in terms of either local region control or disseminated disease control (BERLIN, 1965). The strategy of combining chemotherapeutic agents with radiation – now a major emphasis in cancer management – was based theoretically on the belief that radiation-drug interactions can (1) potentially sensitize cells to the killing effects of radiation and (2) may also kill cells that radiation fails to damage, thus functioning as an adjuvant to radiation. Major experimental programs were initiated as part of the national plan for improved therapy. The preclinical studies rapidly discovered

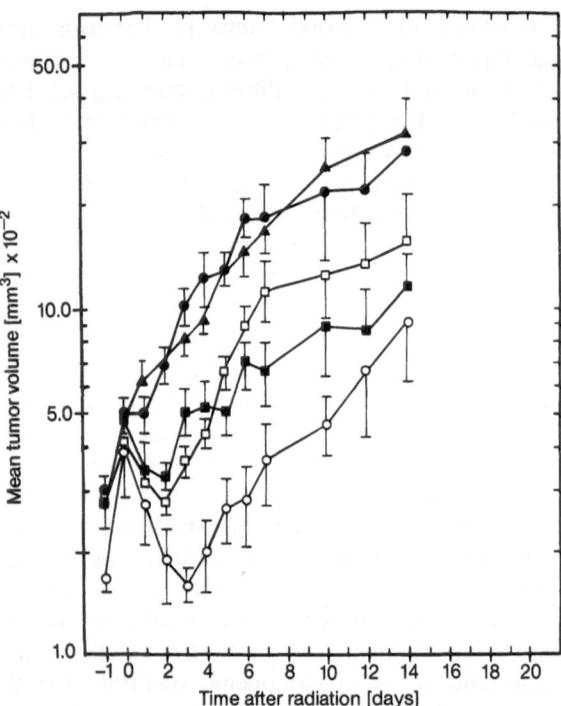

Fig. 1. The effect of acute or fractionated pretreatment with ICRF 159 on the radiation response of the LLca tumor. ●, growth of untreated tumors; ■, 600 rad x-irradiation; □, 100 mg/kg ICRF-159 5 min before 600 R; ○, fractionated (25 mg/kg; 3 hourly × 4) ICRF-159 pretreatment before 600 rad; ▲, fractionated (25 mg/kg; 3 hourly × 4) ICRF treatment alone. Each point represents the mean volume ±s.e. for a group of 10 animals treated on day 7 after tumor inoculation. Reproduced with permission from Kovacs et al., Brit J Cancer 39:516–523, 1979

that combined drug-radiation treatment involved many permutations of the expected response and their conceptual mechanisms. The one concept initially held by advocates of combined mode therapy that remains today is the fact that the interaction of radiation and chemotherapy requires a sensitive balance between antitumor activity and normal tissue toxicity.

Of these two original strategies, the use of chemotherapy as adjunctive treatment both during and following radiation (or surgery) is the more easily interpreted. One of the major failures of oncotherapy after treatment of the primary lesion is a direct result of progressing disseminated disease (Carter, 1976; Bonadonna et al., 1977). Adjuvant therapy, in the form of combined mode has been more effective for some diseases than others (e.g. carcinoma of the breast over lung or colon). However, this may reflect the specific sensitivities of the metastasis for the drugs studied.

During the late 60's and early 70's, an experimental cytostatic drug appeared which was believed to offer a new approach to the major problem of metastatic disease. ICRF-159 {(+)-1,2-bis (3.5 dioxopiperazin-1-yl)propane} was vigorously investigated by Hellman's group in London because of its unique property of preventing metastasis of the experimental Lewis Lung carcinoma (LLca) to the lung of its host (Hellman and Burrage, 1969; Salisbury et al., 1970). The antimetastatic activity, postulated to be the result of drug-induced angiometamorphoses in tumors, resulted from chronic low dose administration having little or no overt influence on the growth of the primary tumor. Furthermore, cytotoxicity when apparent was reported to be schedule-dependent rather than dose-dependent (Stephens and Creighton, 1974), and involved the premitotic (G_2) and early mitotic (M) cells. Unfortunately, the antimetastatic effect was not universally demonstrated in all experimental tumors.

ICRF-159 has also been found to enhance the radiosensitivity (and sensitivity to other drugs) of the LLca tumor provided that the drug is chronically administered at low doses (25 mg/kg; q 3 h × 3-4) prior to a modest acute dose (600 R) of x-radiation (Fig. 1). Similar responses could be generated by daily injections (25 mg/kg; q 24 hr × 7) of the drug prior to irradiation. Acute drug (25–175 mg/kg) given at the time of irradiation (within 5 min) failed to enhance but in fact appeared to protect against the radiation response of the LLca (Fig. 2). Similar studies on the underlying intestinal epithelium suggested that the enhanced radiation response of the tumor did not occur in the normal tissue (Fig. 3) thereby increasing the therapeutic index of this drug/radiation combination in preclinical studies. While this radiopotentiating effect on tumors could result from a reoxygenation of the hypoxic fraction of tumor cells, Peters (1976) has suggested that improved vascularization (angio-metamorphic) cannot fully explain the drugs "radiosensitizing" action. Furthermore, Taylor and Bleehen (1977) have reported ICRF-159 radiopotentiation in vitro where tumor vasculature is of no consequence.

Phase II trials using ICRF-159 unfortunately failed to provide clinical evidence for this enhanced therapeutic ratio. As suggested by the preclinical data, scheduling of drug and radiation in combination plays a major role in the eventual response of the tumor. While not necessarily true for all drugs, the scheduling of ICRF-159 with radiation has been found to be exquisitely sensitive

Fig. 2a–d. The effect of acute ICRF-159 dose on the radiation response of the LL tumor. (a) 25 mg/kg; (b) 50 mg/kg; (c) 100 mg/kg; (d) 175 mg/kg. Dashed line redrawn from the day 7–600 rad radiation response curve. ●, untreated tumors; ○, ICRF-159 5 min before 600 rad. Each point represents the mean tumor volume ±s.e. for a group of 10 animals treated on day 7 after tumor-inoculation. Reproduced with permission from Kovacs et al., Brit J Cancer 39:516–523, 1979

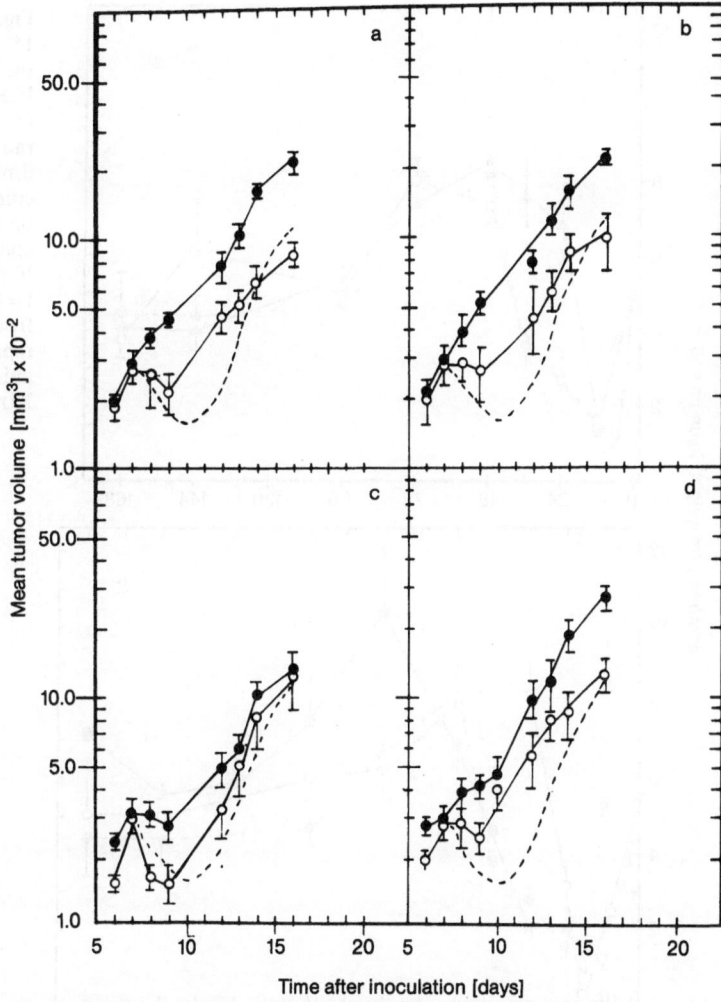

to the biology of the tissue (i.e. cell kinetic characteristics) and may account for its failure in clinical trials.

Unique drugs, such as ICRF-159, are not frequently available for clinical studies. Therefore, the clinician must rely on drugs with potential cytotoxic properties, based on other mechanisms such as analogues of DNA bases and intercalating or alkylating agents, for adjuvant management of metastatic disease. Nonetheless, the time/dose configurations for these drugs cannot be empirically established. Therefore, a continued need exists for additional preclinical, toxicologic and pharmacologic information on existing drugs as well as only newly synthesized and identified potential chemotherapeutic agents. The ultimate goal for effective adjuvant therapy remains the selection of drugs, dose levels and intervals between courses that will kill disseminated cancer cells unaffected by conventional radiotherapy.

We have briefly touched on the second strategy initially governing the approach to combined modality (drug-radiation) treatment. It was assumed that an already sensitive mode could be potentiated by interaction with a second sensitive mode. At the very least, the interaction of two sensitive agents should result in additive effects on cell viability and ultimately on the radiation response of neoplastic and normal tissues. This aspect of combined radiation drug interaction has over the last 25 years resulted in voluminous reports in the literature as one might expect from even a brief consideration of the various permutations of even a single drug, at a single dose, in combination with a single dose of radiation. Expanding this considerations to various dose levels of each agent and adding the additional parameter of intertreatment times renders the entire concept of combined mode incomprehensible. It is not surprising, therefore, that optimal employment of drugs and radiation

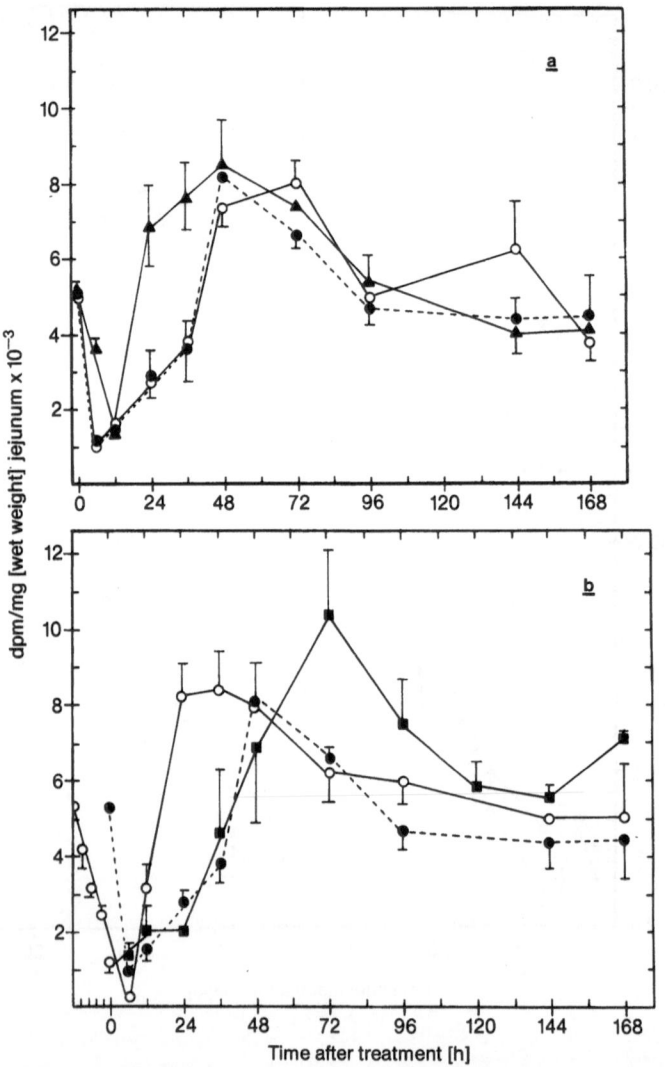

Fig. 3. a The effect of combined acute ICRF-159 and 600 rad on the proliferative activity of the jejunal epithelium. (▲---▲), 100 mg/kg ICRF-159 at t=0; (●---●), 600 rad at t=0; (○---○), 100 mg/kg ICRF-159 (−5 min) +600 rad (t=0). Each point represents the mean d/min/mg±s.e. for 4 animals. **b** The effect of combined fractionated ICRF-159 and 600 rad on the proliferative activity of the jejunal epithelium. (○---○), 25 mg/kg 3 hourly × 4 ICRF-159 from −12 h; (●---●), 600 rad at t=0; (■---■), 25 mg/kg 3-hourly × 4 ICRF-159 from −12 hr +600 rad at t=0. Each point represents the mean d/min/mg±s.e. for 4 animals. Reproduced with permission from KOVACS et al., Brit J Cancer 39:524–530, 1979

to maximize tumor cell kill and minimize normal tissue damage has been somewhat elusive. For this reason a "Conference on Combined Modalities: Chemotherapy/Radiotherapy" was organized in 1978 to collate available information from both clinical and preclinical studies and to firmly establish the nature of the problem and to update the state of the art. The reader is referred to a published summary of the discussions resulting from this conference (PHILIPS, 1979); only a brief consideration of selected reports will be presented here to clarify and identify problems and advances with the overall strategy.

One of the major problems confronted in these studies involves interpretation of the response of tumors (or tumor cells) following radiation/drug combination. When two agents, each with their own effect, are combined a number of possibilities

for the combined effect exists: an enhanced effect, a status-quo, or a reduced effect. Each of these effects are possible as a direct result of the interaction between two therapeutic agents. "Status-quo" is of little consequence to the oncologist. "Reduced effect" will be considered later under the topic of radioprotection. "Enhancement", however, is the obvious goal desired for an improved management of neoplastic disease. Simplistically, the minimum response expected when two agents, each with their own effect, are combined should be equal to the sum of the two effects. Ideally, to establish this "additivity" of effects, both treatments (drug and radiation) must be considered basic treatments and each serve as a control arm of a 3-arm study; (1) drug alone, (2) radiation alone (3) drug + radiation. While this three-arm study is difficult to justify in the clinic if there is reasonable evidence that the combined agent arm will result in increased 5-year survivals, it is appropriate and easily carried out in the laboratory.

In general, the term "enhancement" has been applied to combined mode studies where the net response from drug + radiation studies is greater than the radiation effect alone. "Additivity" has been applied to a net response equivalent to the sum of the drug response and the radiation response. Theoretically, optimal sequencing was reserved for a net response that was in excess of that expected from the sum of the drug and radiation responses. The term synergism or synergistic response, has been freely applied to experimental conditions approaching additivity or in excess of additivity with little consideration of the magnitude. For these reasons, STEEL (1979) has proposed a system of terms to be adopted universally to classify response. These terms, based on isobolograms of experimental data, classify responses as supra-additive or sub-additive not only by type but also on the strength of the experimental data. This consideration of drug/radiation response is well worth the time for both the experimentalist and the oncologist.

A survey of the literature since 1970 unequivocally demonstrates that the response of experimental tumors in rodents to combination radiation/drug treatment is as specific and individual as that observed with human tumors. This is also true if one closely examines the response of individual tumors from a supposedly homogeneous tumor line to a chemotherapeutic agent (LOONEY, W.B., personal communication). To illustrate this point, let us consider the response of a variety of experimental tumors following treatment with cyclophosphamide (CY) and radiation, a combination used extensively for the clinical management of lung disease. TWENTYMAN et al. (1979b) has reported that for three tumor systems, RIF-1, EMT6 and KHT, using a drug dose of 100 mg/kg and a radiation dose of 1,200 R, only the RIF-1 tumor demonstrates a response which tends to be in excess of additivity of the two agents. For intertreatment intervals of drug from (−) 24 hr to (+) 24 hr, pre- and post-irradiation, no consistent dependence upon timing between irradiation and drug administration is observed from system to system. BEGG et al. (1979), using the EMT6/SF tumor has reported apparent "potentiation" of response at minimum doses of 120 mg/kg CY and 800 R and suggests that a marked dose dependence exists for combined mode potentiation of

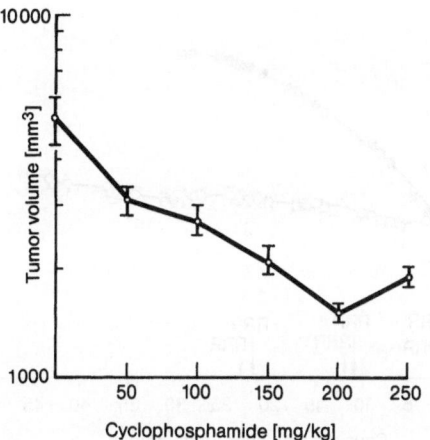

Fig. 4. Mean tumor volume ± standard error for the mean for day 9 after treatment with 50–250 mg/kg of cyclophosphamide. Reproduced with permission from LOONEY et al., Int J Radiat Oncol Biol Phys 5:1461–1465, 1979

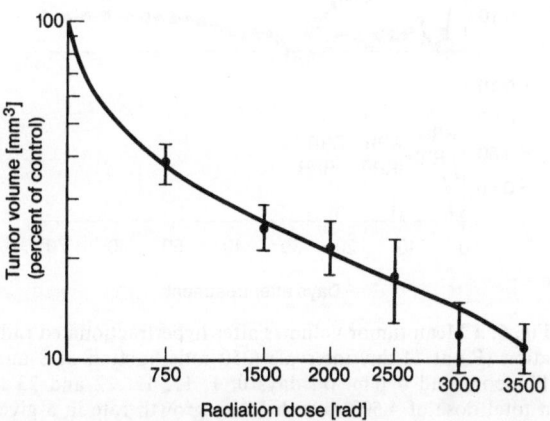

Fig. 5. Mean tumor volume ± standard error of the mean for day 7 after treatment with 750–3,500 R of local tumor irradiation. Reproduced with permission from LOONEY et al., Int J Radiat Oncol Biol Phys 5:1461–1465, 1979

response in this tumor. LOONEY et al. (1979) have also evaluated the dose response of the H-4-II-E tumor to both CY and radiation. The results of this study reproduced in figures 4 and 5 suggest that increasing the CY dose beyond a certain level (150 mg/kg) fails to result in a therapeutic benefit while increasing mortality and morbidity. Furthermore, incremental increases in local tumor radiation doses beyond 2,500 R are less effective than that observed at lower doses and enhance the potential for host toxicity. From the same laboratory HOPKINS et al. (1979), using similar dose levels, but with the 3924A Morris hepatoma, demonstrated that "therapeutic enhancement" results

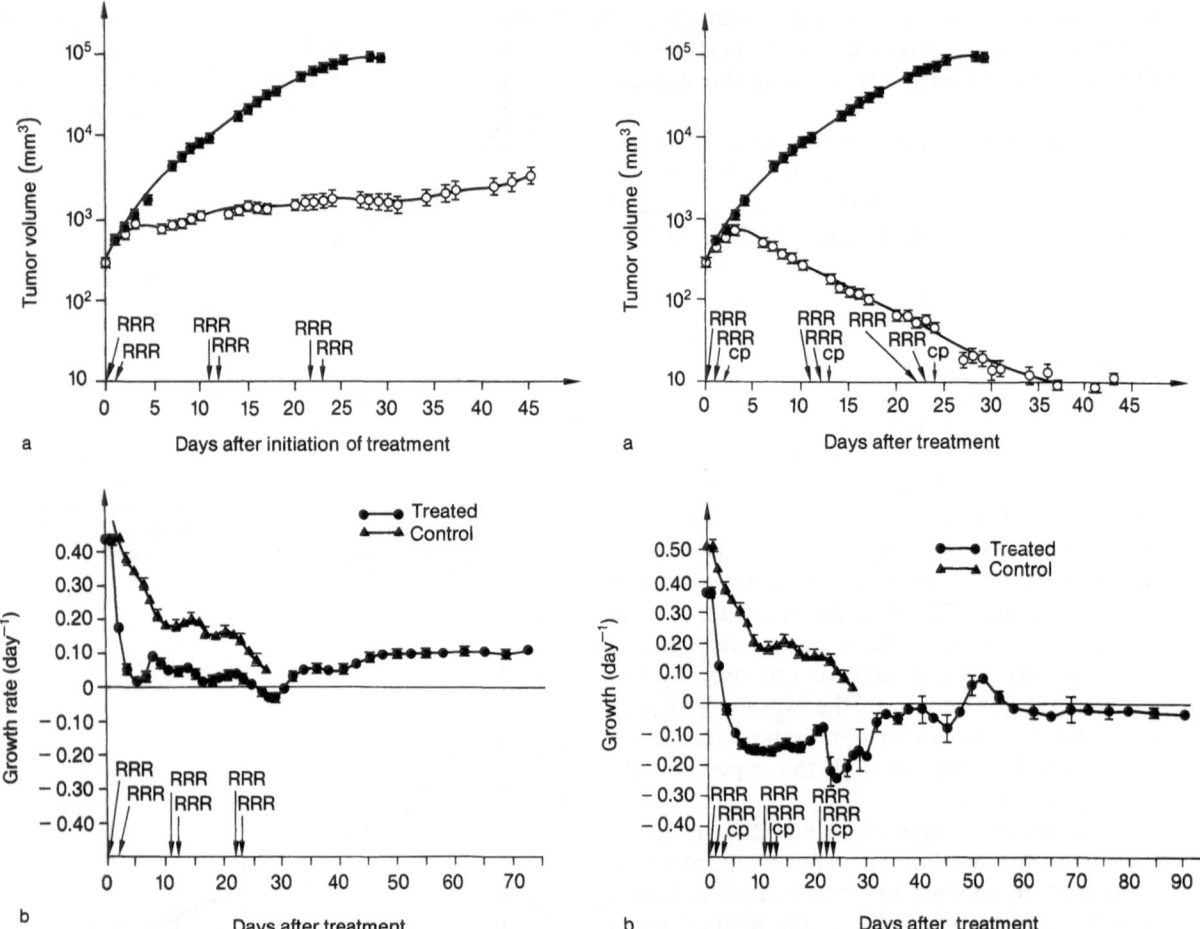

Fig. 6. a Mean tumor volumes after hyperfractionated radiation (R) at 11-day intervals (250 rads/fraction at 8 a.m, 12 noon, and 4 p.m. on days 0, 1, 11, 12, 22 and 23 to a total dose of 4,500 rads. **b** Mean growth rate in **a** given hyperfractionated radiation (R) at 11-day intervals. Bars, S.E. Reproduced from LOONEY et al., Cancer Res, 43:60–67, 1982

Fig. 7. a Mean tumor volumes after combining cyclophosphamide (cp) and hyperfractionated radiation (R) at 11-day intervals (250 rads/fraction at 8 a.m., 12 noon, and 4 p.m. on days 0, 1, 11, 12, 22, and 23, to a total dose of 4,500 rads; cyclophosphamide, 150 mg/kg on days 2, 13 and 24). **b** mean growth rate for tumors in **a** given combined cyclophosphamide (cp) and hyperfractionated radiation (R) at 11-day intervals. Bars, S.E. Reproduced with permission from LOONEY et al., Cancer Res 43:60–67, 1982

when the intertreatment interval between 1,500 R and 150 mg/kg CY is 7-days. No evidence for "potentiation" of response was observed with the 3924A tumor which agreed with the report by STEEL et al. (1978) using the Lewis lung carcinoma. Continuing studies with the 3924A tumor suggested that alternate scheduling of radiotherapy with chemotherapy every 7 days results in a cure rate of 60%; 1,500 R was given 7-days prior to a dose of 150 mg/kg CY and the sequence repeated three times (LOONEY and HOPKINS, 1982). More recently, they have reported on the use of hyperfractionated split-course radiation schedules in combination with CY (LOONEY et al., 1983). A hyperfractionated radiation schedule (250 R × 6) giv-

en 3 times a day for two consecutive days and repeated at 7-day intervals to a total dose of 9,000 R (Fig. 6) results in no tumor cures. The time for tumors to reach 8 times their initial volume $(8 \times V_o)$ was 147 ± 13 days. If the interval between schedules was increased to 11 days, with a total radiation dose of 4,500 R, the 8 V_o was 38.2 ± 3.48. When a 150 mg/kg dose of CY was added 24 hr after each hyperfractionation course (Fig. 7), a continuous decrease in tumor volume, both during and after the 23-day treatment interval was observed. Ultimately, this schedule resulted in a 60% cure rate with median survival of all animals in excess of 384 days as opposed to 73 days for the radiation course alone. Earlier, SCHENKEN et al.

(1976) had observed that while CY in combination with a 600 R dose (days 7, 14, 21) and 400 R dose (days 9, 17 and 24) of x-radiation to the P815X2 mastocytoma had resulted in "better local tumor control", the improved tumor response was accompanied by a dose-dependent increase in radiosensitivity of the gastrointestinal mucosa included in the radiotherapy field.

Normal tissue evaluations, accompanying the hyperfractionation studies of LOONEY et al. (1983), suggested that skin reactions were reduced as the size of the fraction was reduced, and that the addition of CY to the protocol had little effect on these observations. It is not clear whether the results on skin reaction under these conditions will be universally carried over to other dose-limiting normal tissues. Certainly, anyone even remotely involved in either the clinical or experimental area of therapeutics is well aware of the developing proscriptive and prescriptive basis for scheduling based on normal tissue response. In general, it is apparent from available data that normal tissues are more likely to be damaged by combined radiotherapy-chemotherapy. However, the effect of treatment(s) on normal tissues is, and continues to be, better understood than the effect of identical treatment on tumors. Whether this represents a poor selection of the experimental tumors for use in studies aimed toward clinical correlation, or in fact is an inherent ineffectual approach to the treatment of human tumors, is as yet unknown. Nonetheless, the use of chemotherapeutic agents, whether alone or in combination with radiation, appears to present an urgent problem in the clinic; a problem which is more readily solved in the laboratory.

For this reason, the entire concept of combined radiation-chemotherapy effects on normal tissue will not be considered here. Rather, it will appear in the following sections where its emphasis in the treatment arena will be firmly established.

3 Kinetic-Based Therapeutics

Most chemotherapeutic agents were originally recognized as potentially useful drugs for the treatment of cancer because they either interrupted a specific phase of the cell cycle (e.g. hydroxyurea – S phase drug), or were more sensitive to dividing cells than to resting cells. Similar statements could be made for the effects of radiation. That cell kinetics should play a major role in developmental and experimental therapeutics, therefore, is not

surprising. Ideally, it was anticipated that tumor cell kinetics would be markedly different from those of proliferation normal tissues, permitting the rational use of specific agents to result in an enhanced therapeutic ratio. The use of kinetically-based therapy in the clinic has relied on data from preclinical "mouse" studies, where clinical treatment scheduling was a direct extrapolation from "mouse" to "man". While the results of these clinical studies have been less than exciting, and cell kinetics at least academically disclaimed, the use of cell kinetic analysis has been a major tool for establishing schedules that avoid significant normal tissue toxicity. For this reason, the discussion of kinetically-directed therapy to follow will consider tumors separately from normal tissue.

3.1 Predictive Experimental Modeling of Tumors

As early as the 1960's experimental tumors were enthusiastically being explored as potential tools for defining "optimal therapeutic schedules" for the clinician. Inasmuch as rodents have long been known to be a good source for spontaneously-arising neoplasms, there has never been a shortage of "experimental tumors". Unexpected, however, was the observation that tumor cell kinetics for each of the experimental tumors appeared to have little in common with pre-existing laws regulating cell growth and application of classical kinetic methodology; to explain neoplastic growth required the *de novo* establishment of new concepts by LAIRD (1969), MENDELSOHN (1960a, 1960b, 1962) and STEEL (1968) to fully define the proliferative aspects of neoplastic growth. Each tumor was then analyzed to determine the characteristics of the cell proliferative cycle by PLM data would be a major parameter for the area of experimental therapeutics. While these studies resulted in a basic understanding of the laboratory tumor, the PLM curve failed to provide sufficient information or at least successfully achieve its anticipated goal. Today the PLM curve retains little of its former glory. In fact, only the vestigial tritiated thymidine (^{3}H-TdR) labelling index of the PLM remains as a potential tool for the management of cancers (TUBIANA and MALAISE, 1976; MEYER et al., 1978; MEYER and HIXON, 1979; MEYER, 1982).

This is not to say that the efforts of the tumor cell biologists have failed in their attempts to establish effective models for experimental therapeutics. The evolution of tumor models have established specific biological systems to answer specific, clinically relevant questions. More importantly, it has interrelated the parameters associated with tumor growth and while relatively simplistic, has produced a number of well-defined working models.

One of the major accomplishments achieved in tumor modeling has been the definition of a battery of diverse in vivo-in vitro tumor systems. A major goal for the experimentalist has always been the establishment of methods for quantitative assessment of tumor cell survival, a parameter only implied from cell kinetic and growth response data. These "in vivo-in vitro" models have provided opportunities for studies severely limited both technically and ethically in human tumors. ROCKWELL (1977) summarized the characteristics of these tumor systems and pointed out that all were rapidly growing anaplastic tumors carried in inbred rodents where the in vitro cell population doubling time and cell cycle time were generally shorter than in vivo times. While important information has been generated with these tumor systems, the plating efficiencies (ranging from 3–80%), and some of the in vitro methodology have led to inconsistent results and conclusions (TWENTYMAN 1977, 1979a).

As reviewed by DENEKAMP (1979), a number of important considerations should accompany the selection of an appropriate tumor model: (a) the cell of origin, (b) a history of its transplant maintenance, (c) the immunogenicity in its natural host, and (d) the site chosen for transplantation. In general, it would seem wise to select an experimental tumor that retained its primary characteristics for clinical applicability, as opposed to a tumor that markedly progressed (e.g. carcinomatous to sarcomatous) during routine maintenance in the laboratory, Unfortunately, spontaneously-arising tumors suffer from the same drawbacks found with human tumors for predictive modeling (e.g. diversity in histopathology, growth rate, and cell proliferation kinetics). This is also true for the primary tumors resulting from either viral or chemical induction, with the added disadvantage of enhanced artifactual antigenicity. Additional complications of viral-induced, "spontaneously" arising tumors will be discussed in a later section considering the concept of a "tumor stem cell".

More commonly, the experimentalist has concentrated on "in vivo tumor cell lines" which at best represent only a minimum number of transplants into syngeneic animals. Many of the most commonly adopted experimental tumor models, including those used for screening by the National Cancer Institute, have been carried in syngeneic hosts over long intervals (e.g. Lewis lung carcinoma, EMT6 tumor). These tumors, even with a high potential for transplant-induced artifactual immunogenicity, demonstrate a relative stability and uniformity of characteristics from tumor to tumor upon which predictive scheduling can be based. In addition, they provide large sampling sizes for statistical validation of response endpoints such as (a) regrowth delay, (b) local tumor control, (c) animal survival time, and (d) cell kinetic parameters. While all experimental tumor models suffer from some experimental artifact, and by far tumors of "spontaneous" origin and limited passage appear to be the most appropriate, the compromise solution to selecting a model, therefore, is to use a battery of tumors and draw generalities from their respective data.

Methodology in experimental tumor modeling has been relatively slow to evolve, perhaps due to the many set backs resulting from the inherent complexities (and diversities) of the tumor tissue. Kinetic-based predictions to date have been predicated on two characteristics of tumors; the growth response, and the cell kinetic response. The growth response is generally a series of sequential measurements of tumor size. For most experimental tumors, the volume generally approaches that of a hemiellipsoid (LOONEY et al., 1973) where measurements of the height, the width and the length in mm can be used to estimate the tumor volume by the equation $V = 0.5 \times (L \times W \times H)$. More recently, the group at Charlottesville has detailed a method for extracting information on tumor responses to single and combined modality treatment from growth curves. The concept, termed the overall treatment efficiency (OTE), is defined by three general classes of tumor volume response: Class I, Regression; Class II, Pseudoregression; Class III, Slowdown. DENEKAMP (1977) has reported that the degree of shrinkage within a period of fractionated irradiation is a useful prognostic guide to ultimate control of individual tumors. The rate of shrinkage of an individual tumor was not reflective of the number of cells killed, but rather on inherent characteristics of each individual tumor. For these reasons, and while somewhat premature, the concept of OTE may well be applicable to the clinical situation. For details the reader is referred to a treatise of OTE methodology by TREFIL et al. (1978).

The cell kinetic response of tumors has long held promise for predictive modeling of tumors (HELLMAN, 1975), in part due to our knowledge that proliferating cell sensitivity to radiation and drug treatment is markedly influenced by cell age. During treatment, there is a redistribution of cells throughout the cell cycle, a recruitment of non-proliferating cells into the cycle, and an expansion of the growth fraction, each playing a major role in the overall effectiveness of sequential treatment. This information is available in the literature for almost any drug and for almost every experimental tumor and has provided the substantiating basis for the mechanisms of antitumor agents defined in vitro. However, the experimental methods necessary for studies of this type do not lend themselves to clinical application, primarily due to the in vivo administration of isotopes and the long autoradiographic exposure times necessary for data collection. Nonetheless, therapy designs require an understanding of the inherent sensitivity of tumor cells and an application of the magnitude and temporal course of post-treatment recovery. Of particular interest for scheduling is a knowledge of the fluctuations in tumor growth fraction during sequential treatment. Over a number of years, BRAUNSCHWEIGER (BRAUNSCHWEIGER et al., 1976; BRAUNSCHWEIGER and SCHIFFER, 1978) and SCHIFFER (SCHIFFER et al., 1976), in a joint effort, have developed in vitro methods for determining cell kinetic parameters, including the growth fraction, that circumvent the impracticality associated with the classical methods. These in vitro assays have been demonstrated to represent responding indices to various chemotherapeutic agents with the cell kinetic perturbations designating optimal and suboptimal times for further treatment. More recently, BRAUNSCHWEIGER et al. (1979) have employed these in vitro assays to assess a number of radiotherapeutic protocols based on the cytodynamics of underlying intestinal tolerance response kinetics. They were able to conclude from their studies that the most effective schedules for local control and increased animal life span were those in which radiation fractions were given just prior to the initiation of observed proliferative recovery. The least effective schedules were those in which radiation fractions coincided with the time of maximal proliferative activity.

While predictive experimental modeling of experimental tumors has made some advances toward clinical applicability, the major criticisms that remain may very well reside in our own ignorance of the multiplicities of human tumor compartments, their in situ interactions, the stem cell concept, and the role of the host cell on the growth regulation of tumors in general.

4   Toxicity Configuration and Consequences

4.1   Acute Toxicity

As stated earlier, the consequences of more aggressive treatment with new "exotic" drugs and radiotherapy include the possibility of enhanced toxicity. Whether the acute phases of toxicity are life threatening is dependent on the organ specificity of the drug or its radiosensitivity. The response of organs to acute injury by noxious agents usually involves either functional deficiencies (e.g. renal tubular necrosis following the platinum compounds) or transient interruption of steady state cell production of rapidly, dividing tissues (e.g. intestinal epithelium, bone marrow). While function deficiencies may result by themselves, transient interruption of cell production usually leads to functional deficiencies as well. In most cases, the significance of these episodes of acute toxicity are dose dependent. That is, the magnitude and duration of toxicity is directly related to the dose of the agent. In general, however, acute toxicity at most sublethal doses is limited in time to approximately 30 days, depending on the tissue involved (Fig. 8). The $LD_{50/30}$ (50% lethality in 30 days) dose essentially defines the lethal toxicity limitations of the hematopoietic tissue and results from a significant depletion of the cellular elements of the peripheral blood. However, acute toxicity originates either from an irreversible or reversible event occurring much earlier in the hematopoietic compartment of the marrow. The marrow cells, representing a highly organized assemblage of cell hierarchies with different radio- and drug-sensitivities, are either temporarily inhibited from dividing or killed depending on the mechanism of action and/or dose of the toxic agent. In either case, the eventuating result is a function impairment of the red and the white blood cells in addition to those cells involved in the immune defense mechanism.

The $LD_{50/5}$ dose generally defines the lethal toxicity of the intestinal epithelium manifesting either significant crypt progenitor cell (stem cell) killing or prolonged periods of inhibition of crypt cell production. Both of these aspects of insult-recognition lead to a diminished production of

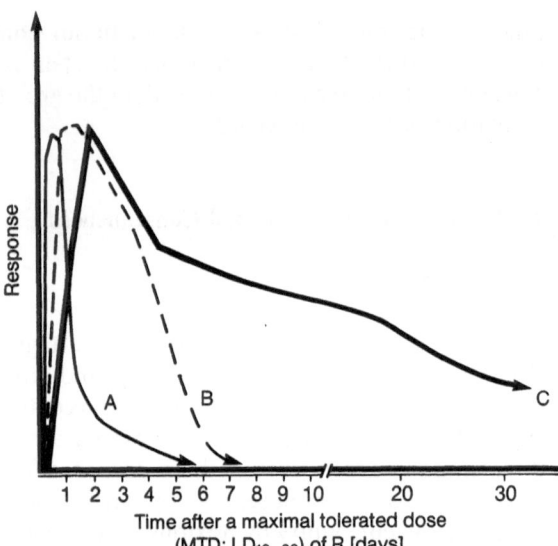

Fig. 8. The temporal response kinetics of (*A*) central nervous system. (*B*) gastrointestinal system, and (*C*) hematopoietic system at sublethal doses of toxic insult

cells, and therefore a diminished cell flux from the proliferative to the differentiated villus compartment. In either case, the end result is a functional impairment of villus (and therefore intestinal) absorptive and metabolic activity. Following acute intestinal damage, there is also evidence that cells produced during recovery, while serving as a villus barrier to invasion by infectious agents, fail to assume normal assimilation activity.

The $LD_{50/1}$ dose defines the lethal toxicity of the central nervous system (CNS) which is manifested by either cytologic damage in neurons and supporting mesenchymal tissues, or at lower doses, functional (biochemical) impairment.

4.2 Delayed Toxicity

Delayed toxicity is associated with the more static, less dynamic components of tissues and organs. While the damage may be realized immediately, expression of the damage to connective tissue, vascular or stromal elements may require periods following treatment where the organ fails to manifest toxicity. One major consequence of delayed toxicity is the response of connective tissue after irradiation and certain drugs. During the early inflammatory phase resulting from small blood vessel damage, an increase in interstitial colloid becomes the site of fibroblastic activity. Depending on dose, sclerotizing of tissue at a later time will severely compromise the function of both the self-renewing

as well as other organ tissues. This interstitial fibrosis, and the fibrosis of small blood vessels, constitutes a premature increase in the histohematic connective tissue barrier, a process that has been suggested to occur gradually during aging.

4.3 Residual Injury or Latent Toxicity

Chemotherapy, unlike radiotherapy, is a relatively new treatment modality and the potential for long-term effects to the cancer patient are not well documented. As experimental therapeutics generate more efficacious time/dose configurations for patient treatment, acute and delayed toxicities gradually diminish with concomitant extension of life for the treated patient. It is at this point that the importance of residual damage (residual injury, RI) resulting from treatment is magnified in comparison to acute and delayed damage. In all probability, clinicians will be forced to concentrate on the eventualities of treatment that are manifested long after "cures" have been achieved. The term "residual damage" refers to a prolonged perhaps permanent impairment of a tissue's function following exposure to either radio- or chemotherapy. Due to the limited considerations of the evolution of effective chemotherapeutics, and the "failures" of treatment, the long-term consequence of treatment has only been marginally imposed on the clinician. Nonetheless, RI has already been observed. For example, persistent bone marrow aplasias after alkylating agents (TRAINOR and MORLEY, 1976; MORLEY, 1980); pulmonary fibrosis after bleomycin (NYGARD et al., 1978); gastrointestinal complications after adriamycin (RANSON et al., 1979); and more recently renal failure after cisdichlorodiammine platinum (ANSAIR et al., 1980) have been reported. RI is presently undergoing extensive preclinical investigation in our laboratories (KOVACS et al., 1981, 1982) as well as in the laboratory of others (HELLMAN and BOTNICK, 1977; BOTNICK et al., 1979). The exact cause of this dysfunction is still unknown, but it has been postulated to result from a compromised ability of the body's cell renewal systems to mount a regenerative response to insult. In many cases, the homeostatic steady-state characteristics appear normal in RI compromised animals. However, when the animals are subjected to an insult of sufficient magnitude to require proliferative regeneration, the renewing systems fail.

Many tissues supporting the mammalian body can be regarded as cell renewal systems since they

Fig. 9a, b. Effect of AdR pretreatment on the jejunal response to 600 R. **a** BDF$_1$, non tumor-bearing mice; **b** BDF$_1$/LLca tumor-bearing mice. (0), 600 R for non-tumor-bearing mice; (●), 600 R for tumor-bearing mice; (■), 10 mg/kg AdR-$^{60\,d}$→600 R. Each point represents the mean ± standard error of the mean (S.E.M.) dpm/mg from 5 animals. The shaded area represents the mean (S.E.M.) intestinal proliferative activity in age and size matched tumor-bearing non-treated control animals. For comparison, the 600 R treated non-tumor-bearing mice data (0) has been produced in **b**. Reproduced with permission from Kovacs et al., Int J Radiat Oncol Biol Phys, 7:1389–1395, 1981

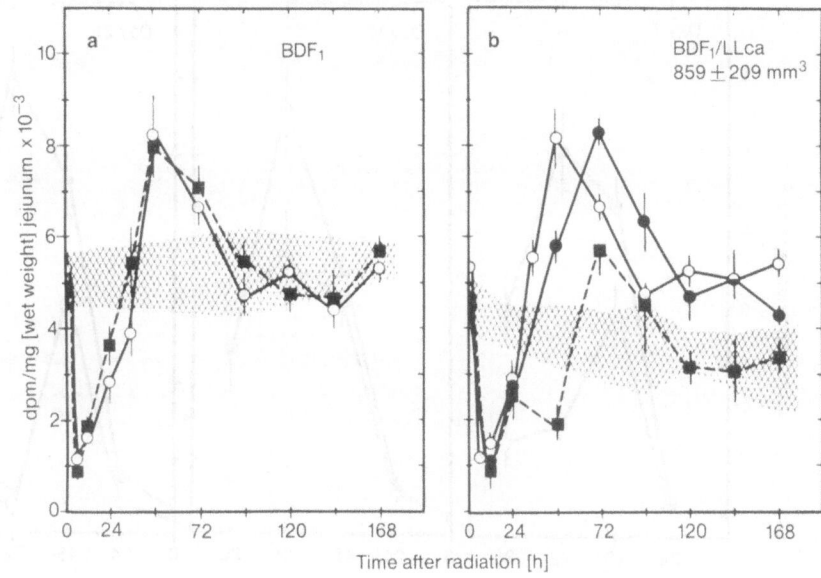

consist of a large population of mature end cells whose numbers are maintained by the proliferation and subsequent differentiation of a small reserve of stem cells. In general, two classes of renewal systems exist: the *active*, such as the gastrointestinal and bone marrow, and the *conditional*, exemplified by the liver or kidney. Normally, the failure of cell renewal systems is rarely a cause of death or disease even in the active self-renewal tissues, for the renewal potential of the stem cell far exceeds the life span of the individual. Exposure to radiation or chemotherapy, while permitting seemingly complete recovery of normal tissues, may cause sufficient depletion of the stem cells or damage to the microenvironment that will subsequently limit the proliferating capacity of the tissues. RI therefore, may be overt (as evidenced by a decreased number of differentiated end cells) or it may be manifested only by suboptimal recovery from a subsequent demonstrable stress.

Of these two possibilities, the latter will eventually be a major concern to the clinician who is either using adjuvant chemotherapy for extended periods following "cures" or is treating recurrent disease after a long period of apparent control. Under both these conditions, subsequent insult will be applied to normal tissues compromised by previous treatment. In modeling for these two situations in the laboratory, we have been made aware of the additional complexities of both primary recurrent disease on normal tissue compromise (discussed later) and the potential problems of RI. To illustrate these concepts we have examined the

radioresponse of the jejunal epithelium in animals pretreated 60 days earlier with a MTD of adriamycin (Fig. 9). The radiation dose (here representing a subsequent insult) selected for these studies (600 R) had been previously found to be insufficient to demonstrate RI in this strain of mouse (Fig. 9a), although at a higher dose (1,000 R), RI was well-documented (Schenken et al., 1979). Fourteen days prior to radiation (46 days after AdR), the Lewis lung carcinoma was implanted on the backs of an experimental group of animals. These date (Fig. 9b) demonstrate the enhanced radiosensitivity of AdR-pretreated mice with simulated recurrent disease and point out the "problem areas" that can be generated in the clinic during a comprehensive treatment protocol involving a drug resulting in RI. Similar data are available for another active self-renewal system, the hematopoietic system.

In addition, examples of RI in conditional self-renewal tissues are also available (Fig. 10a, b). The proliferative reserve capacity of the renal tubule epithelium is assessed by evaluating tritiated thymidine (^{3}H-TdR) uptake following folic acid (FA) – induced tubular necrosis. Following treatment with cis-dichlorodiamine platinum-II (DDP), the proliferative renal response to FA was subnormal. While proliferative reserve appeared to recover between days 7–14, thereafter, a progressive decrease in compensatory proliferative response to FA was observed (day 14-day 45). This limitation on proliferative potential continued through 120 days (Table 1) where the reserve capacity of the renal

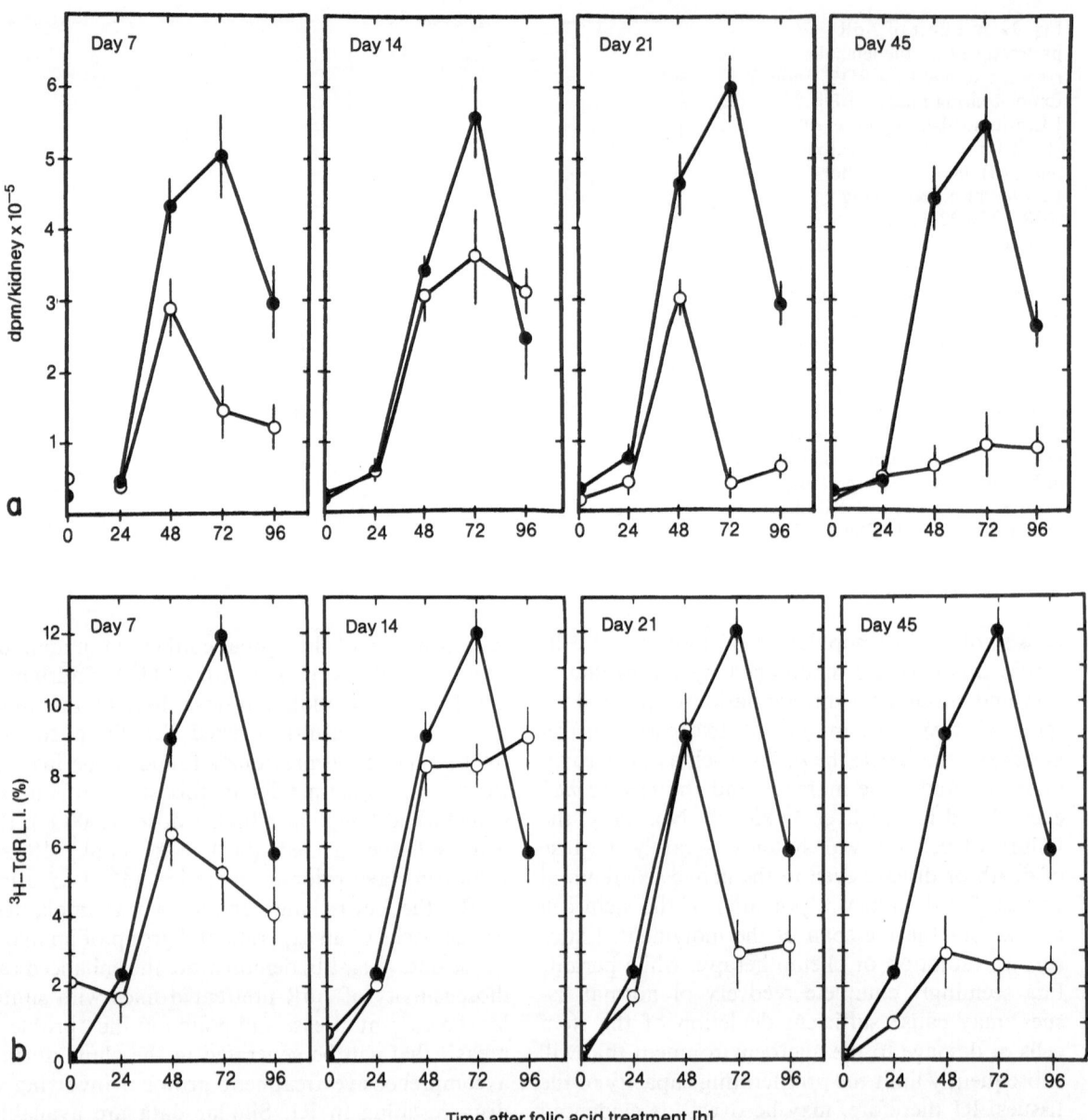

Fig. 10a, b. Response of renal tubular epithelium to folic acid (FA) as a function of time after DDP treatment. **a** ³H-TdR uptake in the kidney after 100 mg/kg FA. **b** renal tubular epithelial cell proliferation (³H-TdR labeling index) following 100 mg/kg FA. (●) untreated animals; (○), animals treated with 8 mg/kg DDP on day 0. Each point represents the mean ± s.e. for 5 animals. Reproduced with permission from Kovacs et al., Brit J Cancer 45:286–294, 1982

tubular epithelium remained severely compromised (a response deficit of 54%). Renal RI resulting from AdR treatment was by far the most severe. Daunomycin-induced RI, on the other hand, was less than either DDP or Adr. However, pathological and physiological assessment of renal damage suggested that the effect of the drugs on renal histology and function was repaired by day 14.

In the future, a rational use of cytotoxic drugs in combination with other drugs and/or radiation will necessarily require an understanding of both their *acute*, *delayed* and *residual* toxicities. At present, documentation of clinical RI is not extensive, and those reports available are seldom comprehensive in their scope. With increased "cures" and five-year survivals resulting from more effective treatment protocols, the concept of residual toxicity will assume a more critical position in considerations of treatment management.

Table 1. Relative renal proliferative response to folic acid in mice pretreated (–120 days) with DNM, AdR and DDP

	Maximum LI[a] / Pre-stress LI	Relative response (% of control)	Integrated cell production (%) (area pretreated/area control)		
			LI[b]	dpm/kidney[c]	RRI[d]
DNM	101	70.6	72.6	77.5	24.8
AdR	46	32.2	29.5	29.5	70.4
DDP	62	43.4	52.8	52.8	54.3
Control	143	100.0	100.0	100.0	0.0

[a] Maximum LI seen at 36 hr for DNM, DDP and control and at 72 hr for AdR.
[b,c] Ratio of area under response curve for pretreated and control expressed in %.
[d] Reproduced with permission from BRAUNSCHWEIGER et al. (1982) Brit J Cancer 45:421–428.

5 Sequencing for Simultaneous Cell Protection and Cell Kill

A major, ongoing emphasis on radiosensitization of tumor cells and, in particular, the hypoxic fraction has had its basis in the biophysical and biochemical characteristics of these cells and in compounds known to be oxygen mimetic. The major radiosensitizer prototype has been misonidazole (Ro 07-0582), a member of the nitroimidozole class of compounds that has demonstrated enhancement ratios (ER) ranging from 1.2–2.1 in experimental systems. Clinically, the overall results with Ro 07-0582 have been inconclusive and, in general, disappointing due both to the failure to achieve consistently high ER's and to toxicity limitations. More recently, experimental programs have been designed to minimize the effects of radiation toxicity on normal tissues. One of the areas of this program has been the investigation of radioprotective drugs with a basis in either tissue selectivity, intercellular thiols or failure to sensitize hypoxic cells. The prototype compound, amino prophylamino-ethylphosphorothioic acid (WR-2721) has also resulted in inconclusive results due primarily to its failure to protect the central nervous system and its increased toxicity with multiple doses. In addition, evidence has accumulated that the selectivity of WR-2721 may not be absolute for normal tissues. Conceptually therefore, radiotherapy is searching for compounds that could advance its effectiveness either by enhancing the radiosensitivity of tumors or by protecting normal tissues from radiation toxicity.

There has been a renewed interest in the effect of cell age distributions as a means of protecting normal tissues. As far back as 1906, the "law"

of BERGONIE and TRIBONDEAU (1906) suggested that radiosensitivity varies (a) directly with the rate of cell proliferation, (b) directly with the number of morphologic and functional differentiation. Since that time, precise method for synchronizing cells in specific phases of the cell cycle have been used to demonstrate the effects of radiation on the cell cycle and its phases both in vitro and, in more limited studies, in vivo. These studies led to a major experimental program designed to establish time/dose schedules for enhanced radiotherapeutic effectiveness when combined with drugs on a cell kinetic basis. The voluminous reports resulting from these studies suggest strongly that applicability of these data to the clinic is more predictive for normal tissues than for neoplastic tissues. Nonetheless, several useful combined mode schedules are available for effective treatment of specific tumor types stemming from these preclinical studies.

In addition, a new direction has been defined based on the combined modality studies of the "70's" suggesting that effective time/dose configurations for combining radiation and certain drugs may also lead to a sparing effect for radiation toxicity in normal tissues, while still maintaining their antitumor effect. Unlike the radiosensitizer/protector program, several laboratories have undertaken the preclinical task of investigating the selection and sequencing of dose levels of radiation and drug treatment regimens that will permit the clinician more freedom to aggressively attack neoplastic tissue, especially those tumors in juxtaposition to, or contiguous with the major dose-limiting hematopoietic and intestinal epithelial tissues.

As far back as the late 1950's, treatment with a wide variety of compounds, some of which themselves are cytotoxic, have been shown to protect against an otherwise lethal dose of radiation. With the advent of the hematopoietic stem cell (BRADLEY and METCALF, 1966; PLUZNIK and SACHS, 1965) and intestinal cryptogenic colony (WITHERS and ELKIND, 1968) assays, the evidence for drug-induced modification of radiosensivity has been confirmed and several mechanisms postulated. The obvious mechanism would be a kinetically-directed induction of age-related radioresistance to the stem cells. However, recent reports on the effect of several drugs on the hematopoietic and intestinal epithelium strongly suggest that the mechanism of action somehow involves an earlier recovery from radiation damage. That cytotoxic agents with a wide variety of chemical properties and modes of action exhibit radioprotection further suggests that a universal biological mechanism, rather than biophysical or biochemical mechanism, is operative.

Of these radioprotecting drugs, the most actively studied have been the mitotic inhibitors vinblastine (VbL) and vincristine (VcR) and cytosine arabinoside (Ara-C). These drugs have been found to afford radioprotection to both the hematopoietic system and the intestinal epithelium of rodents (SMITH et al., 1968; MILLAR et al., 1978; PHELPS and BLACKETT, 1979; HIREOKA et al., 1982), while other drugs (e.g. busulphan and merophan) and radiation itself (doses of 75–150 R) failed to protect against subsequent radiation (lethal dose of 1,000 R). In both biological systems, the major difference observed between drug-pretreated and radiation alone-treated animals was the more rapid onset of proliferative recovery. This enhanced recovery appeared due to the reduction (or elimination) of the post-irradiation lag phase seen in animals receiving radiation alone. Results from these laboratories and from BURHOLT (BURHOLT, D.R., unpublished observation) have demonstrated that following treatment with VcR, lethally-damaged intestinal crypt cells lyse rapidly in situ, causing a more rapid fall in villus height and, therefore, a more rapid entry of cryptogenic cells into proliferation. MILLAR et al. (1982) has suggested that rapid marrow cell lysis may also be responsible for hematopoietic radioprotection. Using the hematopoietic stem cell assay, they have explained drug-induced radioprotection by postulating a two compartment model; one subpopulation (55% of total) having a high self-renewal capability but enhanced radiosensivity, the other a lower self-renewal capacity and radiosensivity. After high dose radiation alone, these two subpo-

pulations are depleted disproportionately (a higher fraction of the high self-renewal cells are destroyed). Drug pretreatment temporarily alters the radiosensivity of this population, increasing it to that of the other subpopulation. Hence, high dose radiation does not selectively kill a greater proportion of the high self-renewal subpopulations of stem cells and thereby advances recovery of this population.

Whether the postulated mechanism will eventually prove satisfactory for explaining the observed radioprotecting nature of these drug is presently unknown. What is obvious is the fact that the mechanism is a complex, biological phenomena involving altered kinetics of proliferative recovery. That this early initiation of recovery results in radioprotection can be best understood by an analysis of the crypt survival of irradiated intestinal tissue. As a general rule, animal survival following intestinal insult is determined by the amount of crypt attrition. Crypt attrition (survival) is generally measured 96 hr post irradiation, a time interval found satisfactory to allow even the most damaged crypts to be well on their way to be repopulated (HAGEMANN and LESHER, 1971; BOARDER and BLACKETT, 1976). It is generally accepted that no drug alone can reduce the cryptogenic "stem" cells to a level that prevents repopulation and crypt survival, and that drugs can only augment (and now protect) and damage resulting from irradiation. That VcR pretreatment provides radioprotection by inducing a more rapid recovery of radiation insult, which eventually leads to less crypt kill, can be seen in Table 2. The magnitude of protection is markedly affected by the radiation dose and is most evident at acute doses $\geq LD_{100/5}$. At present, the maximum radiation dose that can be effectively protected against has not been established. However, information is available for dose ranges with clinical relevance. In addition, these drugs having "radioprotective activity" have also been found to protect against drug toxicity, and it is believed that similar (if not identical) mechanisms are operative.

Whether these radioprotecting drugs will be of significant clinical importance will depend on several factors. First, are the mechanisms similar in mouse and man? Second, if the mechanisms are similar can drug-induced "protection" be provided if the drug is administered only prior to the first dose in a sequence of radiation exposures? And finally, if drug pretreatment must precede each radiation exposure to result in "protection", will a prolonged sequence of these drug/radiation

Table 2. Effect of combined VcR[a] and radiation on intestinal crypt cell survival[b]

Treatment	Crypts per circumference[c]	Percent control
Control	149.37±2.19	100.00
600 R	150.27±3.84	100.60± 2.34
VcR	149.90±1.86	100.02± 0.94
VcR + 600 R	117.05±2.74	78.36± 3.21
VcR → 24 hr → 600 R	148.94±2.58	99.72± 4.21
1,000 R	99.02±2.67	66.28±13.40
VcR + 1,000 R	90.95±2.46	60.89± 2.13
VcR → 24 hr → 1,000 R	126.00±3.39	84.35± 2.27
1,600 R	13.44±4.32	9.27± 6.31
600 R → 24 hr → 1,000 R	85.35±5.18	57.14± 2.01
VcR + 1,600	($>LD_{100/4}$)	($>LD_{100/4}$)
VcR + 600 R → 24 hr → 1,000 R	75.90±1.37	50.81± 1.91
VcR → 24 hr → 600 R → 24 hr	119.30±4.24	79.87± 1.86

[a] VcR administered i.p. at a dose of 1 mg/kg body weight
[b] Each value represents the mean (±S.E.M.) of 20 cross-sections per animal from a group of 4–5 animals
[c] C.J. Kovacs, unpublished data

schedules result in an accumulation of toxicity reducing any accompanying protection from being of clinical value. Certainly, this subject warrants further preclinical experimentation to establish: (a) the mechanism of action, (b) whether these drugs can reduce delayed or residual toxicity, and (c) what magnitude can their "protection" achieve. For the present, however, it is not premature to initiate studies to determine if the sequencing of established "radioprotecting" drugs are of clinical value to the radiotherapist, especially under high dose/fraction radiation conditions.

6 New Markers for Optimal Treatment Sequencing

Clinical experience over the years has generated sufficient information and impressions strongly recommending a need for efficient methods to monitor and predict therapeutic sequencing, both prior to treatment when selection of treatment modalities occurs and also during the actual treatment period. While the information is not readily available, it is generally known that significant numbers of patients entered into defined protocols are either delayed in the sequencing at some point of the protocol, or removed and reentered into other protocols with different agents after their apparent failures are noted. Two major reasons exist for

these recommendations, although numerous others may also be of significance; (1) the diverse sensitivities of tumors in general to specific therapeutic agents (even between tumors of the same cell of origin, histological grade, and prognostic characteristics), and (2) the inherent differences in the magnitude of toxicity realized by individuals to the same therapeutic agent.

Preclinical studies of therapeutic response using tumor cell lines, many of them maintained as clones and carried in inbred animal hosts, have also demonstrated inherent variability, albeit significantly less than that observed for patients. Even under these experimentally controlled conditions, very often data that on the surface appears uniform, must be analyzed by statistical methods before conclusions can be drawn. It is not surprising, therefore, that response patterns in groups of patients under protocol where individuality is markedly expressed cannot be implied at the very best, if at all. Furthermore, multiparametric assays are needed to interpret preclinical tumor responses, and quantitative assessment must also include a consideration of tumor type and size in addition to host physiology, immunology and age. No one end point alone has been found to be completely satisfactory, short of animal survival. Tumor response is best defined by a composite of end points including the tumor regrowth delay (TRD) and TCD_{50} (50% tumor cure dose) assays and the clonogenic cell survival assay. The TRD and TCD_{50} assays can be estimated during closely monitored patient follow-up. The clonogenic tumor cell survival, however, was not available to the clinician until recently due to technical and ethical limitations and will be discussed in detail below.

In addition to monitoring the tumor response, non-invasive methods are needed to determine the magnitude of toxicity associated with specific treatment protocols. More specifically, the advent of more complex, aggressive treatment regimens with an enhanced concurrent potential for life threatening toxicity, must include a consideration of treatment tolerance. Of considerable importance to the clinician, therefore, is an understanding of the kinetics of insult-recognition as "proliferative" recovery as well as an accurate appraisal of the degree of normal tissue integrity. In general, the dose-limiting normal tissues for both radio- and chemotherapy are the hematopoietic organs and the intestinal epithelium. With a few exceptions, the target tissues for toxicity may include other organs in addition to the bone marrow and

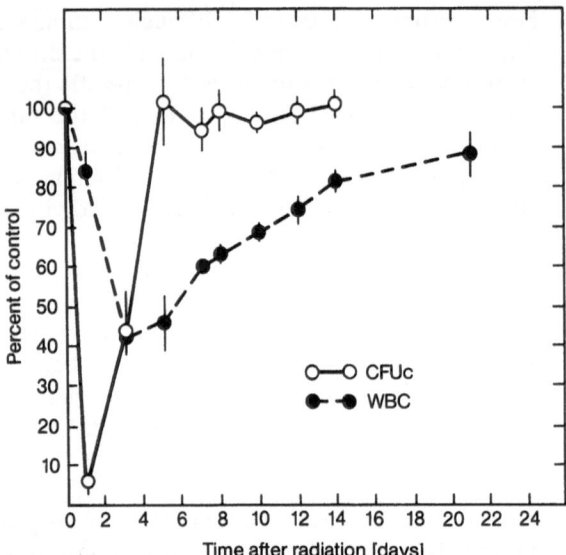

Fig. 11. A comparison of the response of the hematopoietic progenitor cell (CFUc-GM) content of the femoral marrow and the peripheral WBC counts of sequential sampling of New Zealand White rabbits. (R.M. Johnke, unpublished data)

gut. For example, cis-dichlorodiamine platinum and bleomycin, in addition to affecting the bone marrow and gut, are also known to affect renal and lung function respectively. However, many of these complications occurring in other organs are long-term effects and therefore the immediate concern of the clinician is the acute toxicities associated with the marrow and intestinal tissues.

While preclinical, experimental therapeutics established for inbred rodents can define mechanisms and suggest optimal treatment dose and time configurations; even the optimal times established in rodents differ from species to species, and from strain to strain. Treatment scheduling for individual patients, even those on protocols, have been routinely prescribed (or proscribed) by superficial symptomology at the least and by peripheral blood pictures at the best. In most cases, these indices of toxicity are significantly removed both in time and, in some instances, in space from those cells/tissues that are ultimately the discriminators of toxicity. Experimental evidence for rodents, for example, demonstrates conclusively that the insult-recognition and recovery curves for peripheral WBC are significantly delayed when compared to similar curves for the pluripotential (CFUs) and progenitor (CFUc) stem cells of the marrow (Fig. 11). Similar studies are available for intestinal toxicity (Lesher and Bauman, 1969; Rijke, 1980; Hanson et al., 1979). Therefore, markers re-

flecting the biological response of these two treatment-limiting organs to insult would significantly effect the optimal sequencing of effective tumoricidal agents under conditions that minimize the severity of their toxicity.

At present, three potentially important markers are being developed experimentally as guides for the clinician in treating individual patients. Two have demonstrated subjective value for patients, although any conclusions drawn would be premature. The third, in its developmental phase, also appears to be applicable to the patient. A summary of the data available and discussion of their mechanism and future experimental directions should clarify their "therapeutic marker" status.

6.1   Tumor Cell Sensitivity Assays

The idea of using an in vitro assay to determine resistance or sensitivity to drugs is not a new concept. The human tumor clone assay for drug sensitivity has its basis in the plating assay for bacteriological (antibacterial) sensitivity, an assay that has been used successfully by the clinician for many years. The major difference between the two assays, a difference of great consequence, is the cultural requirements of mammalian cells. Tissue culture techniques per se are not new to cancer research, and there has been continued development of new culture techniques and media as well as knowledge regarding the effects of hormones as growth factors on normal and neoplastic cells. As will be discussed later, optimal conditions for all tumor cells have not be established.

The cloning of cells in agar cultures and on plastic has been used for a number of transplantable tumors and tissue culture cell lines (Rockwell, 1977). In addition, methods for clonal assay of hematopoietic progenitor cells have received significant attention, and, at present, is contributing greatly to the definition of the interrelationship of hematopoietic proliferation and differentiation. These two experimental methods have served as the technical framework for quantitation of tumor clonogenic cells and the identification of a controversial "tumor stem cell".

The concept of using clonal assays for identifying human tumor cell sensitivity was first introduced by Bruce et al. (1966, 1969) and others at the Ontario Cancer Institute using mouse lymphoma and myeloma cells. While the cells identified retained the ability to repopulate lethally irradiated recipient animals and, thereby, satisfied one characteristic of the definition of "stem cell", other characteristics related to multipotential differentiation were not addressed. More recently, reports demonstrating prolonged passage of human tumor cells (in vitro and in vivo) have suggested that these cells represent the tumor "stem cells" due to their "infinite" proliferative potential (PAVELIC et al., 1980; CARVEY et al., 1981). By definition, a transformed cell is one that has lost the limited population doubling number associated with normal cells (HAYFLICK, 1965). Therefore, while one criterion of the stem cell has been satisfied, presently the absolute identification of the clonogenic cells of a tumor as the "stem cell" remains incomplete. For these reasons, the term "clonogenic" will be used during the discussions that follow.

During the 1970's SALMON and his group (SALMON and SMITH, 1970; DURIE and SALMON, 1975) reported the development of techniques to quantitate the tumor burden of myeloma patients in vitro. The development of a clonogenic assay for drug sensitivity in myeloma patients followed using techniques comparable to, but requiring environmental culture conditions, those used in the murine myeloma assay system. HAMBURGER (1977) following the work of PARK et al. (1971), first reported the use of mineral oil primed spleen cells (macrophage) of the mouse as a stimulus necessary for quantitative linear growth of the myeloma clonogenic cells in vitro. SALMON (1980a) has reported that this system facilitates the growth of a variety of human tumors and that approximately 70% of all tumors plated under these conditions exhibited colony formation. However, over 50% of these tumors colonized with a cloning efficiency too low for drug sensitivity studies. Since these early reports, many laboratories worldwide have initiated programs attempting to use the human tumor clone assay for clinical predictability (KIMBALL et al., 1978; BRODSKAYA et al., 1981; FRIEDMAN et al., 1981; LABOISSE et al., 1981; SMITH et al., 1981). Fortunately, most of these laboratories have also been interested in developing optimal conditions for the colonization of cells from specific tumor types. This interest may stem from the disappointing growth of clonogenic cells from many tumors and, where growth has occurred, a disappointing plating efficiency. Presently, it appears that no one method will satisfy the requisite growth conditions of all tumor types. Factors influencing the growth of clonogenic cells from different tumors include pH, basic media composi-

tion, oxygen tension and specific growth factors (HILL et al., 1981; ROWBOTTOM et al., 1981; LARSEN and THORLING 1969; RODARO et al., 1980; HUG et al., 1983).

In our laboratories, we have returned to examining the effects of conditions for hematopoietic colony formation on tumor cell clonogenicity. Our initial studies have utilized the mouse mammary tumor (MMT) arising spontaneously in the female C3H/He MMTV+ retired breeder mouse (EMMA et al., 1981). Studies have emphasized (a) media components, (b) matrix, and (c) stimulators for optimal anchorage-independent growth of the clonogenic cells of the tumor (Table 3). In general, all media tested appeared to support tumor colonization equally well, with CMRL or McCoy's 5A media slightly better than others. In all cases, methylcellulose (0.8–2.1%) was far superior to agar as a supportive matrix, as was the inclusion of the components used routinely for hematopoietic colony forming granulocyte-macrophage cultures (CFUc-GM). Growth stimuli, prepared as feeder layers, demonstrated enhanced activity in the following order: no feeder < human lung fibroblast cells < colony-stimulating activity (CSA) < spleen cell conditioned media < burst-promoting activity (BPA). Preparation of single cell suspensions by a tri-enzyme cocktail (0.05% pronase – 0.02% collagenase + 0.02% DNAse I) was far superior to physical mincing.

Obviously BPA, a product of pokeweed mitogen-stimulated spleen T-lymphocytes, has consistently improved both the number of tumors capable of colony formation in vitro as well as their individual plating efficiency. Although preliminary (due to sample size), similar observations have been made for human tumors (Table 4). BPA, a growth factor postulated to trigger a commitment to differentiate by the pluripotential hematopoietic stem cell (colony forming unit spleen; CFUs), also stimulates the subsequent cell (BFU; burst-forming unit) in the hematopoietic hierarchy to divide. While premature, it is exciting to speculate that BPA is a universal growth stimulator of immature or undifferentiated cells, and is involved in the regulation of cell proliferation of both normal and neoplastic cells. We will address this possibility in a later section.

Of equal or even more interest is the marked difference observed between the clonogenic fraction of the spontaneous MMT and its transplant generations. It has been generally accepted that if indeed a tumor "stem cell" exists, it can be recognized by its ability to form anchorage-inde-

Table 3. The effect of overnight incubation with 10% burst promoting activity conditioned medium on the clonogenicity of spontaneous and transplanted mouse mammary tumors *

Feeder	Treatment			
	Transplanted		Spontaneous	
	24 hr T.C.M.[a]	24 hr 10% BPA[b]	24 hr T.C.M.	24 hr BPA
NCM[c]	324.00 ± 4.16[f]	439.67 ± 4.33	917.33 ± 39.75	$1,066.67 \pm 61.81$
S.H.[d]	274.67 ± 10.73	413.33 ± 50.67	$1,018.67 \pm 25.54$	$1,244.00 \pm 50.33$
CSA[e]	234.67 ± 6.36	354.67 ± 17.02	813.33 ± 53.33	881.33 ± 29.24
BPA	240.67 ± 16.18	456.00 ± 7.21	785.33 ± 30.49	$1,318.67 \pm 13.92$
LF[g]	297.33 ± 13.28	350.00 ± 31.79	776.00 ± 15.14	$1,245.33 \pm 56.39$

[a] McCoy's 5A & 10% fetal calf serum
[b] Burst promoting activity conditioned medium $-10\% + 10\%$ fetal calf serum McCoy's 5A
[c] No conditioned medium
[d] Spleen cell conditioned medium (SALMON, S.E., HAMBURGER, A: Science 197:461-463, 1977).
[e] Colony stimulating activity (CFU_{GM}) conditioned medium
[f] Mean & S.E./5×10^5 cells
[g] 1×10^5 Rabbit lung fibroblasts in 0.5% agar feeders
* Reproduced with permission from EMMA et al. (1985) Stem cells, in press

Table 4. The effect of BPA on the clonogenicity of human tumors

Sample	Tumor type	Cloning efficiencies ($\times 10^3$)		
		$(-)$ BPA	(% of control)[a]	$(+)$ BPA
BL	larynx	1.80 ± 0.01	(140)	2.52 ± 0.11
GC	colon	0.24 ± 0.02	(279)	0.67 ± 0.02
NE	liver	0.001 ± 0.002	(331)	0.31 ± 0.001
RA	colon	0.47 ± 0.029	(228)	1.07 ± 0.041
BR	pharynx	0.30 ± 0.017	(1626)	4.88 ± 0.150
GC	colon	0.01 ± 0.001	(300)	0.03 ± 0.001
BD	lung	0.43 ± 0.006	(199)	0.51 ± 0.007
RW	breast	0.029 ± 0.009	(162)	0.47 ± 0.008
MA	teratoma	0.105 ± 0.054	(1571)	1.650 ± 0.021
FF	breast	0.410 ± 0.007	(136)	0.557 ± 0.014
SM	breast	0.000 ± 0.00	$(-)$	0.027 ± 0.015
	$\bar{n}$	0.345 ± 0.047	489.20 ± 58.94	1.12 ± 0.13

[a] (% of Control) is the percent of colony formation in the absence of BPA.

pendent (AI) colonies in vitro. More recently, data from this laboratory and others (RHEINWALD and BECKETT, 1981; BRATTAIN et al., 1981; DEXTER et al., 1981) has accumulated suggesting that the concept of a tumor "stem cell" must include a number of subpopulations within a tumor unlike the stem cell reported for hematopoiesis. The clonogenic (AI) fraction of a well-differentiated spontaneous murine mammary (MMT) tumor decreases in parallel with increasing transplant generation (Table 5). Conversely, there is a simultaneous increase in anchorage-dependent (AD; colony growth by adherence to plastic) colony formation. Both AI and AD subpopulations are tumorigenic; the AD population have a reduced latent period before the appearance of tumors with a reduced tumor doubling time (Td). The Td for spontaneously arising and 1st generation transplants was 12.5 days while the growth rate for 18–25th generation transplants is reduced to 3–4 days. Accompanying these changes in clonogenic fraction and growth rate is a gradual loss of differentiation characteristics and a marked change in cytological phenotypes (Fig. 12a, b). As suggested earlier, the concept of a "tumor stem cell" may have to be modified in as much as tumors appear to have a number of tumorigenic, clonogenic subpopulations. Furthermore, it appears that each of the subpopulations of clonogenic cells referred to as "stem cells" have their own specific sensitivity to chemotherapeutic agents.

There are two major advantages for establishing an in vitro method for growing tumor cells. First, in vitro assays have contributed greatly to our knowledge of cell biology and-vis a-vis would necessarily advance our knowledge of the biology of neoplastic disease. Secondly, and perhaps more obvious, clonogenicity of tumor populations could be used to effectively predict the sensitivity of an individual patient's tumor cells to specific chemotherapeutic agents and radiotherapy which would greatly advance the efforts of the oncologist. From the beginning, the idea of a clonogenic assay for identifying drug sensitivity of human tumors has generated a great deal of interest and excitement in the experimental and clinical oncology communities. Those of us who have had experience with experimental in vivo – in vitro tumor systems looked upon this new clinical area with a jaundiced eye due to reservations drawn from our own observations as well as the criticisms offered by colleagues. Nonetheless, the human tumor cloning assay did represent a "breath of fresh air" to an area that had realized its share of failure. The major reservation stemmed from the low plating efficiencies reported which ranged from 0.001 to 1% and from a suspicion that tumors were heterogeneous "beasts" that were not properly represented by the few cells giving rise to colonies.

Earlier studies on rodent tumours with plating efficiencies of $\cong 25\%$ provided data that failed to agree with, or at least support, other in vivo end points. The controversy was somewhat resolved when it was realized that certain cells damaged in vivo and assayed directly following treatment would express this damage. On-the-other-hand, if these cells were left undisturbed in situ for periods

Table 5. Clonogenicity of mammary tumor cells from different transplant generations: anchorage dependent vs. anchorage independent.[a]

Transplant generation	Methylcellulose[b]	Plastic[b]
SMT[b]	100	100
14	30 ± 1.5	241 ± 27.6
18	–	346 ± 21.3
18	20 ± 2.7	285 ± 20.2
20	10 ± 0.5	–
20	10 ± 0.6	–
25	20 ± 2.3	–
36	29 ± 0.8	569 ± 59.6
40	4 ± 0.2	–
40	4 ± 0.13	–
40	5 ± 0.29	–
40	4 ± 1.78	–
45	7 ± 0.51	–
47		624 ± 42.4

[a] Anchorage independence was measured by determining the colony formation in methylcellulose cultures; anchorage dependence was measured by determining the colony formation on non-treated tissue culture plastic dishes.
[b] Clonogenicity is expressed as a percent of that determined for spontaneous mammary tumor (SMT) under identical culture conditions.

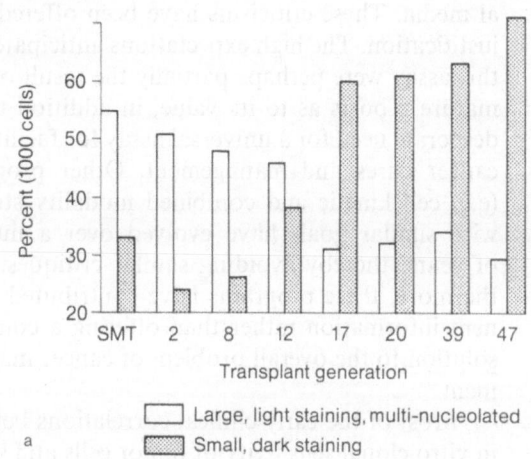

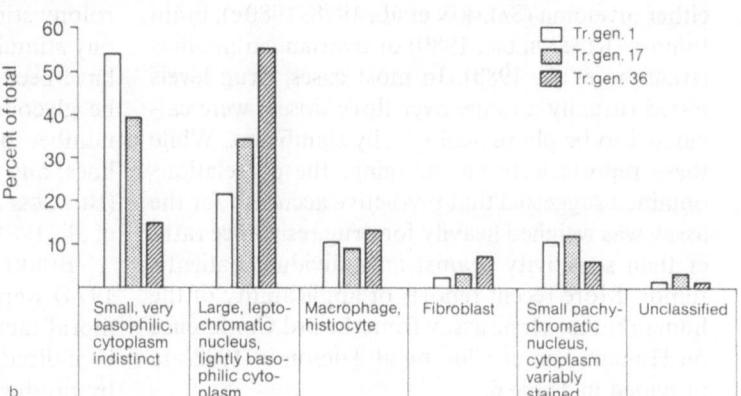

Fig. 12. Cytologic (a) and morphologic (b) changes accompanying the loss of differentiation characteristics of a spontaneous MMT tumor by serial transplantation into C3H/He mice. (J.M. HURST, unpublished data)

approaching 24 hr prior to assaying for clonogenicity, the damage could be repaired and the survival
fraction increased. This concept termed potentially
lethal damage (PLD), while established with the
in vivo – in vitro models, had been recognized
much earlier by radiation biologists during in vitro
studies. Their observations demonstrated that apparently viable cells could both repair sublethal
damage and replicate. Damaged cells, however,
could not repair and replicate simultaneously (LIT-
TLE, 1973; HETZEL and KOLODNEY, 1976; CHAP-
MAN et al., 1970). These considerations of the human tumor clone assay have been and are currently being addressed. It seems obvious that for
the assay to be of significant value to the experimentalist, better growth conditions must be established to permit a more quantitative assessment
of the proliferative status and interrelating events
of neoplastic growth.

What value has the human tumor clone assay
been to the practicing oncologist? Certainly none
of us in either the experimental or clinical oncology communities have escaped the range of criticisms of the human tumor clone assay that have
appeared in both the scientific literature and general media. These criticisms have been offered with
justification. The high expectations anticipated for
this assay were perhaps partially the result of premature reports as to its value, in addition to the
desperate need for a universal assay for facilitating
cancer cures and management. Other programs
(e.g. cell kinetic and combined modality studies)
with similar goals have evolved over a number
of years, thereby avoiding similar critiques. Furthermore, these programs have contributed pertinent information rather than offering a complete
solution to the overall problem of cancer management.

Most of the early clinical correlations between
in vitro clonal sensitivity of tumor cells and subsequent patient response were made on patients with
either myeloma (SALMON et al., 1978, 1980c), brain
tumors (ROSENBLUM, 1980) or ovarian carcinomas
(ALBERTS et al., 1980). In most cases, drug levels
tested (usually a range over three doses) were calculated to be pharmacologically significant. While
these reports were encouraging, the correlations
obtained suggested that predictive accuracy for the
assay was weighed heavily for drug resistance rather than sensitivity against an individual patient's
tumor. More recent reports of applicability of the
human tumor clone assay from the 3rd Conference
on Human Tumor Cloning at Tucson in 1982 are
provided in Table 6.

Table 6. Correlative response (%)

Tumor	Sensi- tivity	Resis- tance	Data source[a]
Small cell lung cancer	75	100	1
Pediatric tumors	71	83	2
Ovarian carcinoma	62	99	3
Leukemia	76		4
Bladder	80	80	5
Human tumors	60–70	95	6

[a]1. D.N. CARNEY et al., MCI-VA Medical Oncology Branch
and NCI-Medical Oncology Branch, DCT/NCI, Beth-
esda, MD. U.S.A.
2. M. PAGANUZZI et al., Gaslini Children's Hospital, Ge-
moa, Italy.
3. D.S. ALBERTS et al., Cancer Center, University of Arizona, Tucson, AZ, U.S.A.
4. B.G.M. DURIE et al., Cancer Center, University of Arizona, Tucson, AZ, U.S.A.
5. T.H. STANISIC and R. OWENS, Arizona Health Science
Center, Tucson, AZ, U.S.A.
6. S.E. SALMON et al., University of Arizona, Cancer
Center, Tucson, AZ, U.S.A.

6.2 Markers for Hematopoietic Toxicity in Serum

Following the independent establishment of an in
vitro method for quantitating the hematopoietic
progenitor cell (CFUc or CFUc-GM) of granulocyte and macrophage production (PLUZNIK and
SACHS 1965) and BRADLEY and METCALF (1966),
the entire area of hematopoietic ontogeny underwent an explosive expansion and has continued
to do so until presently, it represents one of the
most well-defined systems in the mammalian body.
We will forgo until later an indepth consideration
of the regulation of hematopoiesis. It will suffice
at this time to consider a class of growth factors
identified and, in some instances purified, that stimulate the CFUc to proliferate and thereafter differentiate in vitro. These factors, referred to as
colony stimulating activity (CSA; if crude) or colony stimulating factor (CSF; if partially purified),
have been extensively studied and are reported to
be glycoproteins of various sizes produced by a
number of sources (e.g. macrophage, some cell
lines, and tumors) each with target cell specificity
(BURGESS et al., 1977; NICOLA et al., 1979; DAS
et al., 1981).

BURKE and his colleagues (BURKE et al., 1973,
1974) were among the first to recognize that humoral factors capable of stimulating CFUc could
be indiced in the sera of both rodents and humans
by producing marrow aplasia. This induction fol-

lowed a feedback inhibitory pattern (i.e. a reciprocal relationship between neutrophil counts and
CSA activity) and they postulated a cause and effect relationship between the observed changes in
serum CSA and the recovery of the human bone
marrow from drug- (or radiation-) induced aplasia
(BURKE et al., 1973). Furthermore, it was also believed that these changes in CSA following treatment were not derived de novo but rather were
merely an amplification of naturally occurring
feedback regulators of marrow hematopoiesis.

Sera of patients with various neoplastic diseases including leukemias have demonstrated a
cyclic change in the ability to support ^{3}H-TdR
incorporation of both normal and leukemic cells
(BURKE et al., 1974). Unlike the in vitro assays,
the "serum stimulating"assay is a measure of the
^{3}H-TdR uptake and therefore, proliferation of all
marrow elements rather than specific marrow progenitor cells. This cyclic periodicity is related to
the cellularity and morphology of the bone marrow. As depicted in Figure 13, ^{3}H-TdR incorporation by normal human bone marrow cells is maximally stimulated by serum from patients with a
minimal peripheral white blood cell count. Furthermore, cells from the bone marrow from these
"Hi" serum patients are in the proliferative phase
of recovery from profound drug-induced aplasia.
When this compensatory phase is complete and
the marrow cells are maturing, the serum stimulating ability of these patients, as measured by ^{3}H-
TdR incorporation, decreases significantly, reaching minimal levels ("Lo" serum) at the time of
WBC recovery and rebound. Both the serum of
healthy patients and the pretreatment sera of cancer patients may serve as a control for this assay.
Further more, SCHACTER and BURKE (1978) have
observed that the support of ^{3}H-TdR incorporation in a large sampling of normal control serum
is essentially identical ($\pm$ % S.E.M.), and therefore
both control "serum" or 30% phosphate-buffered
saline can be used to normalize test sera. By using
pretreatment patient sera, marrow abnormalities
associated with disease can also be defined. Under
the conditions of this assay, the differences between "normal", "Hi" and "Lo" serum are most
pronounced at a 15–30% range of final serum concentration. At no serum concentration could the
relative abilities of "Hi" or "Lo" sera be reversed.
However, because "Lo" sera reduced the ^{3}H-TdR
uptake levels below that observed in the absence
of any serum, it was suggested that an active inhib-
itor was also present in "Lo" serum. There is some
evidence that a stimulator exists in "Hi" serum.

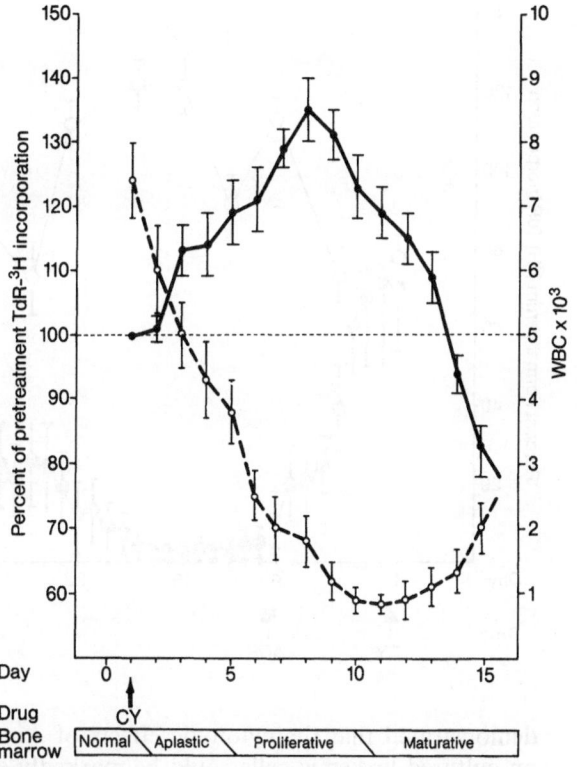

Fig. 13. Relative ability of sera serially collected from patients following a single dose of drug to support ^{3}H-thymi-
dine incorporation by normal human bone marrow cells
(●−−−●). Values are normalized to incorporation in sera
collected prior to any therapy. Figure shows average value
from 4 different patients. Also presented is the average peripheral white blood count in these patients (o−−−o). "Hi"
sera are collected on days 7, 8, 9, 10 and "Lo" sera on
day 14 and later in such patients. The graph extends only
to day 14 because patients are routinely sent home when
the white blood cell counts exceeds 3,000/mm^3. Reproduced
with permission from SCHACTER and BURKE, J Mol Med
3:329–344, 1978

However, only the isolation of this putative stimulator and a demonstration that it is not itself metabolized can distinguish it as a true stimulator.

Despite its rather crude definition, the serum
assay has already proved to be of some value for
the clinician involved in the treatment of hematopoietic neoplasia. Many of these patients have pretreatment sera that inhibit the proliferation of
both normal and neoplastic hematological cells
which may explain the relatively low tumor growth
fraction observed for these diseases. Obviously,
any procedure that could overcome this "potential
inhibition" and increase the growth fraction
should result in enhanced cycle-specific-agent cell
kill, as sufficiently well documented with in vitro
studies. KARP and BURKE (1976) have already

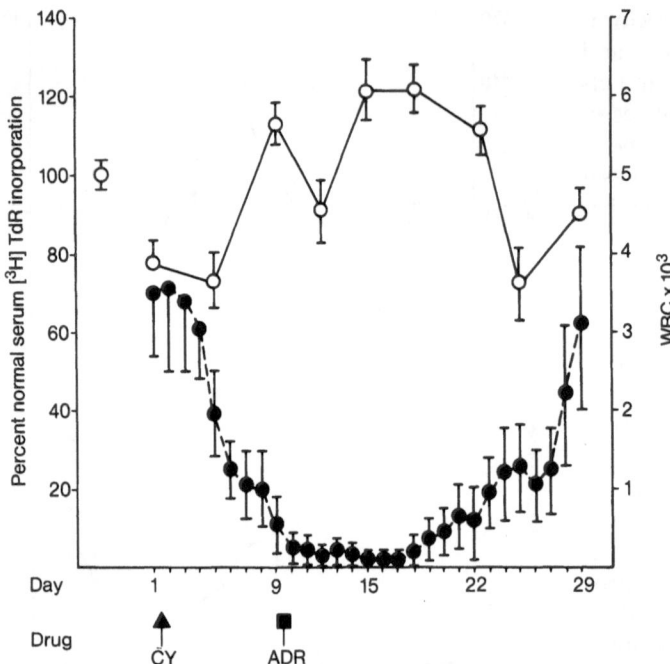

Fig. 14. Mean sequential sera effects on 18 hr normal bone marrow ^{3}H-TdR incorporation (o——o) and peripheral blood WBC (●---●) from the 12 patients treated with Cx given on day 1 (↑) followed by AdR given on day 9 (■) (Cx, Adr). The effect of normal serum is depicted in the upper left portion of the figure (0). Vertical bars represent ±S.E.M. Pretreatment sera inhibited normal marrow cell ^{3}H-TdR incorporation. Sera obtained on day 9 of Cx-induced aplasia had increased activity relative to normal effect. Further HSA increase was detected on days 15–18 of therapy at the time of WBC nadir. The mean duration of granulocytopenia extended from day 7 through 23 (WBC 100/cells/cu mm) with WBC 500/cells/cu mm lasting from day 9 through day 20. Reproduced with permission from KARP et al., Blood 57:468–475, 1981

demonstrated that the cytotoxic effects of Ara-C on cultured leukemic cells could be markedly enhanced if the cells were exposed to humoral factors present in pooled "Hi" serum from leukemic patients undergoing chemotherapy for two days prior to drug treatment. The tumor cell number and labeling index were consistent with a marked recruitment of tumor cells into cycle. Later they observed that similar recruitment (measured by ^{3}H-TdR incorporation) of malignant marrow plasma cells could be brought about by treatment with cytoxan both in vitro and in their patients with a corresponding induction of "Hi serum" (KARP et al., 1977). Similar results were presented for normal hematopoietic cells.

It naturally follows that if "Hi" and "Lo" serum stimulating activity is a direct reflection of the peripheral blood picture and the proliferative status of the marrow progenitor cells, then it also has apparent potential for use as a discriminating assay of acute hematopoietic toxicity of the marrow. Furthermore, the abbreviated time required for estimating serum-stimulating activity ($\cong 18$ hr) also provides a rapid method for determining the temporal marrow response to cytotoxic agents, in advance of the method presently used which is based on the end products rather than on the actual site of hematopoietic toxicity. KARP et al. (1981) have used this to establish a timed sequential chemotherapy protocol for the treatment of cytoxan-refractory multiple myeloma (Fig. 14). In the ex-

perimental model, peak stimulatory serum ("Hi") was detected 9 days following cytoxan treatment. Sequential changes in the ^{3}H-TdR labeling index of the plasma cells were found to parallel changes in serum-stimulating activity. Maximum adriamycin cytotoxicity was observed at 9 days post cytoxan treatment at levels that were significantly higher than observed in pre-cytoxan treated cells. When these observations were taken to clinical trial, patients received cytoxan as a single bolus dose of 2,400 mg/m^2 and were subsequently followed for serum-stimulating activity. Adriamycin was administered (60 mg/m^2) 9 days post cytoxan treatment, or at the time of peak "Hi" serum. The response, measured by a monoclonal protein marker, projected a greater than 8 month median survival which compared favorably with results obtained using AdR in a non-sequenced chemotherapeutic regimen. Furthermore, AdR, used as a single agent, resulted in responses in 10–25% of the patients, while AdR, used in a non-sequenced schedule with other chemotherapeutic agents, resulted in a 25–50% response rate. Using the time sequencing approach with cytoxan, AdR was able to produce responses in 68% of the patients.

In addition to providing a prescriptive definition for combined drug/drug or drug/radiation schedules, the serum-stimulating ^{3}H-TdR assay may have equal or even greater potential for proscriptive definition of combined therapy resulting in reduced hematopoietic toxicity. For non-hematological disease, with little or no marrow involvement, this assay may be used to direct the oncologist in temporal sequencing of therapy. Obviously, a second course of treatment given when the patient has "Hi" serum could result in enhanced morbidity or mortality. At the same time, WBC rebound may delay treatment and result in less effective tumoricidal activity. Using this assay, it is conceivable that the optimal time sequencing for patients could be established by daily monitoring of marrow proliferative activity. Information is then needed that will further clarify the relationships between "Hi" and "Lo" serum, the peripheral WBC counts, and the stem cell, the progenitor cell, and marrow cell differentiation before this assay can be assumed to be a good pre/proscriptive marker of hematologic activity of the patient undergoing aggressive treatment.

6.3 Plasma Diamine Oxidase as an Index of Small Bowel Damage

In the mammalian small intestine, the proliferative cells are organized into discrete units termed crypts, and the maintenance of the integrity of the epithelial lining is dependent on cell renewal from the proliferative compartment of the crypt. Under normal conditions, the intestinal epithelium is considered a steady-state renewal system and, therefore, a prime target for those agents that disrupt cell production. The original description of the small intestine by LEBLOND and STEVENS (1948) has served as the model for steady-state growth in the crypts. Cells produced in the crypt move up the sides of the villi and are eventually sloughed-off at the villus apex. Quantitative cell kinetic and compartmental analysis of steady state conditions in the mouse have provided a basis for the analysis of events occurring in the crypt following cellular insult, as well as other pertubations resulting in steady-state modulation (HAGEMANN, 1980).

The basic response of the intestinal epithelium following acute injury by noxious agents may, for the most part, be considered to be manifested either by crypt progenitor cell (stem cell?) killing (Fig. 15) or by a reduced rate (progression delay) of proliferation of surviving cells or both (Fig. 16). Both of these aspects of insult-recognition lead to a diminished production of cells, and more importantly, a diminished cell flux from the proliferative to the differentiated villus compartment. During

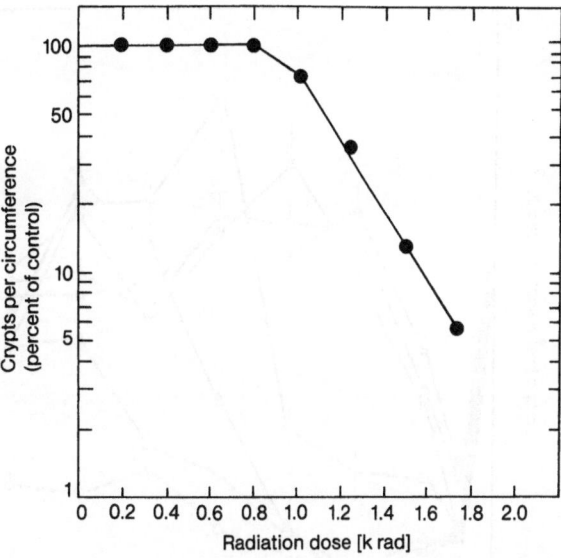

Fig. 15. Radiation vs. intestinal crypt survival for the BDF_1 mouse. The crypts per circumference of a section of jejunal tissue are presented as a percent of non-irradiated control for a radiation dose range from 0–1,700 R. The assay is carried out at 96 hr post irradiation, a time when irradiated crypts are well on their way to recovery. For most experimental studies a dose of 1,000 R is required to place the crypt survival on the exponential phase of generated curves. This large plateau region is the result of crypt multiplicity where even 1 cryptogenic (stem ?) cell can repopulate an entire crypt. (From KOVACS, unpublished data, 1980)

this period of depressed cell production, the functional compartment continues to be depleted by apical cell loss. Recovery from acute insult is rapid, reaching a peak in 3–4 days following treatment. Even with aggressive radiotherapy where, unlike chemotherapy, the surviving crypt progenitor cells can be reduced to a level resulting in significant crypt attrition, recovery can result from a single viable cell. During recovery, there is an increased rate of cell production per surviving crypt (i.e. increased proliferating compartment and abbreviated cell cycle time) and eventually the functional compartment is repopulated. Following this compensatory response, cell proliferation returns to the steady-state value.

The functional compartment can be considered to be the column of maturing enterocytes, dynamically forming the villus structure. In addition to the intestinal enterocyte, the villus components consist of a unique set of immunologically competent cells which presently are receiving a great deal of attention in the laboratory. Mucosal lymphocytes consist of two types, both associated with villus structure: the intra-epithelial (IE) lympho-

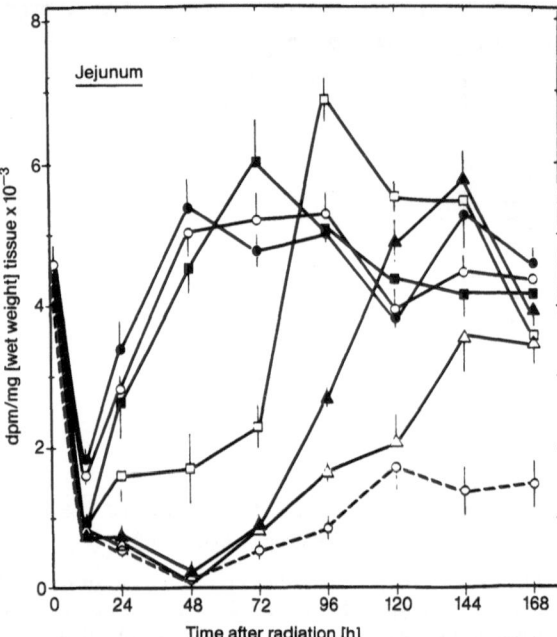

Fig. 16. Proliferative response of the intestinal epithelium of the BDF$_1$ mouse to graded doses of radiation. (●), 200 R; (0) 400 R; (■), 600 R; (□), 1,000 R; (▲), 1,250 R; (△), 1,500 R; (○---○), 1,750 R. Initially, cell production is inhibited ($\cong 24$ hr) by radiation. At lower doses, the magnitude of inhibition is dose-related. The duration of proliferative inhibition is dose-related at all dose levels. The "magnitude" and "duration" are collectively referred to as "insult recognition". The "recovery phase" has essentially three components: the initiation of cell production and return to near control levels; the compensatory response where $\cong 200$–400% increases in cell production are observed; and the stabilizing of cell production at control levels. For comparative purposes, both the insult recognition and kinetics of compensatory response can be of value for determining toxicity

cyte and the lamnia propria (LP) lymphocytes (EARNSHAW et al., 1982). Studies in both mouse and man have demonstrated that the majority of the IE cells are of the suppressor/cytotoxic T-cell phenotype and that the T-cells of the LP are more than likely of the T-helper subclass (SELBY et al., 1981). This unique set of lymphocytes may be responsible for local immunologic responses mediated by activated T-lymphocytes (cell-mediated immunity) and have been postulated to be responsible, via an innocent-bystander function, for a number of pathologic conditions in the gut. More obvious is their role in preventing generalized septicemia by serving a "barrier function" to intestinal pathogens. This "barrier function" of the villus, in addition to its absorptive and metabolic roles, ultimately determines the manifestation of

toxicity, even though the actual target cells of cytotoxic agents are present in the crypt.

The proliferative response of the intestine to multiple (fraction) cytotoxic exposure is determined by both the magnitude (dose) of each fraction as well as the duration of recovery intervals between exposures. Following cytotoxic injury, one consideration that influences the minimum time period between treatment and onset of compensatory hyperplasia in the crypt is the fate of reproductively damaged cells. For example, after irradiation the majority of cells lethally damaged with respect to proliferative potential remain intact and move out into the villi where they perform, at the very least, a "barrier function" thus delaying the fall in villus cellularity. For a number of cell renewal systems including the gastrointestinal system, a feedback control of cell proliferation by the functional cell compartment has been postulated, with supportive data accumulating rapidly. That these "dead" cells serve only a barrier function has been suggested by microchemical analysis during recovery after irradiation. GALJAARD et al. (1970) have observed that following irradiation the migration of crypt enterocyte cells through the villus is accompanied by an insufficient development of certain differentiation characteristics of the epithelial cells, such as non-specific esterase and phosphatase.

Some chemotherapeutic agents, however, result in rapid cell lysis within the crypts as demonstrated in Figure 17. These agents cause a rapid decrease in villus cellularity and necessarily an abbreviated period between damage-recognition and initiation of recovery. Therefore, if compensatory proliferation can be maintained in various treatment schedules, large radiation (or drug) exposures can be accumulated without acute gastrointestinal toxicity. Whether or not toxicity is evident, the question of functionality of the mature villus compartment for periods after either radiation or drug insult remains unanswered. The "barrier function" may be a "built in" protection against bacteremic infection under conditions where severe gastrointestinal toxicity and granulocytopenia could potentially overlap.

As already mentioned, changes in the size of the proliferative population of the crypt markedly influence the responsiveness and tolerance of the intestinal epithelium to treatment. The majority of cytotoxic agents act at the level of the crypt proliferative cells, which is subsequently translated into a functional deficit via depletion of the epithelial cells. During preclinical studies, the concept

Fig. 17. Effect of VcR treatment of crypt cell integrity as measured by proliferation kinetics and ³H-IUdR labeled cell lysis. A comparison between 1 mg/kg VcR (o) and 600 R (●) demonstrates rapid initiation of recovery following VcR treatment. The loss of ³H-IUdR from prelabeled crypt cells of the intestinal epithelium with time (insert) demonstrates that VcR treatment, unlike either 600 R or DDP, results in rapid crypt cell lysis (0–24 hr) and a more rapid depopulation of the villus to initiate an early recovery phase. Data reproduced with permission from Kovacs et al., Brit J Cancer, 1985 (in press)

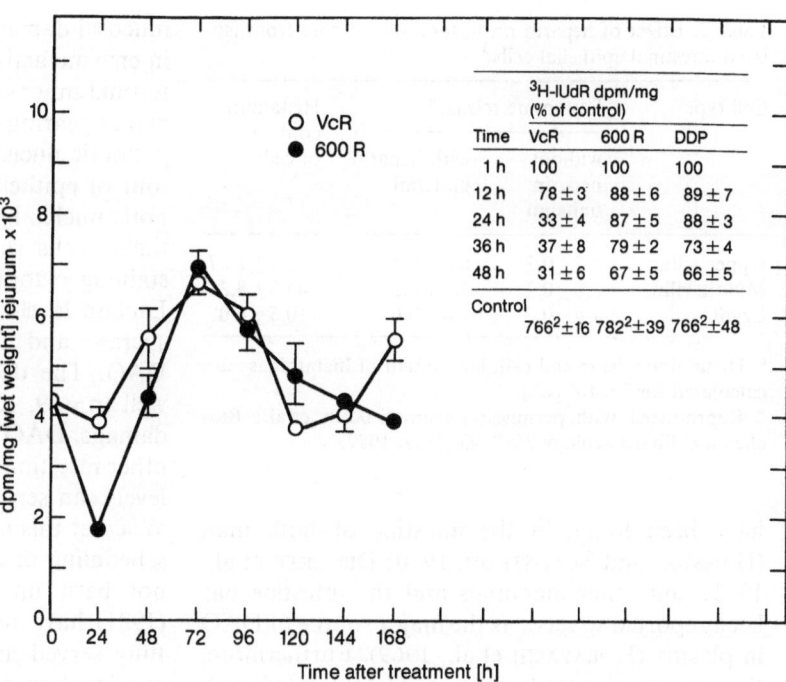

Time	³H-IUdR dpm/mg (% of control)		
	VcR	600 R	DDP
1 h	100	100	100
12 h	78±3	88±6	89±7
24 h	33±4	87±5	88±3
36 h	37±8	79±2	73±4
48 h	31±6	67±5	66±5
Control	766²±16	782²±39	766²±48

of monitoring crypt cell output during treatment schedules as developed by HAGEMANN (1976), has been of great assistance in establishing *pre*- and *pro*scriptive treatment regimens. During any type of continuous, sequential or fractionated treatment to the abdomen, or systemically, the integrity of the epithelial lining is of paramount importance and must be maintained by the continuous production of new cells. The ability of the intestinal epithelium to compensate for damage recognition resulting in a reduced cell flow from the proliferative to the functional compartment is the most important factor for recovery from treatment-associated damage.

Unfortunately, methods used during preclinical studies in rodents to define the temporal course of this recovery are not available for patients, nor would they be of much value for close order treatment schedules due to their lengthy assay times. A non-invasive, rapid sampling method that would measure the functional compartment of the small bowel following and/or during treatment would certainly assist the oncologist, especially for the treatment of primary or disseminated disease involving the abdomen. The search for such "biomarkers" for both diagnosis and treatment efficacy in neoplastic disease has resulted in many reports of compounds that are: a) specific for differentiated tissue, b) are produced by normal tissues in response to tumors during the course of disease, and c) are elevated in blood plasma, se-

rum, or urine during certain states of disease progression. The net result has been a confusing compilation of reports which have not significantly advanced either diagnosis or treatment of neoplastic disease. Of course, this confusion could be the result of the state of the art. However, more realistically, it probably represents the heterogeneity associated with neoplastic disease and the difficulty resulting in interpretation of individual patients.

One such "marker", which more recently has shown promise in permitting a more rational scheduling of treatment, is the enzyme diamine oxidase (DAO). DAO is also referred to as histaminase (EC 1.4.3.6) because histamine serves as one of its substrates. DAO is known to oxidatively deaminate histamine and aliphatic amines such as putrescine and cadaverine, although the physiological role of this enzyme is poorly understood. High levels of DAO activity have been described in three biologic situations: (1) in decidual portions of the placenta in most mammalian species with plasma activity increasing during the course of pregnancy (BEAVEN et al., 1975); (2) in plasma following parenteral administration of heparin (TRYDING, 1965); and (3) in endocrine malignancies (medullary carcinoma) of the thyroid gland (BAYLIN et al., 1972; BAYLIN, 1977), although other reports of a tumor-association are less convincing (BORGLIN and WINERT, 1962; BAYLIN et al., 1975). More importantly, however, high levels of DAO activity

Table 7. Effect of heparin on histaminase release from isolated intestinal epithelial cells*

Cell type	Histamine release[a]		Histamine content of cells
	without heparin units/ml	with heparin units/ml	
Upper villus	5.7 ± 0.3	6.6 ± 0.4	131.0 ± 24.7
Middle villus	3.6 ± 0.2	3.7 ± 0.2	44.0 ± 8.3
Crypt	1.4 ± 0.2	1.4 ± 0.6	10.5 ± 4.0

[a] Histamine release and cellular content of histaminase are calculated for 3×10^6 cells.
* Reproduced with permission from SHAKIR et al.: Biochemical Pharmacology 26:2343–2347, 1977.

have been found in the intestine of both man (HANSSON and SUNDSTROM, 1970; DENCKER et al., 1973) and other mammals and the intestine has been reported to serve as the major source of DAO in plasma (KOBAYASHI et al., 1969). Furthermore, the enzyme is now known to be associated with the mature villus cells of the small bowel (Table 7), increasing sharply from low levels in the cells of the rat crypt region to much higher activity in the villus tips. In studies of intestinal development in the newborn rat, the plasma levels of DAO have been found to be quantitatively proportional to the increasing number of mature villus tip cells (BAYLIN et al., 1978).

DAO, therefore, appeared to satisfy most of the requisites for a potential marker of gastrointestinal integrity and functionality; a) non-invasive, b) specific for a major target tissue of toxicity; and c) quantitative for a dose-limiting functional cell. LUK et al. (1980) have reported that plasma DAO reflected the amount of mucosal damage in rat intestinal loops perfused with hyperosmolar sodium sulfate solutions that selectively damage the villus. At the same time they monitored other intestinal enzymes (Table 8) for comparison of both tissue and plasma enzyme levels. With increasing

mucosal damage, there was a progressive decrease in enzyme activity. Histological grading of the intestinal mucosa was as follows: a) minimal – normal appearing columnar epithelial cells with a few pyknotic nuclei; b) moderate – slight loss of contour of epithelial cells, moderate number of pyknotic nuclei, lymphatic dilatation; c) severe – epithelial cells shortened and cuboidal, with dense staining cytoplasms, many with pyknotic nuclei. Lactase levels fell first, followed by maltase and sucrase and finally both mucosal and plasma DAO. The decrease in plasma DAO correlated well (n=29, D 0.04) with the degree of mucosal damage. DAO activity, therefore, is unique among other intestinal enzymes studied in that circulating levels can serve as a marker of mucosal integrity. Whether this marker can be used clinically for the scheduling of chemotherapy and/or radiation has not been unequivocally established. LUK et al. (1981) have reported that plasma DAO successfully served as a marker of mucosal injury and regeneration after Ara-C treatment of rats. They observed a direct quantitative relationship between the decrease in plasma DAO and the amount of mucosal injury. The relationship appeared to be dose dependent, at least for the magnitude of plasma DAO reduction which was measured on day 4 during a drug exposure schedule of 0.30 g/kg q 8 hr × 6. They also reported that for 3 patients with acute leukemia treated with a 3-day infusion of high dose Ara-C (45 mg/kg) in combination with daunorubicin, DAO appeared to monitor intestinal toxicity, which has been a consistent problem observed both clinically and histologically in leukemic patients sequentially treated with this drug regimen (Fig. 18).

Experimentally, Ara-C at the dose levels tested by LUK et al. (1981) does not result in a significant reduction of plasma DAO if given as a single injection (KOVACS CJ, unpublished observations), although the tissue levels are reduced by 35%. Furthermore, radiation doses on the plateau of an

Table 8. Decreases in mucosal enzyme activities and plasma DAO after selective villus mucosal damage by hypertonic sodium sulfate solution[a]

Perfusion (mosmol × mm)	Histologic injury	Decrease in enzyme activity				
		Lactase	Maltase	Sucrase	Mucosal DAO	Plasma DAO
$1,400 \times 30$	minimal	0	0	0	0	0
$1,400 \times 60$	minimal	10	0	0	0	0
$2,100 \times 30$	moderate	73	62	60	22	12
$2,100 \times 60$	severe	75	65	62	44	42

[a] Reproduced with permission from LUK et al. (J Clin Invest 66:66–70, 1980).

Fig. 18. The effect of systemic combination chemotherapy with Ara-C and daunorubicin (D) on plasma DAO in 3 patients with leukemia. The levels of DAO are plotted as a percentage of pretreatment basal levels and are denoted by a different symbol for each of the 3 patients. The nadir reached on days 9 to 12 is statistically significant (p < 0.05). Reproduced with permission from LUK et al., Cancer Res, 41:2334–2337, 1981

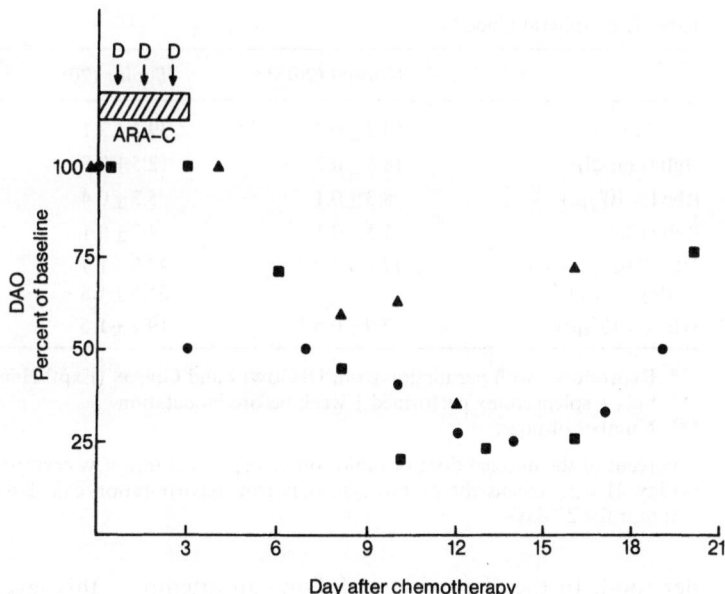

intestinal crypt survival curve, also fail to result in marked reductions of plasma DAO. However, these studies were carried out at a fixed time point (4 days post-treatment), a time at which crypt regeneration is well on its way.

Plasma DAO has the potential to develop into an effective tool for both the medical and radiation oncologist. Information presently available is encouraging concerning its future in the clinic. However, addition pre-clinical, in addition to clinical, studies are needed that will establish the temporal response-relationships between plasma DAO levels and both villus integrity and crypt cell production, following treatment-associated (e.g. radiation and/or drug) or biological (e.g. nutritional) insults. Furthermore, it is also pressing that the change in plasma DAO associated with these insults be correlated with villus functionality. A major question that will ultimately determine optimal time/dose configurations for rational therapy involving the abdominal area is "What is the plasma DAO level for "barrier function" as opposed to complete restoration of villus cell differentiation?". Only after the complete characterization of these relationships has been completed, will the full potential of a "plasma DAO marker" be realized.

7 The Role of the Tumor-host Relationships in the Therapeutic Response

The concept of "tumor host interactions" has been recognized in individual patients, in the laboratory mouse, and more recently in the culture dish. Certainly advances in our knowledge of the treatment of cancer over the last decade has made the oncologist increasingly aware that paraneoplastic syndromes, resulting in dysfunction of organ functions produced at a distance from the primary tumor, but not resulting from space-occupying lesions of metastases, are present or will develop during the course of disease. Altered physiological states in pre-clinical models are well known to the laboratory investigator. While these observations have been well documented, in general, the investigators using experimental animals for therapeutic studies have focused relatively little attention on the "clinical course" of cancer and the mechanisms involved. Clinical investigators are limited ostensibly by the heterogeneity and multiple variables of host response in patients. Herein lies, therefore, the value of studies of the "tumor-host" interactions with preclinical animal models.

The patient with advanced disease exhibits a much narrower safe therapeutic margin for chemotherapy than one in the early stages of metastatic disease. In fact, these patients are often eliminated as candidates for adequate oncologic treatment. Altered metabolism in cancer patients has been the focus of attention in many clinical investigations and it is generally accepted, though poorly understood, that the wasting of body tissue results from a change in the relationship between protein and carbohydrate metabolism which is energy wasteful. Little is known of the response of the dose-limiting tissues to the progression of disease, nor are the relationships between altered metabolism and proliferative activity in these tissues un-

Table 9. Peripheral blood *

	Normal (20) ***	Tumor (20)	Normal/Splx ** (20)	Tumor/Splx (20)
Hct (%)	54.2 ± 0.4	39.3 ± 2.1	49.8 ± 0.7	34.2 ± 0.6
Hgb (Gm/dl)	18.6 ± 0.2	12.5 ± 0.8	17.1 ± 0.3	11.2 ± 0.3
Rbc ($\times 10^6/\mu l$)	8.3 ± 0.1	5.3 ± 0.4	8.1 ± 0.1	4.8 ± 0.2
Retic (%)	1.5 ± 0.1	4.3 ± 0.1	3.0 ± 0.2	4.6 ± 0.4
^{59}Fe Rbc inc. (%)[a]	17.8 ± 1.7	27.9 ± 1.7	30.2 ± 3.2	23.6 ± 1.6
(day 21 wgt)[b]		35.5 ± 1.8		31.3 ± 1.9
Wbc ($\times 10^3/\mu l$)	7.9 ± 0.5	19.2 ± 1.5	7.5 ± 1.0	18.3 ± 1.9

* Reproduced with permission from DeGowin and Gibson (Exptl Hemat 6:568–575, 1978).
** Splx – splenectomy performed 1 week before inoculation.
*** Number of mice.

[a] Percent of the injected dose of radioiron incorporated into new erythrocytes by 18 hr after intravenous injection.
[b] (day 21 wgt) means the erythrocyte radioiron incorporation calculated on the basis of the mice weight after bearing tumor for 21 days.

derstood. In the discussion to follow, an attempt will be made to update the information available from preclinical studies, and to conceptually bridge the gap between empirical clinical observations and changes in treatment tolerance associated with disease-directed normal tissue toxicity.

7.1 Hematopoiesis and Neoplasia

A review of the literature suggests that anemia is a common finding in patients with advanced neoplastic disease, and anemic patients have a lower probability of radiotherapeutic and chemotherapeutic cure than those with normal hematocrits (Hill et al., 1971; Berlin, 1965). This anemia has been linked to a reduced red cell production due to: (1) crowding of erythropoietic stem cells by metastasis, although evidence for crowding outside of the leukemias is not convincing (Shen and Homberger, 1951), (2) hemodilution, although evidence suggests that dilution cannot account for the severe anemia observed in mice with large tumors (Jirtle and Clifton, 1978), and (3) an accelerated random erythrocyte loss due to an intrinsic erythrocyte defect (Jirtle and Clifton, 1978). DeGowin and his colleagues at Iowa have demonstrated a marked compromise of the erythropoietic potential of tumor-bearing mice (De Gowin and Gibson, 1978a, DeGowin et al., 1978b). A normochromic anemia amount of 0.25 or 0.33% of the initial values after 21 days of tumor burden was accompanied by a reticulocytosis of $4.3 \pm 1.0\%$ (Table 9). Erythropoiesis, however, was not suppressed in the spleen which served as a compensating organ. An attempt to ameliorate

this severe anemia by removal of the spleen prior to tumor inoculation failed. However, it did prevent the severe suppression of erythroblast counts in the bone marrow.

In addition to a reduction of red cell components in the peripheral blood, erythropoietic elements were also reduced in the marrow. More importantly, the in vitro assay of marrow stromal cells were found to be reduced to 30% of normal by the presence of the tumor. Later they observed an association between erythropoiesis and partially characterized marrow stromal (fibroblastoid) cells suggesting that, during tumor growth, a marked alteration of the microenvironment of the marrow occurs which limits the proliferation and differentiation of immature erythropoietic progenitor cells (Wertz et al., 1980). Furthermore, it has been suggested that tumor cells produce a substance into conditioned media (Fig. 19) which selectively inhibits the colonization of marrow stromal cells concomitant with excessive secretion of PGE, known to suppress erythropoiesis at high concentrations (De Gowin et al., 1981).

Before proceeding further, a brief consideration of a scheme of hematopoietic differentiation may be helpful (Fig. 20). Within the last 2–3 years, substantial evidence has accumulated suggesting that the hematopoietic stem cell, originally operationally defined in the mouse as the CFUs, was not a uniform population but rather a highly heterogeneous compartment. These stem cells then form a hierarchy or continuum ranging from the earliest, most primitive stem cells with the highest potential for cell renewal and the least likelihood to be found cycling, to the most committed and differentiated stem cells having the lowest renewal

Fig. 19. Suppressive effect of tumor-conditioned media on marrow stromal colony growth per 2×10^6 mouse bone marrow cells. "Percent" means that tumor-conditioned media comprise from 0–50% of the culture media in this figure. Reproduced with permission from DeGowin et al., Exptl Hemat, 9:811–817, 1981

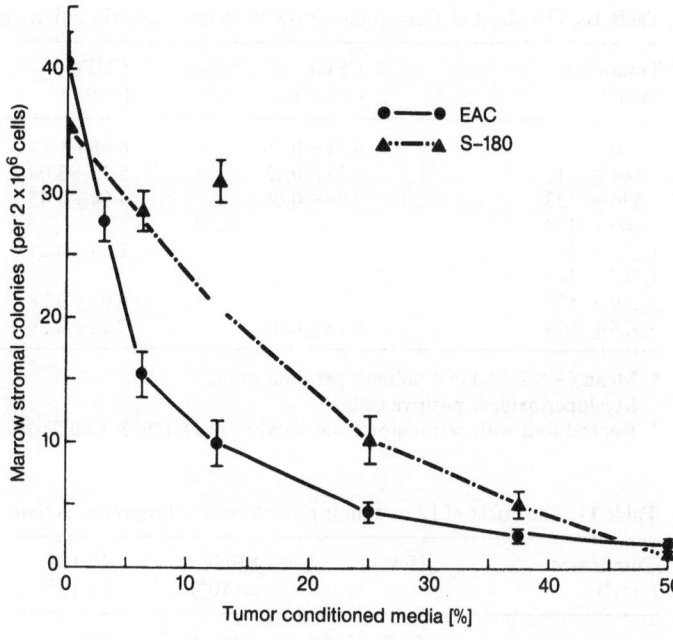

Fig. 20. The hierarchy of hematopoietic differentiation. CFUs, colony forming unit, spleen – a murine pluripotential stem cell assayed as a spleen colony in lethally irradiated mice; BFU, burst forming unit, a less primitive pluripotential stem cell; S_L – lymphoid stem cell giving rise to both a B-cell (S_b) and T-cell (S_t) progenitor. Neither the CFUs nor BFU have been unequivocally established as the progenitors of the S_L. The BFU gives rise to both the CFUc and BFUe, progenitor cells for the myeloid and erythroid lineages. This bifurcation has given rise to a sequence of cell lineages identified by specific in vitro assays and cytological characteristics as the cells approach terminally differentiated mature hematopoietic elements

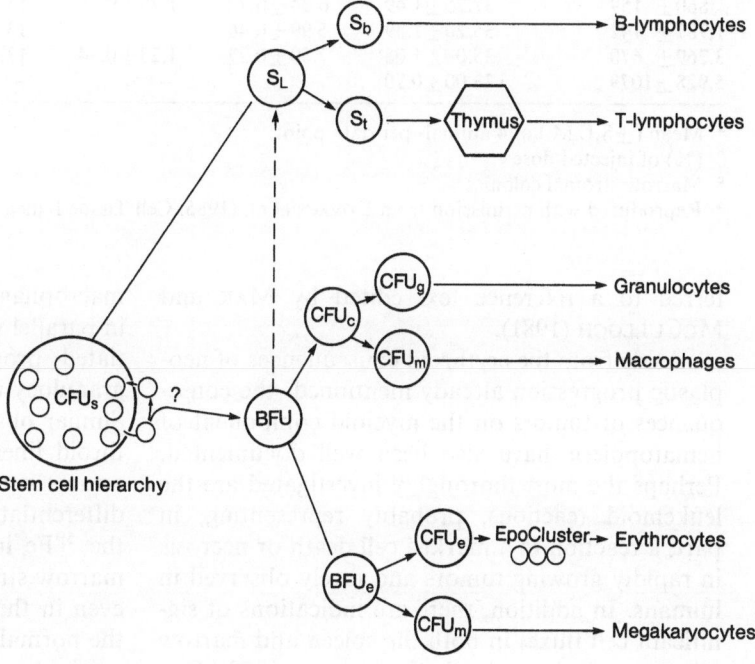

potential, but the greatest likelihood to be found cycling (outside of CFUs circle). These committed CFUs stem cells next proceed to a hypothesized "burst-forming unit" or BFU which is the immediate progenitor to both erythroid and myeloid (and possibly-lymphoid) cell lineages. The in vitro stimulus for this commitment by the CFUs to differentiate is a product of a nitogen stimulated T-lymphocyte. The BFU can then, under the proper

stimulus, commit to either of the differentiated cell lineages. In many cases, the stimulus for the respective steps in the pathways have been identified and partially characterized. Two of the major sources of these stimuli are the macrophage and T-lymphocyte, although increasingly it appears that subsets of these two cell types are actively involved. For a consideration of the activity and characteristics of these stimuli, the reader is re-

Table 10. The effect of LLca tumor growth on myelopoietic activity in the femur of tumor-bearing animals[a][*]

Tumor size (mm³)	CFUs (×10³)	CUFc (×10³)	MPC[b] (×10⁶)	Myeloblasts (%)
0	4.11 ± 0.56	4.96 ± 1.12	9.24 ± 1.37	10.00 ± 1.79
168 ± 12	4.71 ± 0.13	5.72 ± 3.00	9.84 ± 0.28	7.40 ± 0.48
536 ± 23	3.78 ± 0.06	4.34 ± 0.45	2.83 ± 0.22	
860 ± 154			3.82 ± 0.46	5.50 ± 0.98
1,356 ± 141		2.34 ± 0.21	5.62 ± 0.31	
1,787 ± 142				6.20 ± 1.11
3,269 ± 670		6.93 ± 0.28	6.29 ± 1.38	6.25 ± 0.80
5,928 ± 1079	7.28 ± 0.09	7.93 ± 0.29	1.39 ~ 0.05	4.09 ± 1.06

[a] Mean (± S.E.M.) of 4 animals per data point.
[b] Myeloperioxidase positive cells.
[*] Reproduced with permission from KOVACS et al. (1983, Cell Tissue Kinet, in press).

Table 11. The effect of LLca tumor growth on erythropoietic activity in the femur of tumor-bearing animals[a][*]

Tumor size (mm³)	Hct	BFUc (×10⁴)	CFUe (×10⁴)	Erythroblasts (%)	⁵⁹Fe inc[b] (%)	MSC[c]
0	46.20 ± 0.49	4.48 ± 0.37	2.56 ± 0.16	20.40 ± 1.29	0.40 ± 0.00	85.56 ± 2.74
168 ± 2	43.50 ± 1.19	–	–	–	0.36 ± 0.00	–
860 ± 159	37.25 ± 1.49	6.34 ± 0.72	1.78 ± 0.19	13.75 ± 1.11	0.22 ± 0.00	13.48 ± 1.28
1,787 ± 142	35.20 ± 1.39	5.99 ± 0.46	–	13.40 ± 0.80	0.16 ± 0.00	–
3,269 ± 670	35.00 ± 1.08	7.50 ± 0.27	1.23 ± 0.24	13.40 ± 0.52	0.15 ± 0.00	9.50 ± 0.83
5,928 ± 1079	33.00 ± 0.70	–	–	–	0.10 ± 0.00	–

[a] Mean (± S.E.M.) of 4 animals per data point.
[b] (%) of injected dose
[c] Marrow stromal colonies
[*] Reproduced with permission from KOVACS et al. (1985, Cell Tissue Kinet, in press).

ferred to a reference text edited by MAK and McCULLOCH (1981).

Aside from the erythroid consequences of neoplastic progression already mentioned, the consequences of tumors on the myeloid component of hematopoiesis have also been well documented. Perhaps the most thoroughly investigated are the leukemoid reactions, probably representing, in part, a reaction to a marked cell death or necrosis in rapidly growing tumors and rarely observed in humans. In addition, there are indications of significant cell fluxes in both the spleen and marrow of tumor-bearing animals (LALA et al., 1978). One of the major difficulties in interpreting the data in the literature has been the failure of investigators to pay strict attention to both the tumor burden and the degree of tumor differentiation.

During the growth of the Lewis lung tumor in mice, there is evidence for clonal expansion of the immature progenitor cells without further differentiation, suggesting that a feedback regulation of hematopoiesis is interrupted (Table 10 and 11). Both the pluripotential CFUs and granulocyte-

macrophage (CFUc-GM) progenitor cells increase in parallel with tumor burden while their differentiated progeny – the myeloperoxidase-positive granulocytic elements – are markedly suppressed. Similar observations have been made for the erythroid lineage. The early progenitor (BFUe) increases with increasing tumor burden. The more differentiated CFUe and erythroblasts, as well as the ⁵⁹Fe incorporation of the marrow cells and marrow stromal cells, are depressed. Nonetheless, even in the presence of increasing tumor burden the normal humoral modulating factor of at least myeloid proliferation and differentiation is present, suggesting that the tumor prevents these steady-state conditions from functioning effectively, leading to a suppression of terminal differentiation.

7.2 Gastrointestinal Integrity and Neoplasia

A review of the literature reveals that a significant number of reports of malignancy-associated bowel abnormalities exist affecting small bowel morphology, motility and absorptive function (CREAMER, 1964; DELLER et al., 1967; DYMOCK et al., 1967). More recently, the literature focuses on individual case reports with little statistical evaluation. In many of these paraneoplastic syndromes, gastrointestinal symptoms have been tentatively attributed to insufficiencies of pancreatic, liver and bile secretions resulting in maldigestion or malabsorption. In others, syndromes have been linked to tumor released "toxic substances". However, in general, they bear no simple relationship to caloric intake, tumor burden, tumor cell type or anatomical site of involvement. This has been confirmed with experimental data, and, in fact, preliminary studies with the Lewis lung tumor suggest that distant metastatic disease as well as primary tumors influence gastrointestinal steady-state of the host (Table 12).

The growth of cancer leads to profound alterations of host organs and functions which collectively are referred to as the "cachexic syndrome". The association between the wasting of body tissue and the course of advancing disease has been attributed to consequences of impaired food intake or absorption and/or altered metabolism. Host starvation is a common accompaniment to the presence of cancer. While the consequences of starvation on intestinal cell renewal in non-tumor-bearing rodents has been the subject of many investigations, there appears to be significant differences between "uncomplicated starvation" and cachexia-associated starvation. The non-tumor-bearing host has clearly defined mechanisms for conserving lean tissue mass and preserving total body protein, a mechanism which is apparently absent or less effective in the tumor-bearing host (BRENNAN, 1977). Unlike a state of total starvation, the disease state is usually one of semi-starvation with chronic protein malnutrition that has been found to have marked effects on intestinal changes in tumor-bearing rodents which will be discussed below.

A number of tumors including highly undifferentiated, rapidly growing and spontaneous, rapidly growing differentiated models have been found to severely compromise the normal intestinal steady-state conditions of the host, resulting in a marked reduction in the net level of crypt cell output (KOVACS et al., 1981a). Tumors differing in cell or organ, host strain and growth rate, but with a common subcutaneous transplantation site, markedly reduce the proliferative activity of the intestinal epithelium of their host with little corre-

Table 12. Effect of metastatic disease on the gastrointestinal steady state ($BDF_1/LLca$)

	Surgery	Sham surgery
$W(g)$[a]	-0.1 ± 0.066	$+1.0 \pm 0.07$
$Tv(mm^3)$[b]	0	$2,400 \pm 253$
Metastatic disease[c]	$+2.1 \pm 0.5$	$+2.6 \pm 0.7$
^{3}H-TdR dpm/mg		
(a) jejunum	$3,645 \pm 1,014$ (68%)[d]	$1,401 \pm 302$ (26%)[d]
(b) colon	$1,631 \pm 302$ (41%)[d]	702 ± 36 (18%)[d]

[a] Change in animal weight from surgery to sacrifice (day $16 \rightarrow$ day 30)
[b] Change in primary tumor volume from surgery to sacrifice (day $16 \rightarrow$ day 30)
[c] Rated from no lesions (0) to total lung involvement ($+4$)
[d] % of non-tumor-bearing BDF_1 mouse value

lation to absolute tumor size or growth rate. There is some indication that a correlation exists between the relative tumor burden of the host and the level of proliferative depression in the small bowel. These changes have been observed to occur without any changes in the animal weight or food consumption. Similar changes have been observed in an intra-abdominal solid tumor model where both the growth rate of the tumor and the occurrence of the intestinal changes were more rapid.

The cytokinetic changes occurring in the intestinal crypts of tumor-bearing animals suggest an interpretation of the events leading to intestinal compromise. As the tumor burden of the host increases, reductions in both crypt size (cellularity) and the ^{3}H-TdR labelled cells per crypt are reduced (Table 13). However, as the crypts shrink, a compensatory enhancement of crypt proliferation is observed (cells/crypt decrease while proliferating ^{3}H-TdR-labelled cells/crypt increase). The resultant level of cell production in the crypt, however, is not sufficient enough to prevent villus atrophy resulting from continued loss of apical villus cells (Fig. 21). Eventually, crypt cell production and villus exfoliation appear to establish a new "equilibrium" where proliferative activity and villus length appear to stabilize. EVANS et al. (1981) have observed that the migration of cells from the jejunal crypt through the villus in tumor-bearing rodents was reduced in response to a reduction in total cell production in the crypt. However, the life span of the epithelial cell under these conditions was unchanged due to the reduction in villus height. Furthermore, it appears that the epithelial cells fail to mature in their transit from the crypt

Table 13. Lewis lung carcinoma. Survival time: 32 ± 3.4 days. Tumor size at death: $3,277 \pm 343$ mm^3. HOST: BDF$_1$ male mouse. Jejunum[a]

Tissue			Tumor volume [mm^3]	Cellular				
dpm/mg Tissue	dpm/ Crpyt	Crypts/ mg		Cells/ Crypt	˙L. Cells/ Crypt	˙L.I./ Crypt [%]	dpm/ ˙L. Cell	Mitoses/ Crypt
$5,547 \pm 323$	8.90 ± 0.52	628 ± 57	0	199 ± 13	68 ± 7	34 ± 7	0.130 ± 0.011	2.30 ± 0.41
$4,531 \pm 230$	7.56 ± 0.64	602 ± 21	[d 8] 300 ± 22	162 ± 19	56 ± 5	35 ± 4	0.134 ± 0.006	2.07 ± 0.21
$3,741 \pm 189$	6.25 ± 0.79	615 ± 76	[d 13] $1,000 \pm 105$	120 ± 4	49 ± 7	41 ± 5	0.128 ± 0.008	1.31 ± 0.21
$1,819 \pm 636$	2.94 ± 0.79	613 ± 98	[d 22] $3,021 \pm 400$	53 ± 11	30 ± 4	57 ± 3	0.080 ± 0.021	0.95 ± 0.11

˙L = labeled with ^{3}H-TdR for 30 min

[a] Tissue values represent the mean [$\pm$S.E.M.] for 4–5 animals and cellular values represent the mean [$\pm$S.E.M.] for 100 isolated crypts from 4–5 animals. Animals were grouped to provide uniform tumor volume.

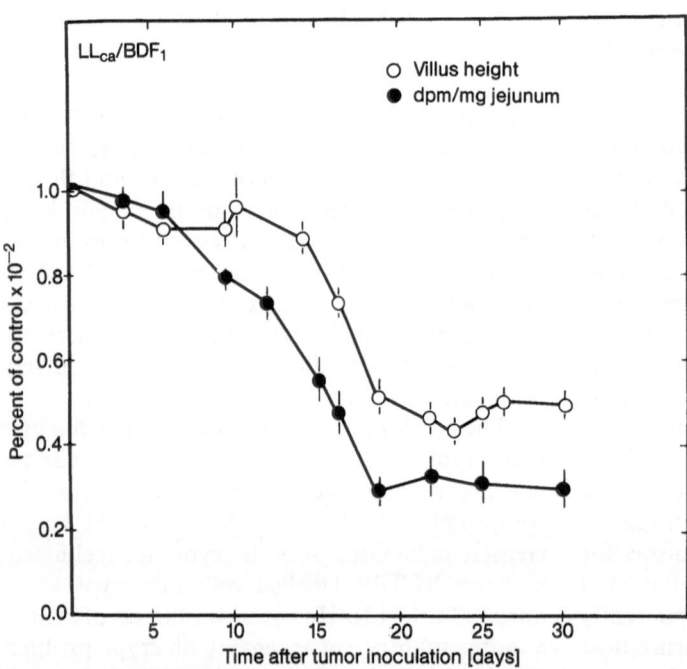

Fig. 21. Villus length and jejunal proliferative activity in tumor-bearing animals. Villus length (o) and dpm/mg jejunal tissue (•) at various times after inoculation of BDF$_1$ mice with 10^6 LLca tumor cells. Control values were determined from six non-tumor-bearing animals. The data points represent the mean ($\pm$S.E.M.) of values obtained from 4–5 animals. Reproduced with permission from Kovacs et al., Cell Tissue Kinet, 14:241–250, 1981

to the villus tip (Evans, personal communication, 1982). These changes in intestinal steady-state have been observed in all experimental tumor models studied. Generally, there is a reduction in the crypt cellularity with a concomitant increase in the proliferative compartment (Fig. 22). For some tumors, the entire crypt population enters the cell cycle. The maturation zone is markedly compromised, resulting in an inhibition of enterocyte differentiation and therefore a loss of villus functionality. The kinetics of crypt cell production, crypt and villus migration and exfoliation are apparently redefined such that immature crypt cell production is optimized, while differentiation of the progeny is minimized.

7.3 Modulators and Their Importance in Tumor/Host Relationships

The broad concept of "biological response modifiers" has been applied to a rapidly developing area of research that has more recently been recognized as having the potential to play a major role in the management of patients through a better understanding of the biology of cancer. The modifier concept has its basis in what was previously called immunotherapy. However, the complexities of the immune response as they are known today, the failure of conventional immunotherapy to be of much value in the clinic, and the evolving recognition that immunoaugmenting, -modulating and

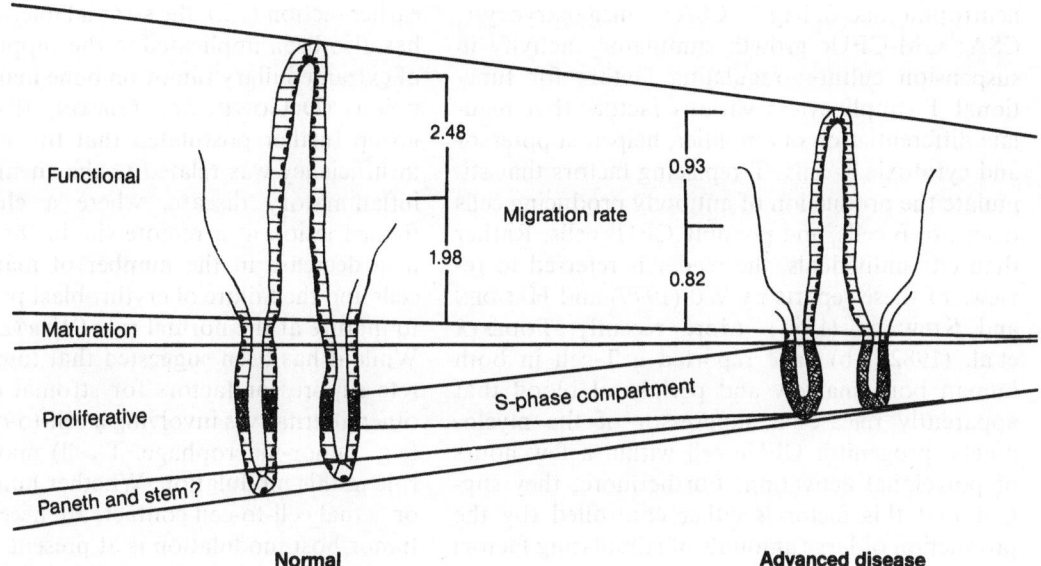

Fig. 22. The effect of tumor growth on the composite zones of the intestinal epithelium of rodents

-restorative factors appear to play roles in the regulation of the other tissues of the host, has led to a major interest in these regulating factors.

Rather than survey the literature on these "factors" over the last ten years, we will approach this topic from a conceptual, and perhaps superficial point of view, and leave other approaches to review articles on specific topics. Briefly, in addition to the modulators associated with the immune reaction, factors designated as lymphokines, cytokines, antigrowth factors, thymic factors, and maturation and differentiation factors are being recognized daily in a complex, cascade-type interrelated regulatory mechanism for normal tissue function. This "new world" of modulator biology is so complicated that those intimately involved have created what appears to be their own language, falling just short of discovering the "barf, snarf and stinkey" factors.

Somewhere at the center of this array of factors lies what, at present, appears to be three major cell types – the T-cell, the macrophage, and the less defined stromal cell. With the exception perhaps of the stromal cell, these cells have long been suspected of performing a dicotomy of functions and only more recently have subpopulations or "subsets" of the major cellular categories been demonstrated to have specific functions. For example, the T-cell category was originally subdivided by functional phenotypes into T-suppressor, T-helper, natural killer (*NK*) and null (*n*) cells. Collectively, these T-cells were held accountable for a major defensive against neoplastic growth, but are now recognized to be effective only during the early phases of tumor establishment (Takei et al., 1977; Bertschmann et al., 1979; Berendt and North, 1980). Furthermore, Thy-1$^+$ T cells isolated directly from an experimental tumor over a range of tumor sizes, have been found to inhibit (Thy-1$^+$, Lyt-1$^-$, 2$^+$) or stimulate (Thy-1$^+$, Lyt 1$^+$, 2$^+$) depending on the tumor size (Mulé et al., 1981). Thus the anti-tumor reactivity that develops in mature T-cells can be abrogated by the activity of separable populations of immature tumor-enhancing T-lymphocytes. These enhancing properties appear very early during the T-cell maturation, suggesting that immature T-cells are not inert cells. Small (1982) has suggested that a premature release of immature T-cells from the thymus occurs when antitumor reactivity of splenic T-cells is cancelled by an accumulation of dominant tumor-enhancing T-cells. These immature T-cells are rapidly dividing cells with a low level of H-2 antigens. They do not undergo blastogenesis when exposed to phytohemagglutin in (PHA). Futhermore, they appear to be independent of a suppressor function, but do require cells expressing Fc receptors.

The T-cell, in response to T-cell mitogens, has also been reported to the source of at least ten functionally distinguishable regulator factor activities, many of which are involved in hematopoietic and "immunopoietic" regulation. These include the following: eosinophil CSA; macrophage CSA;

neutrophil-macrophage CSA; megakaryocytic CSA; GM-CFUc growth stimulatory activity in suspension culture; regulating factors for functional T-lymphocytes; various factors that regulate differentiation of amplifier, helper, suppressor and cytotoxic T-cells; T-replacing factors that stimulate the production of antibody producing cells from pre-B cells, and possibly CFUs cells. Rather than cite individuals, the reader is referred to reviews of these reports by WU (1979) and HADDEN and STEWART (1981). More recently, PODESTA et al. (1982a, b) have reported a T-cell in both human bone marrow and peripheral blood that apparently releases a suppressor of the myelopoietic progenitor CFUc cell within a few hours of polyclonal activation. Furthermore, they suggest that this factor is either controlled (by the production of large amounts of stimulating factor) or is lost with time. These suppressor functions had previously been limited to the regulation of proliferative responses of lymphocytes to soluble antigens, mitogens, mixed lymphocyte reactions and polyclonal immunoglobulin synthesis.

In general, similar bifunctional roles have been ascribed to the macrophage and over the last ten years, reports seemed to point to an existence of relationships between hematopoietic growth factors for myeloid and lymphoid cell differentiation. It would not be unexpected Therefore, if a tumor-induced altered immune competence of the host could also result in a significant altered state of hematopoiesis. More specifically, with tumor progression, the flooding of the host by immune T-cells capable of stimulating undifferentiated tumors may also result in the enhanced production of hematopoietic stem and progenitor cells, while preventing further differentiation as discussed in an earlier section (7.2). This suggestion, in, fact is strengthened by a report implicating a T-cell product released during pokeweed mitogen stimulation that stimulates the growth of both a form of the multipotential hematopoietic stem cell (BFU) and tumor cells as well (EMMA et al., 1981). Furthermore, the work of MACDONALD and FERGUSON (1977) and MOWAT and FERGUSON (1981a, b) suggests that enteropathic lymphokines may very well be responsible for many of the unexplained mucosal pathologies related to altered crypt cells production in the gastrointestinal tract. They have postulated that this immune cell-mediated pathologic effect most probably results from a humoral factor directly influencing the intestinal stroma rather than a direct attack on the intestinal enterocyte. As discussed briefly in an earlier section (7.2), the stromal microenvironment has also been implicated in the suppressive effects of extramedullary tumor on bone marrow erythropoiesis (DEGOWIN and GIBSON, 1978a, b). This group further postulated that this erythropoietic insufficiency was related to the anemia of chronic inflammatory disease, where a chronically inflamed lesion at a remote site in the body results in a decrease in the number of marrow stromal cells and the failure of erythroblast progenitor cells to mature at the normal rate (WERTZ et al., 1980). While it has been suggested that tumors may secrete suppressor factors for stromal cell integrity, other alternatives involving a cell-to-cell mediation (e.g. tumor-macrophage, T-cell) may also play a role in this modulation. Whether humoral factors, or actual cell-to-cell contact, are necessary for this tumor/host modulation is at present unknown.

Obviously, only the very tip of this previously veiled area has surfaced here. The entire concept of biological modifiers is evolving so rapidly that by the time of this reading, new observations may have completely negated the presently accepted postulates. It is increasingly clear, however, that the tumor/host relationship is finally being considered seriously. In the near future, the modulation concept should progress from its previously descriptive state to a critical quantitative pathological state that will have to be reckoned with by both the clinician, the experimentalist, and the theoretician.

Summary

Clinical approaches to the management of cancer has suffered from many unknowns. It appears that many óf these unknowns are related, at least in part, to the marked heterogeneity existing in human tumors, and to the physical diversities that exist from patient to patient. In preparing this manuscript, it became increasingly apparent that the potential solution to these related problems, and as such the "redefining of clinical research" resides in a more inclusive, exact pathological diagnosis that would include a measure of chemo- and radio-responsiveness of individual tumors. In addition, there is a continuing need for the development of non-invasive markers (e.g. NMR, serum, urine) that permit a daily assessment of insult-recognition and recovery of normal tissue stem cell survival and function. This type of marker would provide a method for applying "custom designed" treatments for each individual patient. For the future, serious considerations must also be given to: (1) the concept of drug-induced residual damage – a potential life threatening drug effect independent of suspected carcinogenesis, and (2) to the new area of biological modifiers which may very well provide a better understanding of the tumor/host response presently encompassed by the paraneoplastic syndromes. Individually, these are broad, non-specific directions for the future in clinical research, and each contains more than their fair share of problems. However, preliminary experiences with these directions already available offers optimism to those personally involved.

Acknowledgements. The author wishes to acknowledge those individuals that have kindly furnished personal data for these discussions, the encouragement of Drs. J. VAN'T HOF, W.B. LOONEY and L.L. SCHENKEN, and the assistance of Drs. R.M. JOHNKE and D.A. EMMA and M.J. EVANS and J.R. WHEELING.

References

Abe M, Tahahaski M, Yabumoto E, Adachi H, Yoshii M, Mori L (1980) Clinical experience with intraoperative radiotherapy of locally advanced cancers, Cancer 45:40–48.

Alberts DS, Salmon SE, Chen HSG, et al (1980) In-vitro clonogenic assay for predicting response of ovarian cancer to chemotherapy, Lancet 2:340–342.

Ansair RH, Eishorn LH, Williams SD, et al (1980) Short and long term platinum (DDP) nephrotoxicity in patients (Pts) with testicular cancer. Proc Amer Assoc Cancer Res 21:135. (Abstract 540)

Baylin SB (1977) Histaminase (diamine oxidase) activity in human tumors: an expression of a mature genome, Proc Natl Acad Sci, USA 74:883–887.

Baylin SB, Abeloff Md, Wieman KC, et al (1975) Elevated histaminase (diamine oxidase) activity in small-cell carcinoma of the lung, N Engl J Med 293:1286–1290.

Baylin SB, Beaven MA, Buja LM et al (1972) Histaminase activity: a biochemical marker for medullary carcinoma of the thyroid, Am J Med 523:723–733.

Baylin SB, Stevens SA, Shakir KMM (1978) Association of diamine oxidase and ornithine decarboxylase with maturing cells in rapidly proliferating epithelium, Biochim Biophys Acta 541:415–419.

Beaven MA, Marshall JR, Baylin SB, et al (1975) Changes in plasma histaminase activity during normal early human pregnancy and pregnancy disorders, Am J Obstet Gynecol 123:605–609.

Begg AC, Fu KK, Shrieve DC, et al (1979) Combination therapy of a solid murine tumor with cyclophosphamide and radiation: the effects of time, dose and assay method, Int J Radiat Oncol Biol Phys 5:1433–1439.

Berendt MJ, North RJ (1980) T-cell-mediated suppression of anti-tumor immunity. An explanation for progressive growth of an immunogenic tumor. J Exp Med 141:69–80.

Bergonié J, Tribondeau L (1906) Interpretation de quelques resultats de la radiothérapie et essai de fixation d'une technique rationelle, CR Acad Sci 143:983–985.

Berlin NI (1965) Anemia in cancer, Proc Natl Cancer Conf 5:429–435.

Bertschmann M, Schären B, Lüsher EF (1979) Correlation of in vivo and in vitro immune reactions against the intradermally developing P-815 mastocytoma in the syngeneic mouse, Immunobiology 156:382–399.

Boarder TA, Blackett NM (1976) The proliferative status of intestinal epithelial clonogenic cells: sensitivity to S phase specific cytotoxic agents, Cell Tissue Kinet 9:589–596.

Bonadonna G, Rossi A, Valagussa P, et al (1977) Adjuvant chemotherapy with CMF in breast cancer with positive axillary nodes. In: Salmon SE, Jones SE (eds) Adjuvant Therapy of Cancer, Amsterdam-Oxford, New York, pp 122–141.

Borglin NE, Willert B (1962) Increased histaminolytic power of plasma in endometrial adenocarcinoma, Cancer 15:271–275.

Botnick LE, Hannon EC, Hellman S (1979) A long lasting proliferative defect in the hematopoietic stem cell compartment following cytotoxic agents, Int Radiat Onc Biol Phys 5:1621–1625.

Bradley TR, Metcalf D (1966) The growth of mouse bone marrow cells in vitro, Aust J Exp Biol Med Sci 44:287–300.

Brattain MG, Fine WD, Khaled F, et al (1981) Heterogeneity of malignant cells from a human colonic carcinoma, Cancer Res 41:1751–1756.

Braunschweiger PG, Kovacs CJ, Schenken LL (1982) Renal and haemopoietic proliferative defects as a delayed consequence of cis-platin adriamycin and daunomycin treatment, Br J Cancer 45:421–428.

Braunschweiger PG, Poulakos L, Schiffer LM (1976) In vitro labeling and gold activation autoradiography for determination of labeling index and DNA synthesis time of solid tumors, Cancer Res 36:1748–1753.

Braunschweiger PG, Schenken LL, Schiffer LM (1979) The cytokinetic basis for the design of efficacious radiotherapy protocols, Int J Radiat Oncol Biol Phys 5:37–47.

Braunschweiger PG, Schiffer LM (1978) Cell kinetics after vincristine treatment of C3H/He spontaneous mammary tumors: implications for therapy, JNCI 60:1043–1048.

Brennan MF (1977) Uncomplicated starvation versus cancer cachexia, Cancer Res 37:2359–2364.

Breur K (1966) Growth rate and radiosensitivity of human tumours. II. Radiosensitivity of human tumours, Eur J Cancer 2:173–188.

Brodskaya RM, Stavrovskaya AA, Stromskaya TP, et al (1981) Clonal analysis of the ability of tumor cells to form colonies in semi-solid medium, Int J Cancer 27:689–692.

Bruce WR, Lin H (1969) An empirical cellular approach to improvement of cancer chemotherapy, Cancer Res 29:2308–2310.

Bruce WR, Meeker BE, Valeriote EA (1966) Comparison of the sensitivity of normal hematopoietic and transplanted lymphoma colony-forming cells to chemotherapeutic agents administered in vivo, JNCI 37:233–245.

Burgess AW, Camakares J, Metcalf D (1977) Purification and properties of colony-stimulating factor from mouse lung-conditioned medium, J Biol Chem 252:1998–2003.

Burke PJ, Diggs CH, Owens AH Jr (1973) Factors in human serum affecting the proliferation of normal and leukemic cells, Cancer Res 33:800–806.

Burke PJ, Karp JE, Owens AH (1974) An optimal design for sequential anti-leukemic therapy based on peak serum regulator factors, Proc Am Soc Clin Oncol 15:169.

Carney DN, Gazdar AF, Bunn PA Jr, et al (1981) Demonstration of the stem cell nature of clonogenic tumor cells from lung cancer patients, Stem Cells 1:149–164.

Carter SK (1976) Large-bowel cancer-the current status of treatment, JNCI 56:3–10.

Carter SK, Soper WT (1974) Integration of chemotherapy into combined modality treatment of solid tumors. I. The overall strategy, Cancer Treat Rev 1:1–13.

Chapman JD, Todd P, Sturrock J (1970) X-ray survival of cultured Chinese hamster cells resuming growth after plateau phase, Radiat Res 42:590–600.

Creamer B (1964) Malignancy and the small-intestinal mucosa. Br Med J 2:1435–1436.

Das SK, Stanley ER, Guilbert LJ, et al (1981) Human colony-stimulating factor (CSF-1) radioimmunoassay: resolution of three subclasses of human colony-stimulating factors, Blood 58:630–641.

DeGowin RL, Gibson DP (1978a) Suppressive effects of an extramedullary tumor on bone marrow erythropoiesis and stroma, Exp Hematol 6:568–575.

DeGowin RL, Grund FM, Gibson DP (1978b) Erythropoietic insufficiency in mice with extramedullary tumor, Blood 51:33–43.

DeGowin RL, Gibson DP, Knapp SA, et al (1981) Tumor-induced suppression of marrow stromal colonies, Exp Hematol 9:811–819.

Deller DJ, Murrell TGC, Blowes R (1967) Jejunal biopsy in malignant disease, Aust Ann Med 16:236–241.

Dencker H, Kahlson G, Kockum I, et al (1973) Histamine metabolism in human gastric mucosa, Clin Sci Mol Med 45:225–231.

Denekamp J (1972) The relationship between the 'cell loss factor' and the immediate response to radiation in animals tumours, Eur J Cancer 8:335–340.

Denekamp J (1979) Experimental tumor systems: standardization of endpoints, Int J Radiat Oncol Biol Phys 5:1175–1184.

Denekamp J (1977) Tumour regression as a guide to prognosis: a study with experimental animals, Br J Radiol 50:271–279.

Denekamp J, Thomlinson RH (1971) The cell proliferation kinetics of four experimental tumors after acute x-irradiation, Cancer Res 31:1279–1284.

Deo MG, Ramalingaswami V (1965) Reaction of the small intestine to induced protein malnutrition in Rhesus monkeys-a study of cell population kinetics in the jejunum, Gastroenterology 49:150–157.

Dexter DL, Spremulli EN, Fligiel Z, et al (1981) Heterogeneity of cancer cells from a single human colon carcinoma, Am J Med 71:949–956.

Durie BGM, Salmon SE (1975) A clinical staging system for multiple myeloma. Correlation of measured myeloma cell mass with presenting clinical features, response to treatment, and survival, Cancer 36:842–854.

Dymock IW, MacKay N, Miller V, et al (1967) Small intestinal function in neoplastic disease, Br J Cancer 21:505–511.

Earnshaw P, Busuttil A, Ferguson A (1982) Revelance of colonic mucosal inflammation in aetiology, Recent Results Cancer Res 83:31–44.

Elkind MM, Whitmore GF (1967) The Radiobiology of Cultured Mammalian Cells, Gordon and Breach, New York.

Emma DA, Kovacs CJ, Scarantino CW, et al (1981) Effect of hematopoietic stimuli on tumor cell clonogenicity, Stem Cells 1:281.

Evans MJ, Kovacs CJ, Schenken LL, et al (1981) Modification of the intestinal postirradiation proliferative response by intra-abdominal H-4-II-E_2 tumors, Radiat Res 88:552–564.

Friedman EA, Higgins PJ, Lipkin M, et al (1981) Tissue culture of human epithelial cells from benign colonic tumours, In Vitro 17:632–644.

Galjaard H, Van Durren M, Giesen J (1970) A quantitative histochemical study of intestinal mucosa after x-irradiation, J Histochem Cytochem 18:291–301.

Goldson, AL (1978) Preliminary clinical experience with intraoperative radiotherapy, J Natl Med Assoc, 70:493–495.

Hadden JW, Stewart WE II (1981) The Lymphokines: Biochemistry and Biological Activity. Humana Press, Clifton, NJ

Hagemann RF (1976) Intestinal cell proliferation during fractionated abdominal irradiation, Br J Radiol 49:56–61.

Hagemann RF (1980) The intestinal response to cytotoxic agents. In: Appleton DR, Sunter JP, Watson AJ (eds). Cell Proliferation in the Gastrointestinal Tract. Pitman Medical, Kent, pp. 181–229.

Hagemann RF, Lesher S (1971) Intestinal crypt survival and total and per crypt levels of proliferative cellularity following irradiation: age response and animal lethality, Radiat Res 47:159–167.

Hamburger AW, Salmon SE (1977) Primary bioassay of human tumor stem cells, Science 197:461–463.

Hanson WR, Henninger DL, Fry RJM (1979) Time dependence of intestinal proliferative cell risk vs stem cell risk to radiation or colcemid cytotoxicity following hydroxyurea, Int J Radiat Oncol Biol Phys 5:1685–1689.

Hansson R, Sundström G (1970) Diamine oxidase (Histaminase) and heparin inhibition of gastric secretion in man, Scand J Clin Lab Invest 26:263–269.

Hayflick L (1965) The limited in vitro lifespan of human diploid cell strains, Exp Cell Res 37:614–636.

Hellman S (1975) Cell kinetics, models, and cancer treatment-some principles for the radiation oncologist, Radiology 114:219–223.

Hellman S, Botnick LE (1977) Stem cell depletion: an example of the late effects of cytotoxins, Int J Radiat Oncol Biol Phys 2:181–184.

Hellman K, Burrage K (1969) Control of malignant metastases by ICRF-159, Nature 224:273–275.

Hetzel FW, Kolodny GM (1976) Radiation-induced giant cell formation: the influence of conditions which enhance repair of potentially lethal damage, Radiat Res 68:490–498.

Hill RP, Bush RS, Yeung P (1971) The effect of anaemia on the fraction of hypoxic cells in an experimental tumour, Br J Radiol 44:299–304.

Hill BT, Rupniak HT, Whelan RDH, et al (1981) Improved colony formation with human tumors using the Courtenay clonogenic assay, Stem Cells 1:322.

Hiraoka A, Ohkubo T, Yamagishi M, et al (1982) An accelerated recruitment of CFU_c subpopulations after treatment with vinblastine, Exp Hematol 10:533–543.

Hopkins HA, Ritenour ER, MacLeod MS, et al (1979) The effect of varying the time between irradiation and cyclophosphamide on growth response of hepatoma 3924A, Int J Radiat Oncol Biol Phys 5:1455–1459.

Hug V, Spitzer G, Drewinko B, et al (1983) Effect of diethyl-aminoethyl-dextran on colony formation of human tumor cells in semisolid suspension cultures, Cancer Res 43:210–213.

Jirtle RL, Clifton KH (1978) Erythrokinetics in mice bearing tumors in either preirradiated or unirradiated tissue. Cell Tissue Kinet 11:581–596.

Karp JE, Burke PJ (1976) Enhancement of drug cytotoxicity by recruitment of leukemic myeloblasts with humoral stimulation, Cancer Res 36:3600–3603.

Karp JE, Burke PJ, Humphrey RL (1977) Induction of serum stimulation and plasma cell proliferation during chemotherapy of multiple myeloma, Blood 49:925–934.

Karp JE, Humphrey RL, Burke PJ (1981) Timed sequential chemotherapy of cytoxan-refractory multiple myeloma with cytoxan and adriamycin based on induced tumor proliferation, Blood 57:468–475.

Kimball PM, Brattain MG, Pitts Am (1978) A soft-agar procedure measuring growth of human colonic carcinomas, Br J Cancer 37:1015–1019.

Kobayashi Y, Kupelian J, Maudsley DV (1968) Release of diamine oxidase by heparin in the rat, Biochem Pharmacol 18:1585–1591.

Kovacs CJ, Braunschweiger PG, Schenken LL, et al (1982) Proliferative defects in renal and intestinal epithelium after cis-dichlorodiammine platinum (II), Br J Cancer 45:286–294.

Kovacs CJ, Evans MJ, Burholt DR, et al (1979) ICRF-159 enhancement of radiation response in combined modality therapies. II. Differentiation responses of tumour and normal tissues, Br J Cancer 39:524–530.

Kovacs CJ, Evans MJ, Schenken LL, et al (1979) ICRF-159 enhancement of radiation response in combined modality therapies. I. Time/dose relationships for tumour response, Br J Cancer 39:516–523.

Kovacs CJ, Evans MJ, Schenken LL, et al (1981a) Alterations in gastrointestinal steady-state kinetics associated with the growth of experimental tumours, Cell Tissue Kinet 14:241–250.

Kovacs CJ, Schenken LL, Evans MJ, et al (1981b) Enhanced adriamycin-induced delayed gastrointestinal radiosensitivity in tumor-bearing mice, Int J Radiol Oncol Biol Phys 7:1389–1395.

Kovacs CJ, Evans MJ, Wakefield JA, et al (1977) A comparative study of the response to radiation by experimental tumours with markedly different growth characteristics, Radiat Res 72:455–468.

Laboisse CL, Augeron C, Potet F (1981) Growth and differentiation of human gastrointestinal adenocarcinoma stem cells in soft agarose. Cancer Res 41:310–315.

Laird AK (1969) Dynamics of growth in tumors and in normal organisms, Nat Cancer Inst Monog 30:15–28.

Lala PK, Terrin M, Lind C, et al (1978) Hemopoietic redistribution in tumor-bearing mice, Exp Hematol 6:283–298.

Larsen B, Thorling EB (1969) Inhibitory effect of DEAE-dextran on tumour growth. Action of dextran sulfate after "in vitro" incubation, Acta Pathol Microbiol Scand 75:229–236.

Leblond CP, Stevens CE (1948) The constant renewal of the intestinal epithelium in the albino rat, Anat Rec 100:357–378.

Lesher S, Bauman J (1969) Cell kinetic studies of the intestinal epithelium: maintenance of the intestinal epithelium in normal and irradiated animals, Natl Cancer Inst Monogr 30:185–198.

Little JB (1973) Factors influencing the repair of potentially lethal radiation damage in growth-inhibited human cells, Radiat Res 56:320–333.

Looney WB, Hopkins HA (1982) Solid tumors as a model for the development of antineoplastic therapy, Methods Cancer Res 19:303–384.

Looney WB, Hopkins HA, Longerbeam MB, et al (1983) Comparison of effects of daily versus hyperfractionated split-course radiation schedules with and without cyclophosphamide on median survival, metastatic dissemination, tumor cure, and growth rates, Cancer Res 43:60–67.

Looney WB, Hopkins HA, MacLeod MS, et al (1979) Solid tumor models for the assessment of different treatment modalities-XIV: the evaluation of host and tumor response to cyclophosphamide and radiation, Int J Radiat Oncol Biol Phys 5:1461–1465.

Looney WB, Mayo AA, Allen PM, et al (1973) A mathematical evaluation of tumour growth curves in rapid, intermediate and slow growing rat hepatomata, Br J Cancer 27:341–344.

Luk GD, Bayless TM, Baylin SB (1980) Diamine oxidase (histaminase) a circulating marker for rat intestinal mucosal maturation and integrity, J Clin Invest 66:66–70.

Luk GD, Vaughan WP, Burke PJ, et al (1981) Diamine oxidase as a plasma marker of rat intestinal mucosal injury and regeneration after administration of 1-β-D-Arabinofuranosylcytosine, Cancer Rex 41:2334–2337.

MacDonald TT, Ferguson A (1977) Hypersensitivity reactions in the small intestine. III. The effects of allograft rejection and of graft-versus-host disease on epithelial cell kinetics, Cell Tissue Kinet 10:301–312.

Mak TW, McCulloch EA (1981) Cellular and Molecular Biology of Hematopoietic Stem Cell Differentiation, AR Liss, New York.

Mendelsohn ML (1960a) Autoradiographic analysis of cell proliferation in spontaneous breast cancer of C3H mouse. II. Growth and survival of cells labeled with tritiated thymidine, JNCI 25:485–500.

Mendelsohn ML (1962) Autoradiographic analysis of cell proliferation in spontaneous breast cancer of C3H mouse. III. The growth fraction, JNCI 28:1015–1029.

Mendelsohn ML, Dohan FC Jr, Moore HA Jr (1960b) Autoradiographic analysis of cell proliferation in spontaneous breast cancer of C3H mouse. I. Typical cell cycle and timing of DNA synthesis, JNCI 25:477–484.

Meyer JS (1982) Potential value of cell kinetics in management of cancers of unknown origin, Semin Oncol 9:513–516.

Meyer JS, Bauer WC, Stevens SC, et al (1978) S-phase fractions of breast carcinomas, Bull Cancer 65:449–454.

Meyer JS, Hixon B (1979) Advanced stage and early relapse of breast carcinomas associated with high thymidine labeling indices, Cancer Res 39:4042–4047.

Millar JL, Blackett NM, Hudspith BN (1978) Enhanced post-irradiation recovery of the hemopoietic system in animals pretreated with a variety of cytotoxic agents, Cell Tissue Kinet 11:543–553.

Millar JL, Stephens TC, Wist FA (1982) An explanation for the ability of cytotoxic drug pretreatment to reduce bone marrow related lethality of total body irradiation (TBI), Int J Radiat Onc Biol Phys 8:581–583.

Morley A (1980) Residual marrow damage from cytotoxic drugs. Aust NZ J Med 10:569–571.

Mowat AM, Ferguson A (1981a) Induction and expression of mucosal cell mediated immunity. Current Topics in Veterinary Medical Science 102:107–129.

Mowat AM, Ferguson A (1981b) Hypersensitivity in the small intestinal mucosa. V. Induction of cell mediated immunity to a dietary antigen. Clin Expt Immun 43:574–582.

Mulé JJ, Forstrom JW, George E, et al (1981) Production of T-cell lines with inhibitory or stimulatory activity against syngeneic tumors in vivo. A preliminary report, Int J Cancer 28:611–614.

Nicola NA, Metcalf D, Johnson GR, et al (1979) Separation of functionally distinct human granulocyte-macrophage colony-stimulating factors, Blood 54:614–627.

Nygaard K, Smith-Erichsen N, Hatlevoll R, et al (1978) Pulmonary complications after bleomycin, irradiation and surgery for esophageal cancer, Cancer 17–22.

Park CH, Bergsagel DW, McCullock EA (1971) Mouse myeloma tumor stem cells: a primary cell culture assay, JNCI 46:411–422.

Pavelic ZP, Slocum HK, Rustum YM, et al (1980) Growth of cell colonies in soft agar from biopsies of different human solid tumors, Cancer Res 40:4151–4158.

Peters LJ (1976) Modification of the radiocurability of a syngeneic murine squamous carcinoma by its site of growth, by electron-affinic drugs, and by ICRF 159, Br J Radiol 49:708–715.

Phelps TA, Blackett NM (1979) Protection of intestinal damage by pretreatment with cytarabine (cytosine arabinoside). Int J Radiat Onc Biol Phys 5:1617–1620.

Philips TL (1979) Conference on Combined Modalities: Chemotherapy Radiotherapy, Philips TL (quest ed.) Int J Radiat Oncol Biol Phys 9:1139–1723.

Pluznik DH, Sachs L (1965) The cloning of normal "mast" cells in tissue culture, J Cell Physiol 66:319–324.

Podesta M, Frassoni F, Van Lint MT, et al (1982a) Generation of CFU_c suppressor T cells in vitro. II. Effect of DNA, PWM and Con-A on bone marrow and peripheral blood lymphocytes from healthy donors, Exp Hematol 10:256–262.

Podesta M, Frassoni F, Van Lint MT, et al (1982b) Generation of CFU_c suppressor T cells in vitro. IV. Effect of time on the inhibitory activity of mitogen-primed normal T-lymphocytes, Thymus 4:233–242.

Prehn RT (1977) Immunostimulation of the lymphodependent phase of neoplastic growth, JNCI 59:1043–1049.

Puck TT, Marcus PT (1956) Action of x-rays on mammalian cells, J Exper Med 103:653–666.

Ranson JL, Novak RW, Kumar APM, et al (1979) Delayed gastrointestinal complications after combined modality therapy of childhood rhabdomyosarcoma, Int J Rad Oncol Biol Phys 5:1275–1279.

Rheinwald JG, Beckett MA (1981) Tumorigenic keratinocyte lines requiring anchorage and fibroblast support cultured from human squamous cell carcinomas, Cancer Res 41:1657–1663.

Rijke RPC (1980) Some speculations on control mechanisms of cell proliferation in intestinal epithelium. Appleton DR, Sunter JP, Watson AJ (eds) In: Cell Proliferation in the Gastrointestinal Tract. Pitman Medical, Kent, Great Britain, pp. 57–65.

Rockwell S (1977) In vivo-in vitro tumor systems; new models for studying the response of tumors to therapy, Lab Anim Sci 27:831–851.

Rosemblum ML (1980) Chemosensitivity testing for human brain tumors. In: Salmon SE (ed). Cloning of Human Tumor Stem Cells, AR Liss, New York, pp. 259–276.

Rowbottom LA, Whitehead RH, Roberts GP, Hughes LE (1981) A study of the growth requirements of human tumor cells in tissue culture. AJEBAK 59:91–100.

Salazar OM, Rubin P, Keller B, et al (1978) Systemic (half-body) radiation therapy: response and toxicity, Int J Radiat Oncol Biol Phys 4:937–950.

Salazar OM, Scarantino CW, Rubin P, et al (1980) Total (half-body) systemic irradiation for occult metastases in non-small cell lung cancer, Cancer 46:1932–1944.

Salmon SE (1980a) Background and overview. In: Salmon SE (ed) Cloning of Human Tumor Stem Cells. AR Liss Inc., New York, pp. 3–13.

Salmon SE (1980b) Perspective on future direction. In: Salmon SE (ed) Cloning of Human Tumor Stem Cells. Liss, New York, pp. 315–327.

Salmon SE, Alberts DS, Meyskens FL, et al (1980c) Clinical correlations of in vitro drug sensitivity. In: Salmon SE (ed) Cloning of Human Tumor Stem Cells, AR Liss, New York, pp. 223–245.

Salmon SE, Hamburger AW, Soehnlen B, et al (1978) Quantitation of differential sensitivity of human-tumor stem cells to anticancer drugs, N Engl J Med 298:1321–1327.

Salmon SE, Smith BA (1970) Immunoglobulin synthesis and total body tumor cell number in IgG multiple myeloma, J Clin Invest 49:1114–1121.

Salsbury AJ, Burrage K, Hellmann K (1970) Inhibition of metastatic spread by I.C.R.F. 159: selective deletion of a malignant characteristic, Br Med J 4:344–346.

Schacter LP, Burke PJ (1978) The regulation of bone marrow cell DNA synthesis by human serum, J Mol Med 3:329–344.

Schenken LL, Burholt DR, Kovacs CJ (1979) Adriamycin-radiation combinations: drug induced delayed gastrointestinal radiosensitivity, Int J Radiat Oncol Biol Phys 5:1265–1269.

Schenken LL, Hagemann RF, Burholt DR, et al (1976) Combined-modality oncotherapy with cyclophosphamide (NSC-26271) and radiotherapy: control of murine mastocytoma, JNCI 57:943–949.

Schiffer LM, Markoe AM, Nelson JSR (1976) Estimation of tumor growth fraction in murine tumors by the primer-available DNA-dependent DNA polymerase assay, Cancer Res 36:2415–2418.

Selby WS, Janossy G, Jewell DP (1981) Immunohistological characterisation of intraepithelial lymphocytes of the human gastrointestinal tract, Gut 22:169–176.

Shakir KMM, Margolis S, Baylin SB (1977) Localization of histamine (diamine oxidase) in rat small intestinal mucosa: site of release by heparin, Biochem Pharmacol 26:2343–2347.

Shen SC, Homburger F (1951) The anemia of cancer patients and its relation to metastases to the bone marrow, J Lab Clin Med 37:182–198.

Small M (1982) Tumor enhancing T lymphocytes in mice: further studies on characteristics and mechanism of activity, Int J Cancer 49:465–469.

Smith WW, Wilson SM, Fred SS (1968) Kinetics of stem cell depletion and proliferation: effects of vinblastine and vincristine in normal and irradiated mice, MNCI 40:847–854.

Smith SD, Wood GW, Fried P, et al (1981) In vitro growth

of lymphoma colonies from children with non-Hodgkin's lymphoma, Cancer 48:2612–2623.

Steel GG (1979) Terminology in the description of drug/radiation interactions, Int J Radiat Oncol Biol Phys 5:1145–1150.

Steel GG, Hill RP, Peckham MJ (1978) Combined radiotherapy-chemotherapy of Lewis lung carcinoma, Int J Radiat Oncol Biol Phys 4:49–52.

Stephens TC, Creighton AM (1974) Mechanism of action studies with ICRF 159: effects on the growth and morphology BHK-21 s cells, Br J Cancer 29:99

Strandqvist M (1944) Studien über die kumulative Wirkung der Röntgenstrahlen bei Fraktionierung. Erfahrungen aus dem Radiumhemmet an 280 Haut- und Lippenkarzinomen, Acta Radiol [Suppl] 55:1–293.

Takei F, Levy JG, Kielburn DG (1977) Characterization of suppressor cells in mice bearing syngeneic mastocytoma, J Immunol 118:412–422.

Taylor IW, Bleehen NM (1977) Changes in sensitivity to radiation and ICRF 159 during the life of monolayer cultures of EMT6 tumor line, Br J Cancer 35:587–594.

Todara GJ, Fryling C, De Larco JE (1980) Transforming growth factors produced by certain human tumor cells: polypeptides that interact with epidermal growth factor receptors, Procx Natl Acad Sci (USA) 77:5258–5262.

Trainor KJ, Morley AA (1976) Screening of cytotoxic drugs for residual bone marrow damage, JNCI 57:1237–1239.

Trefil JS, Schaffner JG, Looney WB, et al (1978) Methods for extracting information on tumor responses to single and combined modality treatment from growth curves. In Busch H (ed) Methods in Cancer Research, Vol. XIV Academic Press, New York, pp 324–365.

Tryding N (1965) Heparin-induced diamine oxidase (DAO) activity, Scand J Clin Lab Invest 17:196.

Tubiana M, Malaise E (1976) Comparison of cell proliferation kinetics in human and experimental tumors: response to irradiation, Cancer Treat Rep 60:1887–1895.

Twentyman PR (1977) An artifact in clonogenic assays of bleomycin cytotoxicity. Br J Cancer 36:642–644.

Twentyman PR (1979a) Timing of assays; an important consideration in the determination of clonogenic cell survival both in vitro and in vivo, Int J Radiat Oncol Biol Phys 5:1213–1220.

Twentyman PR, Kallman RF, Brown JM (1979b) The effect of time between x-irradiation and chemotherapy on the growth of three solid mouse tumors-II. Cyclophosphamide, Int J Radiat Oncol Biol Phys 5:1425–1427.

Wert ED, DeGowin RL, Knapp SK et al (1980) Characterization of marrow stromal (fibroblastoid) cells and their association with erythropoiesis, Ex Hematol 8:423–433.

Withers HR, Elkind MM (1968) Dose-survival characteristics of epithelial cells of mouse intestinal mucosa, Radiology 91:998–1000.

Wu AM (1979) Properties and separation of T lymphocyte growth stimulatory activity (TL-GSA) and of granulocyte-macrophage colony stimulatory activity (GM-CSA) produced separately from two human T lymphocyte subpopulations, J Cell Physiol 101:237–250.

Subject Index